Translational Research in Muscular Dystrophy

Shin'ichi Takeda • Yuko Miyagoe-Suzuki •
Madoka Mori-Yoshimura
Editors

Translational Research in Muscular Dystrophy

Springer

Editors
Shin'ichi Takeda
National Institute of Neuroscience
Kodaira, Tokyo
Japan

Yuko Miyagoe-Suzuki
National Institute of Neuroscience
Kodaira, Tokyo
Japan

Madoka Mori-Yoshimura
National Institute of Neuroscience
Kodaira, Tokyo
Japan

ISBN 978-4-431-55677-0 ISBN 978-4-431-55678-7 (eBook)
DOI 10.1007/978-4-431-55678-7

Library of Congress Control Number: 2015957591

Springer Tokyo Heidelberg New York Dordrecht London

Printed on acid-free paper

Springer Japan KK is part of Springer Science+Business Media (www.springer.com)

Preface

Since identification of the DMD (dystrophin) gene as the cause of Duchenne muscular dystrophy (DMD) in 1987, many genes have been found to contribute to muscular dystrophies. In particular, recent next-generation sequencing technology has accelerated the identification of disease-causing genes, especially for α-dystroglycanopathies. In parallel, new research tools for revealing the molecular and cellular mechanisms of muscular dystrophies have been extensively investigated, and new therapeutic strategies for treatment of muscular dystrophy, such as exon skipping therapy using antisense-oligonucleotides or stem cell-based therapy using pluripotent stem cells, have been proposed. To support development of therapies and nationwide and international clinical studies for rare, intractable neuromuscular diseases, the EU started the TREAT-NMD network and the United States started a cooperative international neuromuscular research group (CINRG). In Japan, a patient registry site (registry of muscular dystrophy: REMUDY) (http://www.remudy.jp/) and a muscular dystrophy clinical trial network (http://www.mdctn.jp/network.html) were established. These networks actively communicate with each other to form a worldwide research framework to fight against these devastating neuromuscular disorders.

"Translational research" or "translational medicine" means the transfer of knowledge or technology from bench to bedside, but the interaction should be bidirectional. To accelerate the collaboration between scientists and clinicians, we planned this eBook and asked both talented researchers and clinical physicians who are currently working in the field of muscular dystrophy in Japan to contribute. This book covers cutting-edge studies on muscular dystrophies, e.g., regenerative medicine, next-generation sequencing, and nucleic acid therapies. It also describes the current systems used for clinical trials and patient databases, resources that will support the early realization of clinical application and improve patients' quality of life. Although this eBook might not cover the entire field, we believe that it is informative and useful to all readers who are interested in the neuromuscular diseases.

The editors thank all the authors who have contributed to this eBook and all colleagues who helped us to edit the manuscripts. We also appreciate Dr. Kiyohiko

Takayama and Ms. Tamaki Yamamoto at Springer Japan for their help in both the planning and editing processes.

Tokyo, Japan

Shin'ichi Takeda, M.D., Ph.D.
On behalf of all editors and authors

Contents

Chapter 1
Fukuyama Congenital Muscular Dystrophy: Clinical Aspects

Keiko Ishigaki

Abstract Fukuyama congenital muscular dystrophy (FCMD), the second most common muscular dystrophy in the Japanese population, is an autosomal recessive disorder caused by mutations in the *fukutin* (*FKTN*) gene. *FKTN* encodes a protein involved in the glycosylation of α-dystroglycan (α-DG), which is important for linking the basal lamina to cytoskeletal proteins in muscles, peripheral nerves, and the brain. The main features of FCMD are a combination of infantile-onset hypotonia, generalized muscle weakness, eye abnormalities, and central nervous system involvement with mental retardation and seizures associated with cortical migration defects. The peak motor function is seen between the ages of 2 and 8 years, and maximal motor ability is usually unassisted sitting or sliding on the buttocks. Most patients die of respiratory dysfunction, pulmonary infections including aspiration pneumonia, suffocation, or congestive heart failure. The mean life span is less than 20 years. In managing the FCMD patients, two characteristic complications should be considered. The first is frequent episodes of ketotic hypoglycemia often seen in young lean patients. The second is sudden severe exacerbation of muscle weakness following viral infections, which can be fatal. In this section, the author's extensive experience, gained by managing nearly 200 FCMD patients, will be described.

Keywords α-Dystroglycanopathy • Fukutin • Rhabdomyolysis • Cobblestone lissencephaly

1.1 Introduction

Fukuyama congenital muscular dystrophy (FCMD), characterized by the combination of severe muscular dystrophy and dysgenesis of the eyes and central nervous system (CNS) causing intellectual deficits and epilepsy, was first reported by Fukuyama et al. in 1960 [1]. FCMD is one of the most common autosomal recessive disorders in Japan and is second in prevalence to Duchenne muscular dystrophy (DMD) among Japanese childhood-onset progressive muscular dystrophies, while

K. Ishigaki (✉)
Department of Pediatrics, Tokyo Women's Medical University, School of Medicine,
8-1 Kawada-cho, Shinjuku-ku, Tokyo 162-8666, Japan
e-mail: ishigaki.keiko@twmu.ac.jp

S. Takeda et al. (eds.), *Translational Research in Muscular Dystrophy*,
DOI 10.1007/978-4-431-55678-7_1

it is rarely reported outside of Japan. The annual incidence was reported to be 2.9 of 100,000 live births [2], and the average heterozygous carrier prevalence in various regions of Japan is one in 188 [3].

Toda et al. first reported in 1996 that the locus for FCMD lies on chromosome 9q13 [4]. Kobayashi et al. finally identified the *fukutin* (*FKTN*) gene encoding a 461 amino acid protein and reported a founder mutation, a 3-kb retrotransposal insertion into the 3′ untranslated regions of this gene, to be present in 87 % of FCMD patients [5]. This 3-kb insertion is a hominid-specific, composite noncoding retrotransposon that contains SINE (short interspersed nuclear element sequence), VNTR (variable number tandem repeats), and *Alu* sequences and is thus referred to as an SVA (SINE-VNTR-Alu) retrotransposon. Most patients have at least one copy of this 3-kb SVA retrotransposal insertion. The rate of heterozygosity for this haplotype was reported to be significantly higher in severe than in typical or mild cases [6, 7]. Phenotypically severe FCMD patients appear to be compound heterozygotes for the founder 3-kb insertion mutation and a missense or nonsense mutation at the corresponding allele. The age of the insertion mutation causing FCMD in Japanese patients was calculated to be approximately 102 generations, perhaps slightly less [8]. Taniguchi-Ikeda et al. found that aberrant mRNA splicing induced by SVA exon trapping results in truncating the product of *FKTN* and thereby determined the pathogenic mechanism underlying FCMD [9]. The *FKTN* mutation results in defective *O*-glycosylation of α-dystroglycan (α-DG) leading to disruption of the linkage between the basal lamina and cytoskeleton, known as α-dystroglycanopathy. Recently, α-dystroglycanopathies caused by *FKTN* mutations have been recognized as having a much wider clinical spectrum than previously thought, from the most severe form of congenital muscular dystrophy to the mildest form of limb-girdle muscular dystrophy (LGMD) and can basically be classified into three forms. The first is congenital muscular dystrophy-dystroglycanopathy with brain and eye anomalies (muscular dystrophy-dystroglycanopathy (MDDG) type A4, MDDGA4), previously designated FCMD, Walker-Warburg syndrome (WWS), or muscle-eye-brain disease (MEB). The second is a less severe congenital muscular dystrophy without mental retardation (type B4, MDDGB4), and the third is a limb-girdle muscular dystrophy (LGMD) (type C4, MDDGC4), previously designated LGMD2M. All of the phenotypes of MDDGA4 share the common condition of congenital muscular dystrophy associated with characteristic brain malformations (cobblestone cortical dysplasia and cerebellar malformations) and eye malformations. WWS and MEB are much more severe than FCMD in terms of brain and eye involvement. WWS is a more severe manifestation of the disorder, with death usually in the first year of life and a heterogeneous genetic background. It can be caused by mutations in genes other than *FKTN*, such as *POMT2*, *POMGNT1*, *FKRP*, and *LARGE*. MEB can also be caused by *POMT2* and *POMGNT1* mutations. There are cases that show phenotypic overlapping between FCMD and mild WWS or MEB. FCMD patients are mainly reported in Japan due to the high prevalence of ancestral founder mutation carriers, though some patients with FCMD or *FKTN*-related WWS/MEB have also been reported in China, Turkey, Spain, and Portugal [10–13].

1.2 Clinical Manifestations

FCMD patients can be classified based on maximum motor development. Those who can sit on their own or slide on their buttocks while sitting by extending and flexing the knees with hip rotation are classified as having the typical form, accounting for 75 % of FCMD patients. Those who can walk are classified as having the mild form (15 %) and those lacking head control as having severe FCMD (10 %). All of the severe-type patients have the heterozygous allele, and the typical patients tend to have homozygous alleles of a founder mutation. Mild-type patients can be either heterozygous or homozygous. Saito et al. hypothesized that severe cases have a nonsense mutation of another allele, while typical and milder cases that are heterozygous for the insertion have a missense or silent mutation in another allele [7].

FCMD patients show generalized muscle weakness, hypotonia, and psychomotor retardation from early infancy. Patients are generally brought to the hospital because of floppiness, muscle weakness, poor sucking, poor weight gain, and motor delay as initial symptoms, usually before 9 months of age. In retrospect, mothers sometimes notice less movement or weaker crying than in healthy babies (5 %). Limited hip abduction, as a symptom of contractures, is sometimes mistaken for hip dislocation. Some patients show scoliosis or thoracic deformities such as funnel chest or pigeon chest due to muscle weakness affecting the trunk. Motor delay becomes apparent at the age of 4 months as a lack of head control in typical cases. Most typical cases gain head control from 4 to 12 months of age, sitting from 8 months to 3 years of age, and sliding on the buttocks from 18 months to 7 years of age. Mild cases sometimes show normal motor development by sitting without support, with the delay subsequently becoming apparent. Most mild cases can crawl before 2 years and walk with support before 3 years of age. The muscle power of the upper limbs is rather poor, and most patients can raise their forearms only to the shoulder level, no higher. Most typical patients, when quite young, use a self-propelled manual wheelchair and later switch to using an electric wheelchair. The peak motor function is seen between the ages of 2 and 8 years in all cases, and the deterioration then manifests. Before 15 years of age, typical patients lose the ability to sit without support and become bedridden. Most typical patients die of respiratory dysfunction, pulmonary infections including aspiration pneumonia, suffocation, or congestive heart failure. The mean life span is less than 20 years.

Hypertrophic changes of the calves, forearms, and cheeks are often seen and become evident in late infancy. Facial muscle involvement is a characteristic feature of FCMD, but it is not clear before 1 year of age. Only puffing of the cheeks, shallow nasolabial folds, and a slightly open mouth are recognizable in infancy. After 1 year of age, the myopathic face becomes increasingly apparent as the child grows older [2] (Fig. 1.1a–c). Prognathism and macroglossia become more evident in childhood. After age 6 years, the puffing of the cheeks changes to atrophy and results in the chin having a sharp or pointed shape.

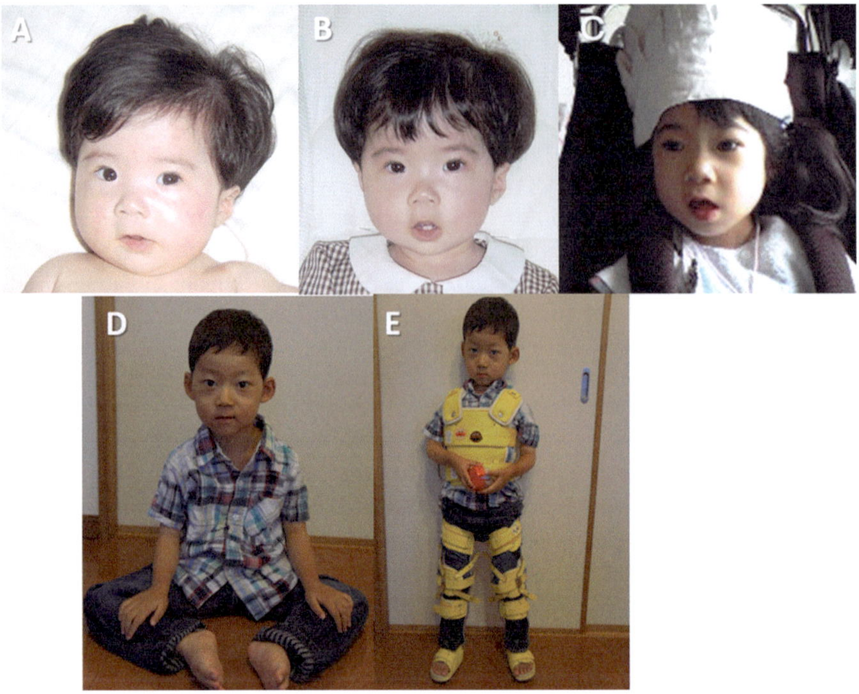

Fig. 1.1 Facial appearance changes with age in a girl with FCMD; images were obtained at 7 months (**A**), at 1 year and 5 months (**B**), and at 8 years of age (**C**). Note that the myopathic face is not evident at 8 months (**A**). At 2 years, puffing of the cheeks and open mouth are evident (**b**). At 5 years, open mouth and a sharp chin are recognizable (**c**). A boy with FCMD at 1 year and at 3 years of age (**D**, **E**). He can sit on his own and is classified as having the typical form. Facial muscle involvement is not evident (**D**). He is training to maintain the standing position with HKAFO (**E**). (These images are shown with permission from the parents)

1.3 Diagnostic Testing

1.3.1 Serum Creatine Kinase (CK)

The level of serum creatine kinase (CK) is usually under 10,000 U/l, not as high as that of DMD patients. Under age 6 years, CK is 10–50 times higher than normal, but it decreases after age 6 years. CK decreases to the normal level when patients become bedridden. The level of CK changes depends on maximum motor development. In patients with the severe phenotype, who are bedridden, the CK level is highest in infancy or early childhood and then decreases linearly. In patients with the typical or the mild phenotype, the CK level increases with motor development, reaching the highest around the time of peak of their motor function, and then decreases with age and deterioration. Aspartate aminotransferase (AST), alanine aminotransferase (ALT), lactate dehydrogenase (LDH), and aldolase are 1.5–3 times higher than normal. FCMD patients are on occasion misdiagnosed as having liver dysfunction because ALT is sometimes higher than AST, a finding that also occurs in young children with DMD.

1.3.2 Neuroimaging

Typical findings of magnetic resonance imaging (MRI) in FCMD patients are cobblestone lissencephaly and cerebellar cystic lesions [14] (Fig. 1.2). Cerebral abnormalities on MRI are mainly classified into two patterns of cerebral cortical dysplasia. Both patterns are usually symmetrical and can be seen at all ages. The first pattern is typical of polymicrogyria showing a slightly thickened cortex with shallow sulci and a bumpy gray-white matter interface at the frontal lobe in all

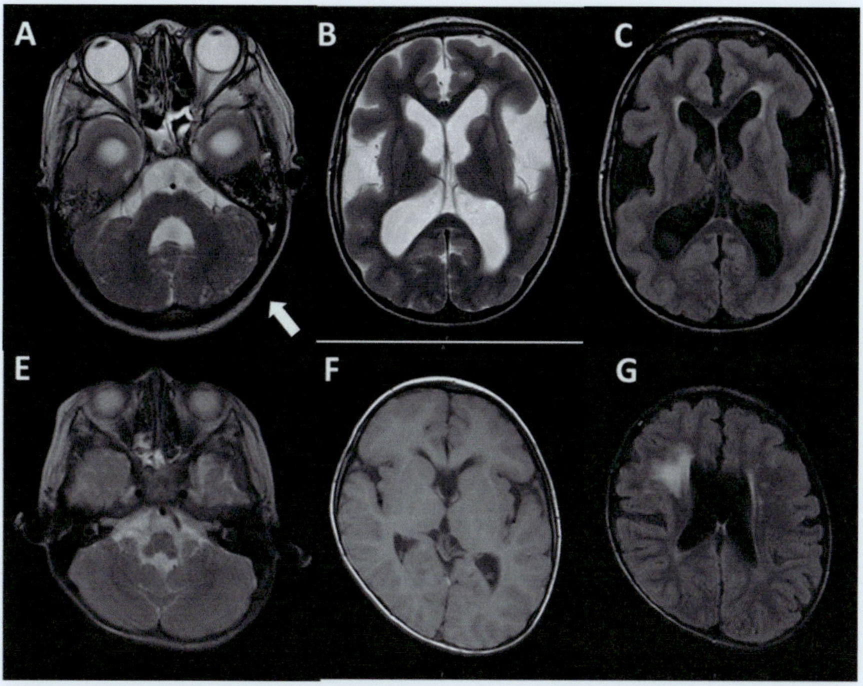

Fig. 1.2 Brain MR images in a 10-year-old girl with severe phenotype (**A**, **B**, **C**) and in a 3-year-old boy with typical phenotype (**D**, **E**, **F**). A T2-weighted image shows several small cysts (*arrow*) in the cerebellum (**A**). Pachygyria with a thickened cortex showing a smooth surface in the frontotemporal lobes can be seen. Wide Sylvian fissures and dilated ventricles are evident on the T2-weighted image. (**B**) The high-intensity area close to the frontal horn of the lateral ventricle in the white matter region was easily demonstrated on FLAIR (**c**). No apparent cysts were detected in the cerebellum on the T2-weighted image (**D**), and pachygyria in the frontal region was very mild on a T1-weighted image (**E**). High-intensity areas were also detected in a typical phenotype case employing FLAIR (**F**)

patients and at the temporoparietal lobes in some cases. Employing sagittal images may facilitate detecting the changes in this cortical dysplasia that were limited to the frontal lobe [14]. The second pattern is pachygyria showing a thick cortex with a smooth surface and a smooth gray-white matter interface in the temporo-occipital lobes. In the cerebellum, polymicrogyria such as disorganized cerebellar foliation with intermingled islands of granular and molecular layers and cerebellar cysts which are intraparenchymal cysts located in the peripheral hemispheres are typically seen in FCMD patients, regardless of age. White matter abnormalities with hyperintensity on T2-weighted images and hypointensity on T1-weighted images are seen especially in younger patients and those with severe phenotypes. Since the signal alteration varies in extent among patients and becomes milder with age, the issue of whether white matter abnormalities suggest delayed myelination, demyelination, dysmyelination, or other problems remains controversial [15–17]. Recent studies with MR spectroscopy indicate delayed myelination rather than dysmyelination [16, 17]. Dilated lateral ventricles are often recognized, and some patients with severe phenotypes may show hydrocephalus similar to that associated with WWS. A thin and rounded corpus callosum and cavities of the septum pellucidum or Berger's space in older patients are often seen. Hypoplasia of the brain stem is sometimes seen, and sagittal views reveal a thin brain stem which is straighter than normal.

In Fig. 1.2, the three upper brain MRIs are from a severe-type patient, and the lower three are from a patient with typical-type FCMD. T2-weighted images show frontal pachygyria, dilated ventricles, and high myelin signals. The cerebellum has numerous pits. These abnormalities are more severe in the severe type.

1.3.3 Skeletal Muscle Imaging (MRI and CT)

Skeletal muscle imaging detecting the patterns of affected muscles specific for each disease is useful for differential diagnosis or assessment of the progression of muscle disease. In FCMD patients, the changes with fatty replacement are more striking and extensive at the calf level (Fig. 1.3). The fatty changes in calf muscles in FCMD patients are already detectable in early infancy and progress rapidly as compared to those in DMD, indicating that this is one reason for FCMD patients never becoming ambulatory [18]. Muscle imaging showed marked involvement of the gastrocnemius and soleus muscles at the calf level, and the biceps femoris, vastus lateralis, and rectus muscles at the thigh level are also secondarily involved. Paraspinal muscles become involved at the early stage. On the other hand, the gracilis, sartorius, and tibialis posterior muscles are relatively preserved. Since there are patients with the mild phenotype who can become ambulant due to preserved soleus muscles, some extent of maximum motor development can be assumed based on skeletal muscle imaging.

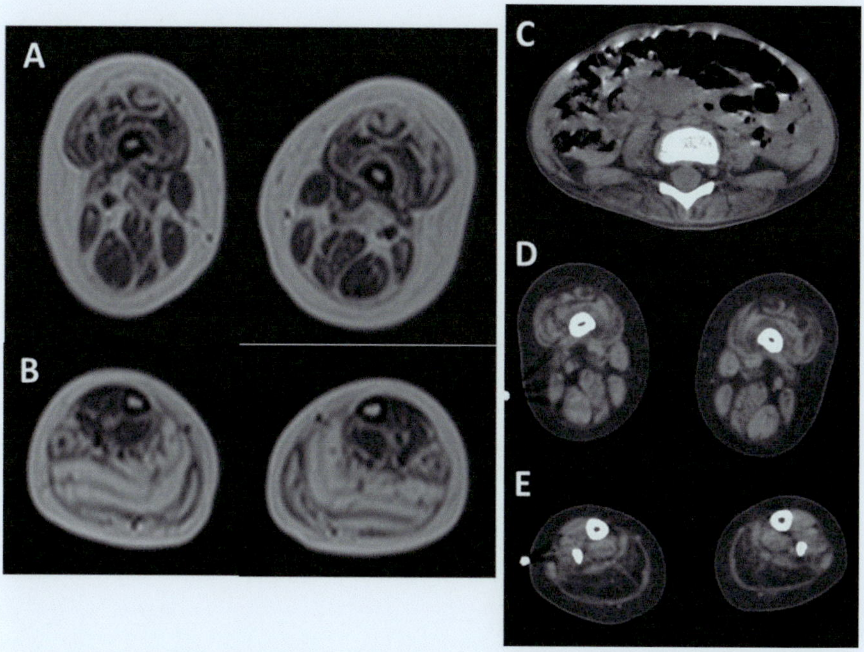

Fig. 1.3 T1-weighted skeletal muscle MRI (**A**, **B**) and CT scans (**C**, **D**, **E**) in a 3-year-old FCMD patient. Reticulated increased intensities were recognized in the rectus femoris and vastus lateralis (**A**) and marked high-intensity areas in the soleus and gastrocnemius muscles. Atrophy and scattered low-density areas were seen in the paraspinal muscles at the T3 level (**C**) and low-density areas in the rectus femoris and vastus lateralis muscles, while the gracilis and sartorius muscles were well preserved (**D**). Low-density changes were seen throughout the soleus and gastrocnemius muscles (**E**)

1.3.4 Muscle Pathology

Findings such as necrosis, regenerating fibers, and increases in connective tissues are seen. Compared with those in DMD cases, all fibers are round and small. Some extremely small fibers (<10 μm) are scattered among other muscle fibers. There is no inflammatory cell infiltration. Hayashi et al. reported a selective deficiency of highly glycosylated α-DG, but not β-dystroglycan (DG), on the surface membranes of skeletal and cardiac muscle fibers in patients with FCMD [19]. Since the diagnosis can be made by genetic analysis and specific clinical features in most cases, muscle biopsy should not necessarily be performed for diagnostic purposes.

1.3.5 Neuropathology

The main central nervous system (CNS) lesion in FCMD patients is cobblestone lissencephaly of the cerebrum and cerebellum. Several studies investigating how fukutin works via α-DG in neurons have been conducted. The basement membrane covers the glia limitans where the glycosylated α-DG is observed. In CNS lesions of the fetus with FCMD, glioneuronal tissues protrude into the leptomeninges through disruption of the glia limitans in which the glycosylation of α-DG is reduced [20–22]. Hence, hypoglycosylation of α-dystroglycan is considered to be one of the main causes of glia limitans disruption, resulting in cobblestone lissencephaly. Astrocytes are also presumably involved in FCMD. As Hiroi et al. suggested, fukutin appears to be important not only simply for migration but also for cell differentiation. Their study demonstrated that the expression of *FKTN* mRNA decreased with maturation in the human cerebrum and raised the possibility that fukutin might be involved in cellular differentiation via glycosylation of α-dystroglycan. Immature neurons remain in an immature state during migration and begin to develop into a mature form once they reach the proper position after migration. Fukutin might be important for preventing inappropriate differentiation during migration [23].

1.4 Complications and Management Strategies

1.4.1 Intellectual Involvement

Mental retardation is seen in most FCMD patients, and the level is moderate to severe [24], with IQs ranging from 30 to 50 [25]. Most typical patients master very little speech, fewer than 20 meaningful words, and are never capable of sentence formation. The severity of mental retardation usually correlates with phenotypes classified by maximum motor development, that is, severe-form patients can learn no or only a few words, while those with the mild form can speak in sentences. Some patients with refractory epilepsy can learn only a few words though they are able to sit without support or slide on the buttocks, showing a discrepancy between speech ability and motor development. There are a few reports on the mild-form FCMD with a mild mental deficit. One report described a mild-form patient, heterozygous for a 3-kb insertion of the ancestral founder mutation, whose IQ on the Tanaka-Binet scale was 97 [26]. Since no mutation was detected in the coding region of the other allele in this patient, the phenotype-genotype correlation remained unclear. Social development is not as severely affected as mental abilities [27]. FCMD patients are shy but enjoy communicating with people and can have positive relationships with other children in kindergarten and primary school. Autistic features are rare in FCMD patients.

1.4.2 Seizures

Because of cortical dysplasia, more than 50 % of FCMD patients exhibit febrile seizures and/or epilepsy beyond 1 year of age [2]. Yoshioka and Higuchi reported seizures in 80 % of their FCMD patients, and the average age at onset was 3 years [28]. Usually, the initial seizures occur with a febrile episode, though one-third of patients had afebrile seizures from the onset [28]. Most patients show generalized tonic or tonic-clonic convulsions, as febrile seizures, early in life. Later, however, the main convulsive disorder becomes complex partial seizures. In most patients, epilepsy is mild and treatable, but some patients develop intractable seizures including Lennox-Gastaut syndrome. West syndrome has also been documented but is rather rare in FCMD patients [29, 30]. Yoshioka et al. reported the correlation between seizure severity and genotype and concluded that mutation analysis of the *FKTN* gene may predict seizure outcomes [30]. In their study, heterozygotes usually developed seizures earlier (the onsets of febrile and afebrile seizures were, on average, 3.6 and 3.7 years) than homozygotes (5.4 and 4.6 years), and some heterozygotes had intractable seizures.

In our recent study, 62 % of patients developed seizures. Among them, 71 % had only febrile seizures, 6 % had afebrile seizures from the onset, and 22 % developed afebrile seizures following febrile seizures. A comparison of seizure prevalences between homozygotes and heterozygotes showed a slightly higher rate in the latter, but the difference did not reach statistical significance. The peak age at febrile seizure onset was 1–2 years and the mean age was 3 years, later than that of febrile convulsions in the normal population. Mean age at afebrile seizure onset was 5.8 years, showing no peak. Most patients have seizures that are controllable with just one type of antiepileptic drug, but 18 % have intractable seizures that must be treated with three medications. Comparison between patients with seizures controllable with one type of antiepileptic drug and those requiring more than two types revealed no statistically significant differences in genotype or phenotype, but there was a tendency for the number of intractable seizures to be lower in homozygotes. There was also a tendency for the total number of seizures and intractable seizures to be lower in homozygotes. In contrast to a previous report, the author's study group found that intractable seizures can manifest in homozygotes, especially those with severe intellectual involvement, despite relatively good motor development and mild abnormalities on brain MR images. Fixed discharges in the F areas tended to be a common feature in the intractable cases. Paroxysmal discharges on electroencephalography did not usually have a fixed location and were independent of the brain MRI abnormalities. Carbamazepine and valproic acid (VPA) are the agents most frequently used and show no statistically significant difference in efficacy. We have experienced a few FCMD patients treated for intractable epilepsy with many types of antiepileptic drugs, including relatively a high dose of VPA, with kidney tubule cell damage progressing to Fanconi syndrome. Instead of high-dose VPA, levetiracetam (LEV), which has recently been administered for intractable epilepsy as a second-line therapy in Japan, is now among the effective choices for seizures complicating FCMD. LEV is effective for both partial and generalized seizures, and we have succeeded in controlling intractable seizures with LEV in some of our FCMD patients. No serious side effects have been reported, and LEV is especially useful for patients with respiratory dysfunction and/or dysphagia since it does not increase oropharyngeal secretion, a common side effect of antiepileptic drugs.

1.4.3 Ocular Abnormalities

Ocular abnormalities including refractive errors and accommodation disorders are seen in almost half of FCMD patients. Retinal abnormalities are mild and focal, but the prevalence is relatively high, being present in 32 % of FCMD patients with the more severe phenotype [2, 31]. Refractive errors (myopia and hypermetropia) are common, and microphthalmia, retinal detachment, and cataracts are seen in patients with the severe phenotype [27]. Hino et al. demonstrated the clinicopathological features of the eyes of FCMD patients in detail [32]. Their histopathological examinations revealed various retinal abnormalities even in FCMD cases without ophthalmological alterations. The authors raised the possibility that the initial changes in retinal dysplasia may occur during the fetal period. Reductions in basement components, cytoskeletal proteins, and glutamate metabolism-related proteins produced by Müller cells in the eyes of FCMD patients implicate defective Müller cell properties in the retinal pathology of FCMD. Fukutin may be highly relevant to the cell-to-cell interaction of retinal blasts with Müller cells, and downregulation of *FKTN* mRNA may thus be responsible for retinal dysplasia [32]. Regular ophthalmologic evaluations are recommended especially for patients with the severe phenotype.

1.4.4 Respiratory Failure

Progressive respiratory failure typically emerges early in the second decade of life and is one of the most common causes of death in FCMD patients. Noninvasive positive pressure ventilation (NPPV) has been used as an effective therapy, although tracheostomy with invasive ventilation (TIV) may be needed in some cases. The author's research group retrospectively studied chronic respiratory failure in genetically diagnosed FCMD patients. In our study, the mean age at the introduction of noninvasive positive pressure ventilation support was 12 years. NPPV is beneficial and well tolerated despite the intellectual impairments. A few patients received tracheostomy with invasive ventilation (TIV) after age 15 years without prior NPPV, because of difficulty with extubation followed by a respiratory infection and some urgently required laryngotracheal separation after episodes of aspiration pneumonia or suffocation. Heterozygotes tended to develop the complication of chronic respiratory failure earlier than homozygotes. Respiratory failure also progressed earlier in the severe-type patients. Though the difference did not reach statistical significance, chronic respiratory failure manifests earlier in those with poor motor function and/or a heterozygous genotype. It is often difficult at the outpatient clinic to detect respiratory dysfunction in FCMD patients. Most patients cannot perform lung function tests mainly due to mental retardation and because they are unable to purse their lips due to facial muscle weakness. Furthermore, the symptoms of chronic respiratory dysfunction such as sleep disturbance or poor intake are difficult to detect since many FCMD patients have had these symptoms since they were quite young. Regular assessments with end-tidal CO_2 monitoring during sleep should be conducted once a year to detect respiratory dysfunction, starting at about age 10 years in typical-form patients and much earlier in those with the severe form.

1.4.5 Cardiomyopathy

Cardiac involvement usually develops very slowly, first appearing after 10 years of age, in FCMD patients. Since Hayashi et al. reported a deficiency of α-DG in the cardiac as well as in the skeletal muscles of FCMD patients [19], it is reasonable that cardiac involvement also manifests in both DMD and Becker muscular dystrophy (BMD). Fibrosis of the myocardium was confirmed at autopsy in several reports [33, 34], and moderate-to-severe multifocal fibrosis was observed throughout the left ventricular (LV) wall, especially in the anterior, lateral, and posterior walls [34]. The degree of fibrosis was greater in patients who died of heart failure than in those who died of other causes such as respiratory problems. Electrocardiographic (ECG) abnormalities are common and similar to those in DMD and BMD. Especially, a tall R wave on V1 with an R/S ratio >1 is observed in most FCMD patients, while deep but narrow Q waves on leads I, aVL, V5, and V6 are not seen as frequently as in dystrophinopathies. In contrast, cardiomegaly on chest radiography is rare. Plasma brain natriuretic peptide is not elevated till the advanced stage of cardiac dysfunction and is not useful for early detection. An echocardiogram is the most useful method of detecting the early stage of cardiac dysfunction. A significant correlation between age and LV fractional shortening (LVFS) was confirmed and LVFS decreased with age. LVSF was normal in most patients under 10 years of age but was reduced in most patients over 15 years of age. Therefore, a regular cardiac evaluation including echocardiograms and follow-up is important in patients aged 10 years and older. It is noteworthy that there was no significant difference in LVFS among the three phenotypes. Also, LV function in heterozygous patients is similar to that in younger children who are homozygous. There is no definite relationship between cardiac dysfunction and either the severity or the genotype of FCMD. Rather, we can say that the frequency of cardiac involvement tends to become higher in mild and typical FCMD cases. There is an involvement discrepancy between cardiac dysfunction and skeletal muscle systems, which is also seen in DMD or BMD. We hypothesized that the greater mobility of mild and typical cases may place more of a burden on the hearts. It is rare, but a few patients rapidly developed serious cardiac dysfunction and died before 15 years of age, and a few patients with the severe form showed LVFS reduction before 5 years. Once the presence of cardiac involvement is recognized, patients are usually treated with angiotensin-converting enzyme (ACE) inhibitors or a combination of ACE inhibitors and β-blockers. These interventions were reported to improve LV function in patients with DMD and BMD [35]. Combination therapy with ACE inhibitors and β-blockers for 2 years was also found to significantly increase LVFS, and this regimen was more efficient than therapy with only ACE inhibitors in several types of muscular dystrophies including FCMD [36].

Only dilated cardiomyopathy was seen, while no patients showed increased wall thickening or a conduction abnormality on ECG. Murakami reported Japanese patients with a compound heterozygous *FKTN* mutation presenting with dilated cardiomyopathy with minimal muscular dystrophy (OMIM # 611615, Cardiomyopathy, dilated, 1X; CMD1X). All of their patients had a compound heterozygous mutation consisting of a 3-kb insertion and a missense mutation in the *FKTN* gene [37]. Elevated serum CK and dilated cardiomyopathy were recognized in all patients with minimal muscle change. A subsequent study detected only one patient who was a compound heterozygote with a 3-kb insertion and a missense mutation among 172 patients with dilated cardiomyopathy and indicated that the compound heterozygous *FKTN* mutation was a rare cause of dilated cardiomyopathy [38]. Among patients with hyper cardiomyopathy, none had mutations in the *FKTN* gene.

1.4.6 Dysphagia

Dysphagia is a serious problem in advanced stage FCMD patients and can, along with respiratory dysfunction or cardiomyopathy, be life-threatening. However, only a few reports have described swallowing problems or therapeutic interventions for dysphagia in FCMD patients [39]. We retrospectively studied dysphagia and therapeutic interventions in genetically diagnosed FCMD patients. No mild-form patients developed dysphagia. All severe-form patients needed tube feeding from infancy, and 67 % underwent gastrostomy in the early stage (0.5–8.5 years). In typical-form patients, dysphagia emerged on average at age 10 (7–14) years, showing double peaks, one at 7–9 years in the group whose maximum ability was sitting and the other at 12–14 years in the shuffling group. Most typical-form patients required gastrostomy, half had early-stage elective surgery before the age of 10 at the family's request, and half had absolute indications. After gastrostomy, the patients were able to maintain their body weights, and the frequency of aspiration decreased significantly. Some patients over 15 years of age underwent urgent tracheostomy or laryngotracheal separation after episodes of aspiration pneumonia or suffocation, though their respiratory dysfunction was not particularly severe. These patients with severe dysphagia tended to have intractable seizures. In

FCMD patients, dysphagia emerged earlier than respiratory dysfunction and required active intervention. Gastrostomy at an early stage was beneficial and well tolerated, though saliva/sputum aspiration remained uncontrollable since mechanical insufflation-exsufflation is occasionally ineffective for uncooperative patients with severe mental retardation.

1.4.7 Sleep Disturbance

Insomnia is well known to occur in other neurodevelopmental disorders, like attention deficit hyperactivity disorder (ADHD), and there is extensive experience with the use of medications for treatment. Alpha-agonists, late-day stimulants, antihistamines, and antidepressants are often prescribed for sleep disturbance in patients with ADHD. Insomnia is often seen in patients with FCMD starting in early childhood and can be a serious problem that bothers their families at home. In our retrospective study [40], the prevalence of insomnia in FCMD patients was 32 %, with difficulty falling asleep (60 %), difficulty staying asleep (33 %), and early waking (7 %), while the insomnia prevalence in the general pediatric or adolescent population ranges between only 0.05 % and 20 %. Most patients showed resistance to medication and a few obtained good results for falling asleep with etizolam or estazolam, and one patient seemed to have a good response to a new narcoleptic, melatonin. We analyzed the relationships between insomnia and other factors, genotype, seizures, maximum motor function, and mental status. However, we identified no statistically significant correlations of any of these clinical factors, even genotype, with insomnia. Thus, insomnia was independent of these factors, and no insomnia-genotype relationship was detected. Ito et al. reported an abnormality of catecholaminergic neurons in the brain stem in FCMD and suggested that it may contribute to brain stem dysfunction and might be related to sleep-wake regulation disorders [41]. Insomnia in FCMD should be considered a central nervous system complication, and medication for insomnia in FCMD should be established in order to improve quality of life for patients and their families.

1.4.8 Severe Muscle Damage Following Viral Infection

We have experienced FCMD patients who showed sudden exacerbation of muscle weakness with marked elevation of serum creatine kinase and urinary myoglobin levels a few days after a febrile episode with a viral infection, occasionally leading to death. To elucidate this characteristic feature of patients with FCMD, we focused on genetically defined FCMD patients who had manifested sudden exacerbation of muscle weakness and retrospectively studied the month in which the episode occurred, age at onset, level of motor function, clinical course, and cause of infection [42]. All of the patients were homozygous for a 3-kb insertion mutation of *FKTN*. The phenotypes of these patients were rather mild, with one-fourth having the mild phenotype with standing or walking with support while others had the typical type. None of the severe phenotype patients were included. The patients developed muscle weakness exacerbations ranging from paralysis to loss of head control, and one-fourth developed severe respiratory failure requiring mechanical ventilator support. The episodes were clustered in the summer, especially in July, and coxsackievirus and enterovirus were most often detected. Most patients were clinically given a diagnosis of herpangina, hand-foot-mouth disease, pharyngitis, or upper respiratory infection. It could happen at any age, of course, but was most often observed in infants. The duration of fever during the viral illness was 1–5 days, a mean of 3.3 days. The interval between the occurrence of symptoms suggestive of viral infection and the exacerbation of muscle weakness was 2–6 days, a mean of 3.3 days. More than half of the patients showed defervescence. Serum CK was markedly elevated, up to 2.7–37.8 times (mean, 10.8 times) the usual level. Urinary myoglobin also showed marked elevation, up to 3000 ng/ml, but none of the patients developed renal failure. The period between the onset of muscle weakness exacerbation and recovery to the previous level was 3–27 days, a mean of 14.8 days. Two-thirds of patients were treated with intravenous prednisolone or methylprednisolone pulse therapy in our study, and there was a tendency for earlier muscle recovery in patients treated with steroids as compared to those not receiving steroid therapy (14 days vs 18.5 days). This phenomenon with exacerbation of muscle weakness associated with viral infection is rarely seen in DMD patients, instead apparently being unique to FCMD patients. In patients with limb-girdle muscular dystrophy 2 M and dilated cardiomyopathy 1X with the *FKTN* gene mutation, transient exacerbations of muscle weakness or heart failure have been reported [37, 43]. Since the patients did not complain of myalgia or muscle swelling and the results of muscle biopsies performed in two patients showed no evidence of myositis [44], we consider this phenomenon to be rather suggestive of rhabdomyolysis. Since the muscle volumes of FCMD patients are decreased from early childhood, the level of myoglobinuria was mild to moderate, thereby not leading to renal failure. The reason for muscle damage being induced by specific viral pathogens such as coxsackieviruses and enteroviruses remains unknown. However, we can hypothesize that changes due to *FKTN* gene abnormalities may increase the affinity for certain viruses, considering the recent discovery that many viruses recognize and bind to carbohydrate chains on host cell membranes serving as specific receptors.

1.4.9 Hypoglycemia

Some patients with FCMD experience repeated episodes of hypoglycemia or ketotic hypoglycemia. Ketotic hypoglycemia is also common in healthy younger children, especially those who are lean. One study focused specifically on glucose metabolism in FCMD [45]. Glucagon, alanine, and glucose tests were performed in four FCMD patients who had episodes of ketotic hypoglycemia, to study hepatic reserve, glycogenosis, and glucose tolerance. The investigators found that glycogenosis and gluconeogenesis did not occur, but ketone metabolism was thought to be accelerated only in one case, while the others showed normal glycogenosis and glucose tolerance. Since hypoglycemia occurred in patients who had a low body mass index (<13), we suspect that the loss of muscle volume, which serves as a site of glycogen storage, is the main reason for hypoglycemia. Hypoglycemia often occurs in the morning after prolonged hunger, for example, in the event of patients missing dinner the day before. The author advises parents to make sure that patients eat regularly and to avoid prolonged periods of hunger, in order to prevent hypoglycemia.

1.4.10 Scoliosis and Contractures

Though some patients show severe multiple contractures from birth, similar to those of patients with congenital arthrogryposis multiplex, most are free of contractures in the neonatal period. Extension limitations of the fingers at the extended position of the wrist due to shortening of the long extensor muscle of the digits are recognized in early infancy and can be the initial symptom. Limited hip abduction is noticed in some patients at 3–4 months of age. By 3 years of age, 70 % of patients have developed hip and knee contractures. Pes equinovarus becomes apparent in typical phenotype cases whose maximum motor function is sitting without support or sliding on the buttocks. Beyond 5 years of age, flexion contractures of the elbows and toes, pronation contractures of the forearm, limited neck anteflexion, and malocclusion become marked. To prevent contractures, physical therapy and stretching exercises are essential. Maintaining the standing position with a hip-knee-ankle-foot orthosis (HKAFO) and wearing an ankle-foot orthosis (AFO) are also useful.

Scoliosis is another serious problem that can cause pain, gastrointestinal difficulties, and respiratory dysfunction. Unlike idiopathic scoliosis with a thoracic curve, FCMD patients often have thoracolumbar curve scoliosis like that in DMD patients. Kyphosis and lumbar lordosis are common, and lumbar lordosis especially often causes pain and breakdown of the skin in bedridden patients. Scoliosis is present even in early childhood in patients with severe to typical phenotypes. We speculate that this is due to sitting in the baby buggy despite their trunk muscles not being strong enough to maintain the sitting position. It is important to monitor patients for the presence of spinal deformity and refer them to an orthopedic specialist, if surgical correction is needed. Pedicle-screw-alone fixation and fusion to L5 were reported to be safe and effective in congenital muscular dystrophy patients free of respiratory dysfunction, and the satisfaction of patients and their families was high [46]. However, they must be warned that cardiomyopathy might be a risk factor for mortality, and surgery in these patients should thus generally be avoided.

1.5 Genetic Counseling

Genetic counseling is recommended for the parents of FCMD patients, who want another child. Carrier testing is available after the mutation has been identified in the proband. In Japanese cases, detection of the 3-kb insertion of the ancestral founder mutation can facilitate the prenatal diagnosis of FCMD. For the purposes of family planning, the optimal time for determination of genetic risk and clarification of carrier status, as well as the discussion of prenatal testing, should be completed before pregnancy [47].

1.6 Future Treatments

To date, no definitive and effective treatment for FCMD patients has been developed. Multidisciplinary management such as respiratory support, medications for cardiac dysfunction, nutritional control, and physical therapy are important and can prolong survival. Recently, Taniguchi-Ikeda et al. reported an important insight into the pathogenic mechanism of FCMD and suggested splicing modulation therapy with antisense oligonucleotides (AONs) [9]. They showed that aberrant mRNA splicing induced by SVA exon trapping resulted in truncation of the fukutin gene product and the addition of unnecessary amino acids encoded by SVA. Introduction of AONs has the potential to restore normal *FKTN* mRNA expression and protein production in FCMD patients and in a model mouse, by preventing pathogenic exon trapping by SVA. This revolutionary treatment is now under preparation with clinical trials being planned for the near future.

As another possible treatment, Kanagawa et al. suggested gene therapy with adeno-associated virus (AAV) [48]. In their study, AAV successfully rescued fukutin expression that was limited in myofibers with severe pathology, and, surprisingly, this was achieved even after disease progression.

1.7 Conclusion

FCMD was first reported by Fukuyama et al. in 1960. Thus, global recognition has taken a long time, since patients were rarely reported outside of Japan. After Toda et al. localized a responsible gene at 9q31-33 in 1993 and Kobayashi identified the *FKTN* gene, FCMD was accepted as a new entity, and contributions by non-Japanese researchers have since increased dramatically. In 2012, there was the aforementioned report suggesting a possible treatment for FCMD using ASO. We believe that major steps will be taken to solve the problems of our patients in the near future.

References

1. Fukuyama Y, Kawazura M, Hamura H (1960) A peculiar form of congenital muscular dystrophy. Report of fifteen cases. Paedoatr Univ Tokyo 4:5–8
2. Osawa M, Sumida S, Suzuki N et al (1997) Fukuyama type congenital muscular dystrophy. In: Fukuyama Y, Osawa M, Saito K (eds) Congenital muscular dystrophies. Elsevier Science, Amsterdam, pp 31–68
3. Watanabe M, Kobayashi K, Jin F et al (2005) Founder SVA retrotransposal insertion in Fukuyama-type congenital muscular dystrophy and its origin in Japanese and Northeast Asian populations. Am J Med Genet A 138:344–348
4. Toda T, Miyake M, Kobayashi K et al (1996) Linkage-disequilibrium mapping narrows the Fukuyama-type congenital muscular dystrophy (FCMD) candidate region to <100 kb. Am J Hum Genet 59:1313–1320
5. Kobayashi K, Nakahori Y, Miyake M et al (1998) An ancient retrotransposal insertion causes Fukuyama-type congenital muscular dystrophy. Nature 394:388–392
6. Kondo-Iida E, Kobayashi K, Watanabe M et al (1999) Novel mutations and genotype-phenotype relationships in 107 families with Fukuyama-type congenital muscular dystrophy (FCMD). Hum Mol Genet 8:2303–2309
7. Saito K, Osawa M, Wang ZP et al (2000) Haplotype-phenotype correlation in Fukuyama congenital muscular dystrophy. Am J Med Genet 29:184–190
8. Colombo R, Bignamini AA, Carobene A et al (2000) Age and origin of the FCMD 3-′-untranslated-region retrotransposal insertion mutation causing Fukuyama-type congenital muscular dystrophy in the Japanese population. Hum Genet 107:559–567
9. Taniguchi-Ikeda M, Kobayashi K, Kanagawa M et al (2011) Pathogenic exon-trapping by SVA retrotransposon and rescue in Fukuyama muscular dystrophy. Nature 478:127–131
10. Godfrey C, Clement E, Mein R et al (2007) Refining genotype-phenotype correlations in muscular dystrophies with defective glycosylation of dystroglycan. Brain 130:2725–2735
11. Cotarelo RP, Valero MC, Prados B et al (2008) Two new patients bearing mutations in the fukutin gene confirm the relevance of this gene in Walker-Warburg syndrome. Clin Genet 73:139–145
12. Tunc BT, Mungan IA, Okulu E et al (2009) Hyperekplexia in a neonate: a novel finding in Fukuyama type congenital muscular dystrophy. Genet Couns 20:275–279
13. Vuillaumier-Barrot S, Quijano-Roy S, Bouchet-Seraphin C et al (2009) Four Caucasian patients with mutations in the fukutin gene and variable clinical phenotype. Neuromuscul Disord 19:182–188
14. Aida N, Tamagawa K, Takada K et al (1996) Brain MR in Fukuyama congenital muscular dystrophy. AJNR Am J Neuroradiol 17:605–613
15. Kato T, Funahash M, Matsui A et al (2000) MRI of disseminated developmental dysmyelination in Fukuyama type of CMD. Pediatr Neurol 23:385–388
16. Kato Z, Saito K, Isogaki K et al (2006) Magnetic resonance imaging and spectroscopy in Fukuyama-type congenital muscular dystrophy. J Pediatr Neurol 4:261–264
17. Kato Z, Morimoto M, Orii KE et al (2010) Developmental changes of radiological findings in Fukuyama-type congenital muscular dystrophy. Pediatr Radiol 40:127–129
18. Arai Y (1993) Characteristic of muscles involvement evaluated by CT scans in early stages of progressive muscular dystrophy: comparison between Duchenne and Fukuyama types (in Japanese). J Tokyo Wom Med Univ 63:1089–1103
19. Hayashi YK, Ogawa M, Tagawa K et al (2001) Selective deficiency of alpha-dystroglycan in Fukuyama-type congenital muscular dystrophy. Neurology 57:115–121
20. Nakano I, Funahashi M, Takada K et al (1996) Are breaches in the glia limitans the primary cause of the micropolygyria in Fukuyama-type congenital muscular dystrophy (FCMD)? Pathological study of the cerebral cortex of an FCMD fetus. Acta Neuropathol 91:313–321
21. Yamamoto T, Kawaguchi M, Sakayori N et al (2006) Intracellular binding of fukutin and alpha-dystroglycan: relation to glycosylation of alpha-dystroglycan. Neurosci Res 56:391–399

22. Saito Y, Yamamoto T, Mizuguchi M et al (2006) Altered glycosylation of alpha-dystroglycan in neurons of Fukuyama congenital muscular dystrophy brains. Brain Res 1075:223–228
23. Hiroi A, Yamamoto T, Shibata N et al (2011) Roles of fukutin, the gene responsible for Fukuyama-type congenital muscular dystrophy, in neurons: possible involvement in synaptic function and neuronal migration. Acta Histochem Cytochem 44:91–101
24. Fukuyama Y, Osawa M, Suzuki H (1983) Congenital progressive muscular dystrophy of the Fukuyama type – clinical, genetic and pathological considerations. Brain Dev 3:1–29
25. Osawa M, Suzuki N, Arai Y et al (1993) Fukuyama-type congenital progressive muscular dystrophy (FCMD)-special comment on the relationship between case reported by Nakayama et al and FCMD. Neuropathologica 13:259–268
26. Hino-Fukuyo N, Haginoya K, Hayashi YK et al (2006) A case of Fukuyama-type congenital muscular dystrophy with a very mild mental deficit. Neuromuscul Disord 16:274–276
27. Saito K, Kobayashi M (2001) Fukuyama congenital muscular dystrophy. In: Emery AEH (ed) Muscular dystrophies. Oxford Press, Oxford, pp 39–54
28. Yoshioka M, Higuchi Y (2005) Long-term prognosis of epilepsies and related seizure disorders in Fukuyama-type congenital muscular dystrophy. J Child Neurol 20:385–391
29. Akiyama T, Ohtsuka Y, Takata T et al (2006) The mildest known case of Fukuyama-type congenital muscular dystrophy. Brain Dev 28:537–540
30. Yoshioka M, Higuchi Y, Fujii T et al (2007) Seizure-genotype relationship in Fukuyama-type congenital muscular dystrophy. Brain Dev 30:59–67
31. Tsutsumi A, Uchida Y, Osawa M et al (1989) Ocular findings in Fukuyama type congenital muscular dystrophy. Brain Dev 11:413–419
32. Hino N, Kobayashi M, Shibata N et al (2001) Clinicopathological study on eyes from cases of Fukuyama type congenital muscular dystrophy. Brain Dev 23:97–107
33. Miura K, Shirasawa H (1987) Congenital muscular dystrophy of the Fukuyama type (FCMD) with severe myocardial fibrosis. A case report with postmortem angiography. Acta Pathol Jpn 37:1823–1835
34. Nakanishi T, Sakauchi M, Kaneda Y et al (2006) Cardiac involvement in Fukuyama-type congenital muscular dystrophy. Pediatrics 117:e1187–e1192
35. Jefferies JL, Eidem BW, Belmont JW et al (2005) Genetic predictors and remodeling of dilated cardiomyopathy in muscular dystrophy. Circulation 112:2799–2804
36. Kajimoto H, Ishigaki K, Okumura K et al (2006) Beta-blocker therapy for cardiac dysfunction in patients with muscular dystrophy. Circ J 70:991–994
37. Murakami T, Hayashi YK, Noguchi S et al (2006) Fukutin gene mutations cause dilated cardiomyopathy with minimal muscle weakness. Ann Neurol 60:597–602
38. Arimura T, Hayashi YK, Murakami T et al (2009) Mutational analysis of fukutin gene in dilated cardiomyopathy and hypertrophic cardiomyopathy. Circ J 73:158–161
39. Mizuno T, Komaki H, Sasaki M et al (2012) Efficacy and tolerance of gastrostomy feeding in Japanese muscular dystrophy patients. Brain Dev 34:756–762
40. Sato T, Ishigaki K, Kajino S et al (2013) Insomnia in patients with Fukuyama congenital muscular dystrophy. J Tokyo Wom Med Univ 83:42–46
41. Itoh M, Houdou S, Kawahara H et al (1996) Morphological study of the brainstem in Fukuyama type congenital muscular dystrophy. Pediatr Neurol 15:327–331
42. Murakami T, Ishigaki K, Shirakawa S et al (2012) Severe muscle damage following viral infection in patients with Fukuyama congenital muscular dystrophy. Brain Dev 34:293–297
43. Godfrey C, Escolar D, Brockington M et al (2006) Fukutin gene mutations in steroid-responsive limb girdle muscular dystrophy. Ann Neurol 60:603–610
44. Ikenaka H, Kawahara M, Yanagaki S et al (2000) Transient exacerbation of muscle weakness induced by febrile illness in patients with congenital muscular dystrophy. J Tokyo Wom Med Univ 70:40–46
45. Komine S, Kodaira K, Ikeya K et al (2013) Glucose metabolism in patients with congenital muscular dystrophy (in Japanese). J Tokyo Wom Med Univ 83:25–35

46. Takaso M, Nakazawa T, Imura T et al (2010) Surgical correction of spinal deformity in patients with congenital muscular dystrophy. J Orthop Sci 15:493–501
47. Saito K (2006) Prenatal diagnosis of Fukuyama congenital muscular dystrophy. Prenat Diagn 26:415–417
48. Kanagawa M, Yu CC, Ito C et al (2013) Impaired viability of muscle precursor cells in muscular dystrophy with glycosylation defects and amelioration of its severe phenotype by limited gene expression. Hum Mol Genet 22:3003–3015

Chapter 2
α-Dystroglycanopathy

Motoi Kanagawa and Tatsushi Toda

Abstract α-Dystroglycanopathy encompasses a group of congenital and limb-girdle-type muscular dystrophies that are caused by abnormal glycosylation of α-dystroglycan. α-Dystroglycanopathy is often associated with brain abnormalities including type II lissencephaly and mental retardation. Currently, around 15 genes have been identified in which mutations cause abnormal glycosylation of α-dystroglycan resulting in disease. Dystroglycan is a highly glycosylated peripheral membrane protein that functions as a cell-surface receptor for proteins in the extra-cellular matrices and synapses. Unique *O*-mannosyl glycosylation is necessary for the ligand-binding activities of dystroglycan, and some of α-dystroglycanopathy gene products are involved in the process of α-dystroglycan glycosylation. Studies using animal and cell models for α-dystroglycanopathy have contributed to understanding the pathogenesis of this disease and to establishing therapeutic strategies. In this chapter, we review the structure, modification pathways, and physiological roles of dystroglycan glycosylation, as well as their involvement in human diseases, disease pathogenesis, and therapeutic strategies.

Keywords Dystroglycan • Glycosylation • *O*-Mannose • Fukutin • Fukuyama congenital muscular dystrophy • Gene therapy

2.1 What Is α-Dystroglycanopathy?

α-Dystroglycanopathy (α-DGpathy) is a muscular dystrophy disease entity that is caused by the abnormal glycosylation of α-dystroglycan (α-DG). Dystroglycan (DG) was originally identified from skeletal muscle as a component of the

M. Kanagawa (✉)
Division of Molecular Brain Science, Kobe University Graduate School of Medicine,
7-5-1 Kusunoki-cho, Chuo-ku, Kobe, Hyogo 650-0017, Japan
e-mail: kanagawa@med.kobe-u.ac.jp

T. Toda
Division of Molecular Brain Science, Kobe University Graduate School of Medicine,
7-5-1 Kusunoki-cho, Chuo-ku, Kobe, Hyogo 650-0017, Japan

Division of Neurology, Kobe University Graduate School of Medicine, 7-5-1 Kusunoki-cho,
Chuo-ku, Kobe, Hyogo 650-0017, Japan

S. Takeda et al. (eds.), *Translational Research in Muscular Dystrophy*,
DOI 10.1007/978-4-431-55678-7_2

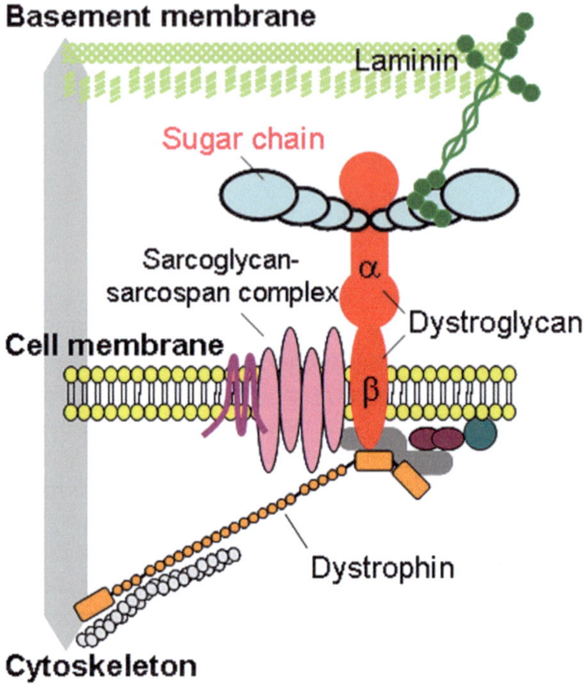

Fig. 2.1 Schematic representation of the dystrophin-glycoprotein complex and dystroglycan

dystrophin-glycoprotein complex (DGC) [1]. DGC is a large glycoprotein complex containing dystrophin in the muscle plasma membrane and forms a structural linkage between the basement membrane and actin cytoskeleton [2]. One of the functions of the DGC is to provide physical strength to the skeletal muscle cell membrane. Within the DGC, DG functions as a central axis by anchoring the dystrophin underneath the cell membrane and binding to basement membrane proteins such as laminin on the outside of the cell (Fig. 2.1).

Mutations in components of the DGC, such as dystrophin and sarcoglycans, were identified to be associated with Duchenne/Becker and limb-girdle type-muscular dystrophies in the late 1980s to the mid-1990s. Although mutations in the *DAG1* gene, which encodes DG, were not identified until 2011 [3], there was a unique route leading to the establishment of the disease entity called α-DGpathy. In 2001, Hayashi and colleagues reported that the reactivity of the monoclonal antibody IIH6 that recognizes a portion of the *O*-glycan structure of α-DG is dramatically reduced in patients with Fukuyama congenital muscular dystrophy (FCMD) [4]. Subsequently, Campbell and colleagues confirmed that the α-DG proteins from patients with FCMD, Walker-Warburg syndrome (WWS), and muscle-eye-brain disease (MEB) were abnormally glycosylated and had lost their ligand-binding activities [5]. Abnormal α-DG glycosylation was subsequently also found in patients with congenital muscular dystrophy (CMD) and limb-girdle muscular dystrophy (LGMD) [6–8]. In this way, the concept of α-DGpathy was established [9, 10]. Currently, there are around 15 known α-DGpathy genes, all of which are

Table 2.1 Dystroglycanopathy genes and their functions

Dystroglycanopathy genes	Gene functions	MDDG number
POMT1	*O*-mannosyltransferase (POMT1/POMT2 complex)	1
POMT2	*O*-mannosyltransferase (POMT1/POMT2 complex)	2
POMGNT1	Protein *O*-mannose β1,2-GlcNAc transferase	3
FKTN	Unknown, likely involved in post-phosphoryl modification	4
FKRP	Unknown, likely involved in post-phosphoryl modification	5
LARGE	Synthesis of Xyl-GlcA repeating units	6
ISPD	Unknown	7
GTDC2/POMGNT2	Protein *O*-mannose β1,4-GlcNAc transferase	8
DAG1	Dystroglycan, reduced interaction with LARGE	9
TMEM5	Unknown	10
B3GALNT2	β1,3-GalNAc transferase	11
SGK196/POMK	*O*-Man kinase	12
B3GNT1(B4GAT1)	β1,4-GlcA transferase	13
GMPPB	GDP-mannose pyrophosphorylase B	14
DPM1	Dol-P-Man synthesis	–
DPM2	Dol-P-Man synthesis	–
DPM3	Dol-P-Man synthesis	–
DOLK	Dolichol phosphate synthesis	–

involved either directly or indirectly in the glycosylation of α-DG (Table 2.1). However, some unidentified causative genes for α-DGpathy could possibly be identified in the near future.

FCMD is an autosomal recessive muscular dystrophy that is the most common CMD in Japan. FCMD is also the most common childhood muscular dystrophy, next to Duchenne muscular dystrophy (DMD), in Japan [11]. The incidence of FCMD is around 3 per 100,000 persons, and one in about 90 persons is expected to be a heterozygous carrier. FCMD is characterized by CMD in combination with abnormalities of the central nervous system (brain malformations characterized by micropolygyria of the cerebrum and cerebellum and type II lissencephaly) and the eye (severe myopia, cataracts, optic nerve hypoplasia, retinal dysplasia, etc.) [12]. Severe mental retardation is observed in all cases. Most patients are never able to work, and they die by the age of 20 years.

MEB is a severe autosomal recessive disease characterized by CMD, ocular abnormalities, and brain malformations and is seen mainly in Finland. As with FCMD, hypoglycosylation of α-DG is commonly seen in MEB patients [5, 13]. WWS is the most severe form of α-DGpathy, with most patients living only a year or less. Similar to FCMD and MEB, this disease is characterized by CMD, structural brain defects, and eye malformations. WWS patients show a high degree of genetic heterogeneity, and several genes have been implicated in this disease.

All of these disorders are biochemically characterized by abnormal glycosylation of α-DG and are clinically associated with severe CMD and brain abnormalities. On the other hand, a considerable number of patients who show only mild muscular dystrophy without brain malformations have been also reported [14, 15]. A number of studies on large cohorts of α-DGpathy patients confirmed that there is a wide clinical spectrum, and there is no clear genotype-phenotype correlation [16, 17]. It is thought that effects of mutation on the gene function, rather than types of disease-causing gene, affect disease severity. The most severe end of the spectrum is characterized by CMD with extensive structural abnormalities in the brain and eyes, which usually results in early infantile death. Patients at the mildest end of the spectrum may present in adult life with LGMD, without the involvement of the brain or eyes.

In 2007, Muntoni and colleagues proposed a clinical classification system comprising seven broad phenotypic categories [16]. They first categorized α-DGpathy into four groups: (a) WWS/WWS-like, (b) MEB/FCMD-like, (c) CMD, and (d) LGMD. Categories (c) and (d) were further classified into subgroups: (c-1) CMD with mental retardation and cerebellar involvement as the only structural brain abnormality, (c-2) CMD with mental retardation and a structurally normal brain, (c-3) CMD with no abnormal cognitive development, (d-1) LGMD with mental retardation, and (d-2) LGMD without mental retardation. Later, new Online Mendelian Inheritance in Man (OMIM) entries created a simplified classification scheme for α-DGpathy (MDDG; muscular dystrophy dystroglycanopathy) by combining three broad phenotypic groups and gene defects. First, α-DGpathy was divided into three groups: (A) CMD with brain/eye abnormalities, (B) CMD with milder brain structural abnormalities, and (C) LGMD. Second, the causative gene was indicated numerically (e.g., *POMT1* is "1" and *fukutin* is "4"). From this classification, typical FCMD is named "MDDG type A4." For more information, please refer to Godfrey et al. [17].

2.2 Sugar Chain Structure and Modification Mechanisms of α-DG

Glycosylation is a posttranslational modification that attaches sugar moieties to proteins or lipids and plays crucial roles in a wide range of biological processes. Glycosylation of α-DG also plays a central role in the functional maturation of α-DG as well as in the pathogenesis of α-DGpathy. In this section, the structure of sugar chain and mechanisms by which it is modified are reviewed.

DG consists of α and β subunits, both of which are expressed from a single mRNA and cleaved into α-DG and β-DG during posttranslational modifications [18]. α-DG is a highly glycosylated extracellular protein that functions as a ligand-binding subunit for several ligand proteins that commonly contain laminin G (LG) domain-like modules. β-DG is a transmembrane subunit that anchors α-DG on the

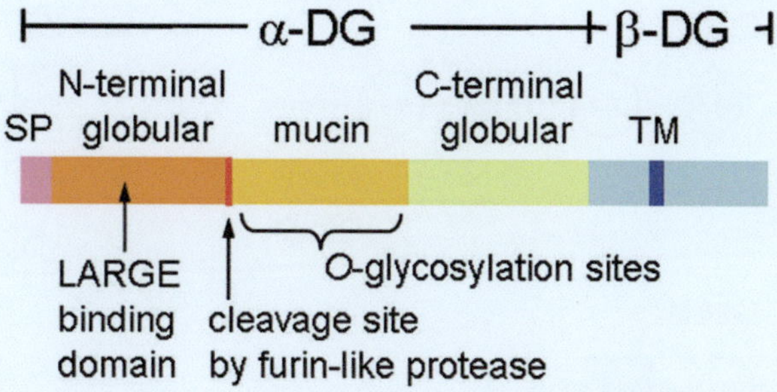

Fig. 2.2 Schematic representation of dystroglycan. The domain structure of dystroglycan. *SP* signal peptide, *TM* transmembrane

cell surface and binds to dystrophin inside the cell. α-DG consists of three domains, two globular domains at the N- and C-termini and an intervening mucin-like domain (Fig. 2.2). The mucin-like domain contains more than 40 Ser/Thr residues that form *O*-glycan clusters. The N-terminal globular domain is essential for *O*-glycosylation to proceed in the mucin-like domain. However, the N-terminal domain is cleaved and shed from the α-DG core portion after the completion of glycosylation and is therefore not present in mature α-DG [19]. The significance of this cleavage is not understood. Because glycosylation, which is necessary for ligand binding, takes place a few amino acids downstream of the cleavage site, it may provide a stereochemically efficient structure for interaction with the ligands [20]. Among heterogeneous groups of *O*-linked sugar chains on the mucin-like domain of α-DG, a unique *O*-mannose (*O*-Man) type sugar chain is important for the ligand-binding activity.

O-Mannosyl glycan structures of α-DG that are currently known are shown in Fig. 2.3. Core M1 (Siaα2–3Galβ1–4GlcNAcβ1–2Man), which was the first *O*-Man type glycan found in mammals, was originally identified from the bovine peripheral nerve by Endo and colleagues [21]. The structure of Core M2 is currently presumed based on the finding that *N*-acetylglucosaminyltransferase IX (GnT-IX) can transfer GlcNAc to *O*-Man [22]. Core M3 (GalNAcβ1–3GlcNAcβ1–4Man) was identified in recombinant α-DG proteins expressed in HEK293 cells [23]. In 2010, Campbell and colleagues reported the presence of a novel moiety that is modified on *O*-Man via a phosphodiester linkage and proposed that this moiety forms a ligand-binding domain [23]. Because its complete structure has not yet been elucidated, this structure has been tentatively termed as the "post-phosphoryl moiety" or "post-phosphoryl modification." It is likely that this post-phosphoryl moiety contains repeat units consisting of xylose (Xyl) and glucuronic acid (GlcA) and that these units are assembled through the enzymatic activity of LARGE (like-acetylglucosaminyltransferase) [24]. Enzymatically synthesized Xyl-GlcA repeats bind to laminin, and their ligand-binding capacity is associated with the length of the repeats [25]. Overexpression of LARGE produces hyperglycosylated α-DG that has increased ligand-binding activity [19, 26]. This activity is likely due to the formation of longer and/or more repeating units. Taken together, it appears that the repeating Xyl-GlcA units function as the ligand-binding epitopes of α-DG. Details of the linker structure between the phosphorylated Man (Man-P) and the Xyl-GlcA

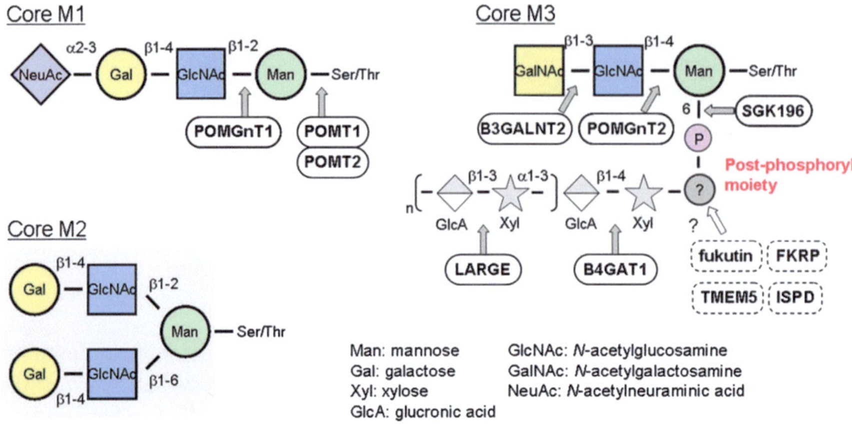

Fig. 2.3 Sugar chain structures of α-dystroglycan. Unique *O*-mannose glycans of α-dystroglycan and enzymes involved in their synthesis are illustrated

repeats remain unknown. Currently, more than 15 genes have been identified in which mutations cause abnormal glycosylation of α-DG resulting in human disease (Table 2.1). The enzymatic or putative functions of these gene products are described in the following paragraphs.

Protein *O*-mannosyltransferase (*POMT*) *1* and *POMT2* were originally identified as the genes responsible for WWS [27, 28]. POMT1 and POMT2 localize to the endoplasmic reticulum (ER) and form a POMT1/POMT2 heterocomplex [29]. This POMT complex catalyzes the transfer of a mannosyl residue from dolichol-phosphate mannose (Dol-P-Man) to the Ser and Thr residues of α-DG.

Protein *O*-linked mannose β1,2-*N*-acetylglucosaminyltransferase 1 (*POMGNT1*) was cloned from a cDNA sequence that is homologous to *N*-acetylglucosaminyl-transferase I (GnT-I, encoded by *MGAT1*) and was identified as a causative gene for MEB [30]. POMGnT1 is a glycosyltransferase that catalyzes the formation of the GlcNAcβ1–2Man linkage by transferring GlcNAc from UDP-GlcNAc to *O*-Man. The enzymatic removal of NeuAc, Gal, and GlcNAc from Core M1 does not affect the ligand-binding activity of α-DG [31]. This suggests that Core M1 may not directly serve as a ligand-binding domain. However, in POMGnT1-deficient mice, and fibroblasts from MEB patients, the post-phosphoryl modification is partially disrupted, raising the possibility that the structure of Core M1 may influence the biosynthesis of the Core M3/post-phosphoryl moiety [23, 32].

Glycosyltransferase-like domain containing 2 (*GTDC2*, *POMGNT2*), β1,3-*N*-acetylgalactosaminyltransferase 2 (*B3GALNT2*), and *SGK196* (*POMK*) are newly discovered α-DGpathy genes that are involved in the synthesis of Core M3 [33–36]. GTDC2 (alternatively called AGO61) is localized in the ER and catalyzes the formation of the GlcNAcβ1–4Man linkage by the transfer of GlcNAc from UDP-GlcNAc to the *O*-mannosyl peptide derived from α-DG. B3GALNT2 is also localized in the ER and catalyzes the formation of the GalNAcβ1–3GlcNAc linkage by transferring GalNAc from UDP-GalNAc. SGK196 catalyzes the addition of a phosphate group from ATP to position 6 on the *O*-Man residues in the Core M3 structure. Mutations in any molecule that participates in the synthesis of Core M3 result in α-DGpathy. Therefore, highly ordered and sequential actions of the POMT complex, GTDC2, B3GALNT2, and SGK196 are required for subsequent post-phosphoryl modifications. It is not known whether Core M1 and Core M3 can be simultaneously modified on the same *O*-Man residues. In addition, because defects in either Core M1 or Core M3 synthesis result in the loss of the ligand-binding activities of α-DG, it is necessary to uncover the nature of their relationship in the biosynthetic pathway and/or in the state of ligand binding.

LARGE was originally discovered as a gene that was defective in meningiomas [37] and was later shown to be causative for spontaneous muscular dystrophy in *Large*^{myd} mice [38] and CMD 1D (MDC1D) in humans [8]. LARGE possesses both xylosyltransferase and glucuronyltransferase activities that produce repeating units of [−3Xylα1–3GlcAβ1–] using UDP-GlcA and UDP-Xyl as donor substrates [24]. In addition to the enzymatic activities of LARGE, a physical interaction between LARGE and the α-DG N-terminal domain is required for the functional maturation of α-DG [19]. Thus, the N-terminal domain serves as a recognition motif for LARGE, thereby providing substrate specificity for this unique modification. As mentioned previously, a missense mutation in the *DAG1* gene was identified in an α-DGpathy patient. The mutation was located within the N-terminal globular domain of α-DG, which leads to reduced interactions with LARGE and consequently impairs the formation of Xyl-GlcA repeating units [3].

Mutations in *B3GNT1* were identified in WWS patients [39], and its gene product was thought to be required for LARGE-dependent glycosylation of α-DG [40]. Recently, it has been revealed that B3GNT1 encodes for a β1,4-glucuronyltransferase to form a GlcAβ1–4Xyl disaccharide and thus proposed to rename the enzyme B4GAT1 [41, 42]. The GlcAβ1–4Xyl acts as an acceptor primer that can be elongated by LARGE (Fig. 2.3).

Fukutin (*FKTN*) was identified as the gene responsible for FCMD [43]. Fukutin-related protein (FKRP) was identified based on sequence homology to fukutin [6]. Both fukutin and FKRP are localized in the Golgi apparatus and are involved in the post-phosphoryl modifications of α-DG [23, 32], although their exact functions remain unknown. It is expected that mutations in fukutin or FKRP reduce the activities of these proteins in α-DG glycosylation. Interestingly, however, several disease-causing point mutations cause misfolding of the fukutin protein resulting in changing its cellular localization from the Golgi apparatus to the ER, which also triggers abnormal glycosylation of α-DG [44]. A database retrieval study showed that there is a region in the fukutin protein that is homologous to bacterial proteins involved in polysaccharide/phosphorylcholine modifications and to a yeast protein involved in the mannosyl phosphorylation of oligosaccharides [45]. Another report proposed that fukutin and FKRP belong to the nucleotidyltransferase (NTase) fold protein superfamily [46].

TMEM5 is a newly discovered α-DGpathy gene that encodes transmembrane protein 5 [35, 47]. The TMEM5 protein contains the exostosin family domain found in EXT1, a glycosyltransferase required for the biosynthesis of heparan sulfate. The exact function of TMEM5 is unknown, but it is expected to be a glycosyltransferase.

The isoprenoid synthase domain-containing protein (ISPD) belongs to the 4-diphosphocytidyl-2C-methyl-D-erythritol (CDP-ME) synthase family, and mutations in the *ISPD* gene were found in WWS patients [48, 49]. ISPD contributes to the synthesis of isoprenoid precursors in the methylerythritol phosphate (MEP) pathway in *Escherichia coli*. However, it is postulated that the MEP pathway is absent in mammals. Therefore, specific roles for ISPD, especially in relation to α-DG glycosylation, are still unknown in humans. It has been proposed that the function of ISPD is crucial for efficient POMT-dependent *O*-mannosylation or synthesis of a novel nucleotide sugar that is required for α-DG glycosylation.

Defects in the synthesis pathway of Dol-P-Man are associated with α-DGpathy. Dol-P-Man is a Man donor in reactions that include *N*-glycosylation, *O*-mannosylation, and glycophosphatidylinositol (GPI) anchor biosynthesis in the ER lumen. Dol-P-Man is synthesized from GDP-Man and dolichol phosphate by the DPM complex, which consists of the catalytic component DPM1 and the ER-localized transmembrane proteins, DPM2 and DPM3. Mutations in *DPM1*, *DPM2*, or *DPM3* have been identified in patients that show α-DGpathy with a type I congenital disorder of glycosylation (CDG) [50–52]. CDG is a heterogeneous group of rare genetic disorders that were originally defined as defects in the *N*-glycosylation process and are now reclassified to include *O*-linked and lipid glycosylation defects. In addition, mutations in the gene for dolichol kinase (*DOLK*) that is responsible for the formation of dolichol phosphate were discovered in patients with CDG and dilated cardiomyopathy [53]. Heart tissues from these patients showed abnormal *O*-mannosylation of α-DG. Mutations in the GDP-Man pyrophosphorylase B (*GMPPB*) gene that is responsible for the formation of GDP-Man were also reported in α-DGpathy patients [54]. Presumably, mutations in GMPPB result in a decrease in GDP-Man and consequently Dol-P-Man levels. Taken together, defects in the Dol-P-Man synthesis pathway are expected to perturb *O*-mannosylation of α-DG. However, it is also expected that defects in the synthesis of Dol-P-Man would affect *O*-mannosylation, *N*-glycosylation, and GPI anchor formation of other proteins. In fact, defects in *N*-glycosylation were found in patients with DPM mutations [50–52]. It is possible that defects in reactions using Dol-P-Man, other than *O*-mannosylation of α-DG, may also contribute to the pathology of these diseases. Thus, it remains controversial whether or not gene mutations in the Dol-P-Man biosynthesis pathway can be attributed to a cause of α-DGpathy.

2.3 Pathophysiological Function of DG

Several extracellular matrix and synaptic proteins such as laminins [55–58], agrin [59, 60], perlecan [61], neurexin [62], pikachurin [63], and slit [64] are ligands of α-DG. All of these ligand proteins commonly contain LG domain-like modules that function as binding sites for α-DG. Because *O*-mannosylations and post-phosphoryl modifications are required for the ligand-binding activities of α-DG, the DG-ligand interactions are dramatically reduced in patients with α-DGpathy.

Laminin is a major component of the basement membrane and is composed of three subunits (α, β, and γ) [65]. The expression pattern of each laminin isoform (currently, more than 15 different isoforms are known) differs among different tissues and cells. In the skeletal muscle basement membrane, the laminin α2 subunit of the main laminin isoform (laminin-211, composed of α2, β1, and γ1 subunits) interacts with α-DG on the surface of muscle cells. This interaction establishes a physical link between the basement and plasma membranes.

Agrin is a heparan sulfate proteoglycan and agrin-DG interactions play important roles in the structural maintenance and stabilization of neuromuscular junctions [66]. Perlecan is also a heparan sulfate proteoglycan and one of the major components of basement membranes. The relatively high binding affinities in perlecan-DG interactions possibly indicate that there are specific roles for these interactions [56].

Neurexins are transmembrane proteins that are expressed in the nervous system. There are two families of neurexins, α- and β-neurexins, and both can bind to α-DG. The significance of the neurexin-DG interaction is unclear, but it may be involved in the formation and/or maintenance of synapses because neurexins are located on the presynaptic membranes, and α-DG is expressed on the postsynaptic membranes [67].

Pikachurin is expressed in the synaptic clefts of the photoreceptor ribbon synapses. Interactions between pikachurin and DG play important roles in the maintenance of retinal synapse structures, synaptic signal transmissions, and visual functions [63, 68]. Slit is a protein widely referred to as a repulsive axon guidance cue, and Robo is its known transmembrane receptor. Slit-DG interactions are required for the proper localization of Slit, suggesting a new function for α-DG as an extracellular scaffold for controlling axon guidance [64].

Several mouse models for α-DGpathy have been established, and studies using these models have helped reveal pathophysiological roles of α-DG glycosylation (Table 2.2). Targeted disruptions of α-DGpathy genes resulted in embryonic lethality (*POMT1*, *fukutin*) [69, 70] or early postnatal lethality (*GTDC2*) [71]. POMGnT1 knockout (KO) mice are viable but show variable life spans [72, 73]. To bypass these issues, chimeric mice, knock-in (KI) mice, or conditional KO (cKO) mice have been generated. Fukutin-deficient chimeric mice, generated using embryonic stem cells targeted for both *Fktn* alleles, develop severe muscular dystrophy and display brain and eye anomalies [74]. Fukutin KI mice carrying the most prevalent FCMD mutation (retrotransposal insertion) confirmed that the retrotransposal insertion leads to abnormal post-phosphoryl modification of α-DG [32, 75]. Skeletal muscle-selective fukutin-cKO mice recapitulate features of α-DGpathy [76, 77]. Ablation of the putative functional domain from *Fkrp* (E310 to the TGA stop) results in embryonic lethality; the mutant homozygous embryos die before reaching embryonic day 12.5 [78]. Homozygous KI mice carrying the missense P448L mutation develop muscular dystrophy as well as a wide range of structural

Table 2.2 Summary of dystroglycanopathy mouse models introduced in this chapter

Model mice	Gene	Phenotypes	References
Knockout (KO)			
POMT1 KO	*POMT1*	Embryonic lethal	[69]
Fukutin KO	*FKTN*	Embryonic lethal	[70]
GTDC2 KO	*GTDC2*	Postnatal lethality Brain abnormality	[71]
POMGnT1 KO	*POMGNT1*	Variable life span Brain abnormality	[72, 73]
Chimeric mice			
Fukutin chimera	*FKTN*	Severe muscular dystrophy Brain and eye abnormality	[74]
Knock-in (KI)			
Fukutin KI (retrotransposon)	*FKTN*	No obvious phenotype	[75]
FKRP E310del homozygous	*FKRP*	Embryonic lethal	[78]
FKRP P448L homozygous	*FKRP*	Muscular dystrophy Brain and eye abnormality	[78]
FKRP-Neo^{Tyr307Asn} homozygous	*FKRP*	Postnatal lethality Reduced muscle mass Brain and eye abnormality	[79]
Conditional KO (cKO)			
Fukutin-cKO (muscle precursor cell)	*FKTN*	Severe muscular dystrophy	[76, 77]
Fukutin-cKO (myofiber)	*FKTN*	Mild muscular dystrophy	[76, 77]
POMT2-cKO (brain)	*POMT2*	Brain abnormality	[80]
Spontaneous mutant			
Large^{myd}	*Large*	Muscular dystrophy Brain and eye abnormality	[38, 81]

abnormalities in the central nervous system that are characteristic of neuronal migration defects [78]. Abnormal phenotypes in skeletal muscle and the central nervous system have been described in another FKRP mutant KI mouse (FKRP-Neo^{Y307N}) [79]. Abnormal brain development was shown in GTDC2-KO, POMTGnT1-KO, and brain-selective POMT2-cKO mice [71–73, 80]. These models are genetically engineered mice, but there is a spontaneous Large mutant mouse (*Large*^{myd}) that exhibits abnormal α-DG glycosylation and shows skeletal muscle pathology and neuronal migration defects that recapitulate α-DGpathy phenotypes [38, 81]. This is probably the most used model of α-DGpathy.

In α-DGpathy, the loss of α-DG ligand-binding activity leads to disruption of the linkage between the basement membrane and the plasma membrane. Indeed, an ultrastructural abnormality, in which the basement membrane was detached from the muscle plasma membrane, was shown in skeletal muscle from skeletal muscle-selective DG-deficient mice as well as the *Large*^{myd} mouse [82]. These structural abnormalities likely render muscles prone to contraction-induced injuries, eventually leading to necrosis of muscle cells. By using myofiber-selective fukutin-cKO

(MCK-fukutin-cKO) mice, membrane weakness was shown to precede the onset of disease and that membrane fragility triggers manifestation of the disease [77].

MCK-fukutin-cKO mice exhibited only mild muscular dystrophy, indicating that membrane fragility is not sufficient to explain the severe muscle pathology of α-DGpathy. When myofibers are damaged, muscle-specific stem cells, called satellite cells, are activated for differentiation into muscle precursor cells (MPCs), followed by myoblasts and eventual fusion into myotubes. In this way, the skeletal muscle can regenerate. In contrast to MCK-fukutin-cKO mice, MPC-selective Myf5-fukutin-cKO mice showed severe muscular dystrophy with reductions in the number of satellite cells, proliferation/differentiation activities of MPCs, and muscle regeneration activity [77]. All of these abnormalities become more severe as the disease progresses. Thus, properly glycosylated α-DG likely plays important roles in the maintenance of satellite cell viability and MPC activities, and defects in their functions correlate with the severity of the disease. It is also possible that the absence of α-DG glycosylation during postnatal/juvenile muscle growth and development has a high impact on muscle degeneration and/or dystrophic pathology in later stages [76]. In FCMD and *Large*^{myd} mice, the aberrant formation of neuromuscular junctions, and the presence of many immature muscle fibers, suggests that impaired differentiation signals from these aberrant neuromuscular junctions, and maturational delays in muscle fibers, underlie the etiology of α-DGpathy [83]. Together, in addition to muscle membrane fragility, it appears that muscle maturation and regeneration processes are involved in the pathogenesis of α-DGpathy.

α-DGpathy is often associated with brain abnormalities, and abnormal glycosylation of α-DG is considered one of the main causes of brain malformation. The surface of the cerebral cortex is covered by the glia limitans/basement membrane complex, which prevents the over-migration of neurons. In FCMD [84] and other α-DGpathy models [5, 85], there is a breakdown in the basement membrane resulting in protrusion of neurons into the subarachnoid space through breaches in the basement membrane. These abnormalities may be the underlying causes of cortical dysplasia and type II lissencephaly.

α-DG is expressed in radial glia and presumably plays a role in the physical connection of the glia limitans to the basement membrane [85, 86]. During the developmental growth of embryonic brain, abnormally glycosylated α-DG may be unable to maintain sufficient physical strength and/or plasticity of the glia limitans-basement membrane complex against an expanding cortical surface area. Furthermore, the neuron-selective DG-cKO (NEX-DG-cKO) and *Large*^{myd} mice show impairment of long-term potentiation at CA3–CA1 synapses [87], suggesting that α-DG glycosylation is also involved in synaptic plasticity, although the precise mechanism is unknown.

2.4 Therapeutic Strategies for α-DGpathy

In spite of recent progress in identifying α-DGpathy disease-causing genes, and a deeper understanding of the underlying pathological mechanisms, effective therapies for α-DGpathy have not yet been established. Several genetically engineered KI or cKO mice for α-DGpathy genes have been used to develop treatment strategies for α-DGpathy. In this section, we introduce ongoing therapeutic studies using model animals and cells with a main focus on fukutin-deficient α-DGpathy.

A transgenic fukutin KI mouse model carrying a retrotransposal insertion in the *fukutin* gene (*fukutin*$^{Hp/Hp}$, *fukutin*$^{Hp/-}$) exhibited hypoglycosylation of α-DG but did not show any signs of muscular dystrophy due to the presence of minor levels of intact α-DG with residual laminin-binding activities [75]. This indicates that even a small amount of intact α-DG is sufficient for maintaining skeletal muscle function and suggests that an effective treatment of α-DGpathy will not require a full recovery of glycosylation. In addition, considering the pathological mechanisms revealed by analyses of the fukutin-cKO mice, any therapeutic strategy must involve the prevention of myofiber membrane weakness and/or the rescue of the substantial loss and dysfunction of MPCs [77].

Because frequent cycles of degeneration and regeneration of myofibers accelerate the substantial and/or functional loss of MPCs, it is expected that protection from disease-triggering myofiber degeneration will provide therapeutic benefits even in skeletal muscles that have MPC defects. Therefore, the therapeutic benefits of rescuing fukutin expression in myofibers were tested. This gene therapy study was conducted by using recombinant adeno-associated virus 9 (AAV9) vectors containing the mouse fukutin cDNA under the control of the MCK promoter, which allowed fukutin expression in differentiated myofibers [77]. Systemic gene delivery via the tail vein into adolescent Myf5-fukutin-cKO mice, which exhibit early stage of muscular dystrophy, dramatically ameliorated the dystrophic phenotype and restored muscle function to the same level, as seen in the wild-type mice.

In addition to fukutin gene therapy, other successful gene therapies to newborn *Large*^{myd} and adolescent FKRP mutant mice have been reported [26, 88, 89]. Many genes associated with α-DGpathy code for enzymes, and therefore it is expected that even small quantities of exogenously delivered genes that express normal proteins can compensate for the mutant genes. In fact, therapeutic effects from the *fukutin* gene transfer were achieved with much lower AAV titers than those used in other types of muscular dystrophy models that had defects in structural proteins. Importantly, therapeutic benefits can be attained even after manifestation of the disease. Therefore, gene therapy is a feasible treatment for the wide range of α-DGpathies. However, the glycosylation status of α-DG varies during myogenesis and muscle regeneration, suggesting that expression patterns and activities of genes involving α-DG glycosylation are strictly controlled. In order to achieve an effective therapeutic intervention, it is thus important to consider the timing of the intervention, the nature of the targeted cells, and the types of promoters used for driving gene expression.

When LARGE is overexpressed, α-DG is hyperglycosylated and its laminin-binding activity is increased in wild-type and α-DGpathy cells derived from fukutin-deficient or POMGnT1-deficient patients [26]. This unique characteristic of LARGE led to the development of a novel treatment strategy by involving overexpressing or increasing the activity of LARGE, which could enhance or bypass the DG-ligand linkage in genetically distinct α-DGpathy. Viral vector-mediated gene transfers of *LARGE* into POMGnT1-deficient mice and $FKRP^{P448L}$ mice improve their motor performance [88] and dystrophic pathology [90], respectively. In contrast, transgenic overexpression of LARGE in FKRP mutant mice or MCK-fukutin-cKO mice resulted in a worsening of the muscle pathology [91, 92]. This adverse effect may have resulted from constitutively hyperglycosylated α-DG and/or an overdose of LARGE having a negative impact in skeletal muscle pathologies. In addition, LARGE-dependent hyperglycosylation requires *O*-mannosyl phosphorylation and therefore does not always occur in all types of α-DGpathies [49, 71]. Currently, whether overexpression of LARGE possesses any therapeutic benefits is inconclusive.

Finally, we introduce a novel antisense oligonucleotides therapeutic strategy that is based on the pathogenesis of FCMD [93]. The major mutation in FCMD is a SINE-VNTR-*Alu* (SVA) retrotransposon insertion in the 3' noncoding region of the *fukutin* gene, which accounts for approximately 90 % of the FCMD chromosome [43]. This insertion contains a strong splice acceptor site that induces a rare alternative donor site in the last exon, thus causing abnormal mRNA splicing (exon trapping). This abnormal mRNA splicing produces an aberrantly spliced fukutin protein that lacks 38 amino acids from the C-terminus but contains 129 amino acids derived from the SVA sequence [93]. This mutant fukutin protein localizes to the ER, and it is thought that this mislocalization and/or lack of a portion of the C-terminal sequence leads to disruption in the activity of fukutin. Introduction of antisense oligonucleotides that target the splice acceptor, the predicted exonic splicing enhancer, and the intronic splicing enhancer prevents the pathogenic exon trapping by SVA in cells from FCMD patients as well as from fukutin KI mice ($fukutin^{Hp/Hp}$ and $fukutin^{Hp/-}$ mice). Importantly, this treatment restores normal *fukutin* mRNA expression, protein production, and consequently α-DG glycosylation and laminin-binding activity both in vitro and in vivo. This treatment strategy can potentially be applied to almost all FCMD patients in Japan and has the potential to be the first radical clinical treatment for α-DGpathies.

2.5 Conclusions

More than a decade has passed since the discovery of α-DGpathy. During this period, there have been advances in identifying the genes responsible for this disorder and in understanding the functions of these genes, the molecular and cellular pathogeneses of this disorder, and the structure and modification pathway of α-DG. In general, α-DGpathy is a grouping of CMD and LGMD disorders that is characterized by abnormal glycosylation of α-DG. More than 15 genes have been identified in which mutations are implicated in the abnormal glycosylation of α-DG and α-DGpathy. There is a wide variation in the clinical spectrum of α-DGpathy. Studies using cell or animal models of this disease revealed that myofiber membrane fragility, as well as impairments of muscle precursor cell and regeneration activity, is associated with disease pathogenesis. Finally, based on the pathological mechanism, several therapeutic strategies for α-DGpathy, such as antisense and gene replacement therapies, have been proposed and examined in animal systems. We are reaching at the beginning of translational stage from basic research to therapeutic approaches. International registry for α-DGpathy has been established and FCMD registry has also started in Japan since 2011. The issues that remain unresolved include obtaining a more complete understanding of the post-phosphoryl structures and functions of any unknown α-DGpathy genes. Hopefully, clarifying these issues in the future will contribute to a deeper understanding of α-DGpathy and also establish more specific diagnosis and possible cures for α-DGpathy.

References

1. Ervasti JM, Ohlendieck K, Kahl SD et al (1990) Deficiency of a glycoprotein component of the dystrophin complex in dystrophic muscle. Nature 345:315–319
2. Barresi R, Campbell KP (2006) Dystroglycan: from biosynthesis to pathogenesis of human disease. J Cell Sci 119:199–207
3. Hara Y, Balci-Hayta B, Yoshida-Moriguchi T et al (2011) A dystroglycan mutation associated with limb-girdle muscular dystrophy. N Engl J Med 364:939–946
4. Hayashi YK, Ogawa M, Tagawa K et al (2001) Selective deficiency of alpha-dystroglycan in Fukuyama-type congenital muscular dystrophy. Neurology 57:115–121
5. Michele DE, Barresi R, Kanagawa M et al (2002) Post-translational disruption of dystroglycan-ligand interactions in congenital muscular dystrophies. Nature 418:417–422
6. Brockington M, Blake DJ, Prandini P et al (2001) Mutations in the fukutin-related protein gene (FKRP) cause a form of congenital muscular dystrophy with secondary laminin alpha2 deficiency and abnormal glycosylation of alpha-dystroglycan. Am J Hum Genet 69:1198–1209
7. Brockington M, Yuva Y, Prandini P et al (2001) Mutations in the fukutin-related protein gene (FKRP) identify limb girdle muscular dystrophy 2I as a milder allelic variant of congenital muscular dystrophy MDC1C. Hum Mol Genet 10:2851–2859
8. Longman C, Brockington M, Torelli S et al (2003) Mutations in the human LARGE gene cause MDC1D, a novel form of congenital muscular dystrophy with severe mental retardation and abnormal glycosylation of alpha-dystroglycan. Hum Mol Genet 12:2853–2861
9. Toda T, Kobayashi K, Takeda S et al (2003) Fukuyama-type congenital muscular dystrophy (FCMD) and alpha-dystroglycanopathy. Congenit Anom (Kyoto) 43:97–104
10. Michele DE, Campbell KP (2003) Dystrophin-glycoprotein complex: post-translational processing and dystroglycan function. J Biol Chem 278:15457–15460
11. Fukuyama Y, Osawa M, Suzuki H (1981) Congenital progressive muscular dystrophy of the Fukuyama type – clinical, genetic and pathological considerations. Brain Dev 3:1–29
12. Toda T, Kobayashi K, Kondo-Iida E (2000) The Fukuyama congenital muscular dystrophy story. Neuromuscul Disord 10:153–159

13. Kano H, Kobayashi K, Herrmann R (2002) Deficiency of alpha-dystroglycan in muscle-eye-brain disease. Biochem Biophys Res Commun 291:1283–1286
14. Murakami T, Hayashi YK, Noguchi S et al (2006) Fukutin gene mutations cause dilated cardiomyopathy with minimal muscle weakness. Ann Neurol 60:597–602
15. D'Amico A, Tessa A, Bruno C et al (2006) Expanding the clinical spectrum of POMT1 phenotype. Neurology 66:1564–1567
16. Godfrey C, Clement E, Mein R et al (2007) Refining genotype phenotype correlations in muscular dystrophies with defective glycosylation of dystroglycan. Brain 130:2725–2735
17. Godfrey C, Foley AR, Clement E et al (2011) Dystroglycanopathies: coming into focus. Curr Opin Genet Dev 21:278–285
18. Ibraghimov-Beskrovnaya O, Ervasti JM, Leveille CJ et al (1992) Primary structure of dystrophin-associated glycoproteins linking dystrophin to the extracellular matrix. Nature 355: 696–702
19. Kanagawa M, Saito F, Kunz S et al (2004) Molecular recognition by LARGE is essential for expression of functional dystroglycan. Cell 117:953–964
20. Hara Y, Kanagawa M, Kunz S et al (2011) Like-acetylglucosaminyltransferase (LARGE)-dependent modification of dystroglycan at Thr-317/319 is required for laminin binding and arenavirus infection. Proc Natl Acad Sci U S A 108:17426–17431
21. Chiba A, Matsumura K, Yamada H et al (1997) Structures of sialylated O-linked oligosaccharides of bovine peripheral nerve alpha-dystroglycan. The role of a novel *O*-mannosyl-type oligosaccharide in the binding of alpha-dystroglycan with laminin. J Biol Chem 272: 2156–2162
22. Inamori K, Endo T, Gu J et al (2004) *N*-Acetylglucosaminyltransferase IX acts on the GlcNAc beta 1,2-Man alpha 1-Ser/Thr moiety, forming a 2,6-branched structure in brain *O*-mannosyl glycan. J Biol Chem 279:2337–2340
23. Yoshida-Moriguchi T, Yu L, Stalnaker SH et al (2010) *O*-mannosyl phosphorylation of alpha-dystroglycan is required for laminin binding. Science 327:88–92
24. Inamori K, Yoshida-Moriguchi T, Hara Y et al (2012) Dystroglycan function requires xylosyl- and glucuronyltransferase activities of LARGE. Science 335:93–96
25. Goddeeris MM, Wu B, Venzke D et al (2013) LARGE glycans on dystroglycan function as a tunable matrix scaffold to prevent dystrophy. Nature 503:136–140
26. Barresi R, Michele DE, Kanagawa M et al (2004) LARGE can functionally bypass alpha-dystroglycan glycosylation defects in distinct congenital muscular dystrophies. Nat Med 10: 696–703
27. Beltrán-Valero de Bernabé D, Currier S, Steinbrecher A et al (2002) Mutations in the *O*-mannosyltransferase gene POMT1 give rise to the severe neuronal migration disorder Walker-Warburg syndrome. Am J Hum Genet 71:1033–1043
28. van Reeuwijk J, Janssen M, van den Elzen C (2005) POMT2 mutations cause alpha-dystroglycan hypoglycosylation and Walker-Warburg syndrome. J Med Genet 42:907–912
29. Manya H, Chiba A, Yoshida A et al (2004) Demonstration of mammalian protein *O*-mannosyltransferase activity: coexpression of POMT1 and POMT2 required for enzymatic activity. Proc Natl Acad Sci U S A 101:500–505
30. Yoshida A, Kobayashi K, Manya H et al (2001) Muscular dystrophy and neuronal migration disorder caused by mutations in a glycosyltransferase, POMGnT1. Dev Cell 1:717–724
31. Combs AC, Ervasti JM (2005) Enhanced laminin binding by alpha-dystroglycan after enzymatic deglycosylation. Biochem J 390:303–309
32. Kuga A, Kanagawa M, Sudo A et al (2012) Absence of post-phosphoryl modification in dystroglycanopathy mouse models and wild-type tissues expressing non-laminin binding form of α-dystroglycan. J Biol Chem 287:9560–9567
33. Manzini MC, Tambunan DE, Hill RS et al (2012) Exome sequencing and functional validation in zebrafish identify GTDC2 mutations as a cause of Walker-Warburg syndrome. Am J Hum Genet 91:541–547

34. Stevens E, Carss KJ, Cirak S et al (2013) Mutations in B3GALNT2 cause congenital muscular dystrophy and hypoglycosylation of α-dystroglycan. Am J Hum Genet 92:354–365
35. Jae LT, Raaben M, Riemersma M et al (2013) Deciphering the glycosylome of dystroglycanopathies using haploid screens for lassa virus entry. Science 340:479–483
36. Yoshida-Moriguchi T, Willer T, Anderson ME et al (2013) SGK196 is a glycosylation-specific *O*-mannose kinase required for dystroglycan function. Science 341:896–899
37. Peyrard M, Seroussi E, Sandberg-Nordqvist AC et al (1999) The human LARGE gene from 22q12.3-q13.1 is a new, distinct member of the glycosyltransferase gene family. Proc Natl Acad Sci U S A 96:598–603
38. Grewal PK, Holzfeind PJ, Bittner RE et al (2001) Mutant glycosyltransferase and altered glycosylation of alpha-dystroglycan in the myodystrophy mouse. Nat Genet 28:151–154
39. Buysse K, Riemersma M, Powell G et al (2013) Missense mutations in β-1,3-*N*-acetylglucosaminyltransferase 1 (B3GNT1) cause Walker-Warburg syndrome. Hum Mol Genet 22: 1746–1754
40. Bao X, Kobayashi M, Hatakeyama S et al (2009) Tumor suppressor function of laminin-binding alpha-dystroglycan requires a distinct beta3-*N*-acetylglucosaminyltransferase. Proc Natl Acad Sci U S A 106:12109–12114
41. Willer T, Inamori KI, Venzke D et al (2014) The glucuronyltransferase B4GAT1 is required for initiation of LARGE-mediated α-dystroglycan functional glycosylation. Elife (in press). doi: 10.7554/eLife.03941
42. Praissman JL, Live DH, Wang S et al (2014) B4GAT1 is the priming enzyme for the LARGE-dependent functional glycosylation of α-dystroglycan. Elife (in press). doi: 10.7554/eLife.03943
43. Kobayashi K, Nakahori Y, Miyake M et al (1998) An ancient retrotransposal insertion causes Fukuyama-type congenital muscular dystrophy. Nature 394:388–392
44. Tachikawa M, Kanagawa M, Yu CC et al (2012) Mislocalization of fukutin protein by disease-causing missense mutations can be rescued with treatments directed at folding amelioration. J Biol Chem 287:8398–8406
45. Aravind L, Koonin EV (1999) The fukutin protein family – predicted enzymes modifying cell-surface molecules. Curr Biol 9:R836–R837
46. Kuchta K, Knizewski L, Wyrwicz LS et al (2009) Comprehensive classification of nucleotidyltransferase fold proteins: identification of novel families and their representatives in human. Nucleic Acids Res 37:7701–7714
47. Vuillaumier-Barrot S, Bouchet-Séraphin C, Chelbi M et al (2012) Identification of mutations in TMEM5 and ISPD as a cause of severe cobblestone lissencephaly. Am J Hum Genet 91: 1135–1143
48. Roscioli T, Kamsteeg EJ, Buysse K et al (2012) Mutations in ISPD cause Walker-Warburg syndrome and defective glycosylation of α-dystroglycan. Nat Genet 44:581–585
49. Willer T, Lee H, Lommel M et al (2012) ISPD loss-of-function mutations disrupt dystroglycan *O*-mannosylation and cause Walker-Warburg syndrome. Nat Genet 44:575–580
50. Yang AC, Ng BG, Moore SA et al (2013) Congenital disorder of glycosylation due to DPM1 mutations presenting with dystroglycanopathy-type congenital muscular dystrophy. Mol Genet Metab 110:345–351
51. Barone R, Aiello C, Race V et al (2012) DPM2-CDG: a muscular dystrophy-dystroglycanopathy syndrome with severe epilepsy. Ann Neurol 72:550–558
52. Lefeber DJ, Schönberger J, Morava E et al (2009) Deficiency of Dol-P-Man synthase subunit DPM3 bridges the congenital disorders of glycosylation with the dystroglycanopathies. Am J Hum Genet 85:76–86
53. Lefeber DJ, de Brouwer AP, Morava E et al (2011) Autosomal recessive dilated cardiomyopathy due to DOLK mutations results from abnormal dystroglycan *O*-mannosylation. PLoS Genet 7, e1002427
54. Carss KJ, Stevens E, Foley AR et al (2013) Mutations in GDP-mannose pyrophosphorylase B cause congenital and limb-girdle muscular dystrophies associated with hypoglycosylation of α-dystroglycan. Am J Hum Genet 93:29–41

55. Ervasti JM, Campbell KP (1993) A role for the dystrophin-glycoprotein complex as a transmembrane linker between laminin and actin. J Cell Biol 122:809–823
56. Talts JF, Andac Z, Göhring W et al (1999) Binding of the G domains of laminin alpha1 and alpha2 chains and perlecan to heparin, sulfatides, alpha-dystroglycan and several extracellular matrix proteins. EMBO J 18:863–870
57. Ido H, Harada K, Futaki S et al (2004) Molecular dissection of the alpha-dystroglycan- and integrin-binding sites within the globular domain of human laminin-10. J Biol Chem 279: 10946–10954
58. Yoon JH, Chandrasekharan K, Xu R et al (2009) The synaptic CT carbohydrate modulates binding and expression of extracellular matrix proteins in skeletal muscle: partial dependence on utrophin. Mol Cell Neurosci 41:448–463
59. Gee SH, Montanaro F, Lindenbaum MH et al (1994) Dystroglycan-alpha, a dystrophin-associated glycoprotein, is a functional agrin receptor. Cell 77:675–686
60. Bowe MA, Deyst KA, Leszyk JD et al (1994) Identification and purification of an agrin receptor from Torpedo postsynaptic membranes: a heteromeric complex related to the dystroglycans. Neuron 12:1173–1180
61. Peng HB, Ali AA, Daggett DF et al (1998) The relationship between perlecan and dystroglycan and its implication in the formation of the neuromuscular junction. Cell Adhes Commun 5:475–489
62. Sugita S, Saito F, Tang J et al (2001) A stoichiometric complex of neurexins and dystroglycan in brain. J Cell Biol 154:435–445
63. Sato S, Omori Y, Katoh K et al (2008) Pikachurin, a dystroglycan ligand, is essential for photoreceptor ribbon synapse formation. Nat Neurosci 11:923–931
64. Wright KM, Lyon KA, Leung H et al (2012) Dystroglycan organizes axon guidance cue localization and axonal pathfinding. Neuron 76:931–944
65. Yurchenco PD (2011) Basement membranes: cell scaffoldings and signaling platforms. Cold Spring Harb Perspect Biol 3:a004911
66. Singhal N, Martin PT (2011) Role of extracellular matrix proteins and their receptors in the development of the vertebrate neuromuscular junction. Dev Neurobiol 71:982–1005
67. Zaccaria ML, Di Tommaso F, Brancaccio A et al (2001) Dystroglycan distribution in adult mouse brain: a light and electron microscopy study. Neuroscience 104:311–324
68. Kanagawa M, Omori Y, Sato S et al (2010) Post-translational maturation of dystroglycan is necessary for pikachurin binding and ribbon synaptic localization. J Biol Chem 285: 31208–31216
69. Willer T, Prados B, Falcón-Pérez JM et al (2004) Targeted disruption of the Walker-Warburg syndrome gene Pomt1 in mouse results in embryonic lethality. Proc Natl Acad Sci U S A 101: 14126–14131
70. Kurahashi H, Taniguchi M, Meno C et al (2005) Basement membrane fragility underlies embryonic lethality in fukutin-null mice. Neurobiol Dis 19:208–217
71. Yagi H, Nakagawa N, Saito T et al (2013) AGO61-dependent GlcNAc modification primes the formation of functional glycans on α-dystroglycan. Sci Rep 3:3288
72. Liu J, Ball SL, Yang Y et al (2006) A genetic model for muscle-eye-brain disease in mice lacking protein *O*-mannose 1,2-*N*-acetylglucosaminyltransferase (POMGnT1). Mech Dev 123:228–240
73. Miyagoe-Suzuki Y, Masubuchi N, Miyamoto K et al (2009) Reduced proliferative activity of primary POMGnT1-null myoblasts in vitro. Mech Dev 126:107–116
74. Takeda S, Kondo M, Sasaki J et al (2003) Fukutin is required for maintenance of muscle integrity, cortical histiogenesis and normal eye development. Hum Mol Genet 12:1449–1459
75. Kanagawa M, Nishimoto A, Chiyonobu T et al (2009) Residual laminin-binding activity and enhanced dystroglycan glycosylation by LARGE in novel model mice to dystroglycanopathy. Hum Mol Genet 18:621–631
76. Beedle AM, Turner AJ, Saito Y et al (2012) Mouse fukutin deletion impairs dystroglycan processing and recapitulates muscular dystrophy. J Clin Invest 122:3330–3342

77. Kanagawa M, Yu CC, Ito C et al (2013) Impaired viability of muscle precursor cells in muscular dystrophy with glycosylation defects and amelioration of its severe phenotype by limited gene expression. Hum Mol Genet 22:3003–3015
78. Chan YM, Keramaris-Vrantsis E, Lidov HG et al (2010) Fukutin-related protein is essential for mouse muscle, brain and eye development and mutation recapitulates the wide clinical spectrums of dystroglycanopathies. Hum Mol Genet 19:3995–4006
79. Ackroyd MR, Skordis L, Kaluarachchi M et al (2009) Reduced expression of fukutin related protein in mice results in a model for fukutin related protein associated muscular dystrophies. Brain 132:439–451
80. Hu H, Li J, Gagen CS et al (2011) Conditional knockout of protein *O*-mannosyltransferase 2 reveals tissue-specific roles of *O*-mannosyl glycosylation in brain development. J Comp Neurol 519:1320–1337
81. Holzfeind PJ, Grewal PK, Reitsamer HA et al (2002) Skeletal, cardiac and tongue muscle pathology, defective retinal transmission, and neuronal migration defects in the Large (myd) mouse defines a natural model for glycosylation-deficient muscle-eye-brain disorders. Hum Mol Genet 11:2673–2687
82. Han R, Kanagawa M, Yoshida-Moriguchi T et al (2009) Basal lamina strengthens cell membrane integrity via the laminin G domain-binding motif of alpha-dystroglycan. Proc Natl Acad Sci U S A 106:12573–12579
83. Taniguchi M, Kurahashi H, Noguchi S et al (2006) Aberrant neuromuscular junctions and delayed terminal muscle fiber maturation in alpha-dystroglycanopathies. Hum Mol Genet 15: 1279–1289
84. Nakano I, Funahashi M, Takada K et al (1996) Are breaches in the glia limitans the primary cause of the micropolygyria in Fukuyama-type congenital muscular dystrophy (FCMD)? Pathological study of the cerebral cortex of an FCMD fetus. Acta Neuropathol 91:313–321
85. Moore SA, Saito F, Chen J et al (2002) Deletion of brain dystroglycan recapitulates aspects of congenital muscular dystrophy. Nature 418:422–425
86. Myshrall TD, Moore SA, Ostendorf AP et al (2012) Dystroglycan on radial glia end feet is required for pial basement membrane integrity and columnar organization of the developing cerebral cortex. J Neuropathol Exp Neurol 71:1047–1063
87. Satz JS, Ostendorf AP, Hou S et al (2010) Distinct functions of glial and neuronal dystroglycan in the developing and adult mouse brain. J Neurosci 30:14560–14572
88. Yu M, He Y, Wang K et al (2013) Adeno-associated viral-mediated LARGE gene therapy rescues the muscular dystrophic phenotype in mouse models of dystroglycanopathy. Hum Gene Ther 24:317–330
89. Xu L, Lu PJ, Wang CH et al (2013) Adeno-associated virus 9 mediated FKRP gene therapy restores functional glycosylation of α-dystroglycan and improves muscle functions. Mol Ther 21:1832–1840
90. Vannoy CH, Xu L, Keramaris E et al (2014) Adeno-associated virus-mediated overexpression of LARGE rescues α-dystroglycan function in dystrophic mice with mutations in the fukutin-related protein. Hum Gene Ther Methods 25:187–196
91. Whitmore C, Fernandez-Fuente M, Booler H et al (2014) The transgenic expression of LARGE exacerbates the muscle phenotype of dystroglycanopathy mice. Hum Mol Genet 23:1842–1855
92. Saito F, Kanagawa M, Ikeda M et al (2014) Overexpression of LARGE suppresses muscle regeneration via down-regulation of insulin-like growth factor 1 and aggravates muscular dystrophy in mice. Hum Mol Genet 23:4543–4558
93. Taniguchi-Ikeda M, Kobayashi K, Kanagawa M et al (2011) Pathogenic exon-trapping by SVA retrotransposon and rescue in Fukuyama muscular dystrophy. Nature 478:127–131

Chapter 3
Myotonic Dystrophy

Masayuki Nakamori and Masanori P. Takahashi

Abstract Myotonic dystrophy (DM) is the most common form of muscular dystrophy in adults, caused by unstable genomic expansions of simple tandem repeats. Myotonic dystrophy type 1 (DM1) results from expansion of a CTG repeat in the 3′ untranslated region of *DMPK*. In myotonic dystrophy type 2 (DM2), the expanded repeat is a CCTG tetramer in intron 1 of *CNBP/ZNF9*. The mRNA transcripts containing expanded repeats form ribonuclear inclusions, thereby retained in the nucleus. The mutant RNA gives rise to a toxic gain of function by perturbing splicing factors, resulting in misregulation of alternative pre-mRNA splicing that may underlie the multisystemic symptoms of DM. Although no curative treatment exists, recent advances in basic and translational research and pharmacological approaches provide clues for therapeutic intervention in DM. In this review, we describe the RNA-dominant mechanism in DM and summarize potential therapeutic approaches that address RNA toxicity and current progress toward translational research.

Keywords Trinucleotide • Toxic RNA • Repeat instability • Alternative splicing • Spliceopathy

3.1 Myotonic Dystrophy

Myotonic dystrophy (DM) is the most common type of muscular dystrophy in adults, with a prevalence of 1 per 8,000 individuals [1]. DM is a dominantly inherited multisystemic disorder caused by the expansion of CTG (myotonic dystrophy type 1, DM1) or CCTG (myotonic dystrophy type 2, DM2) repeats [2, 3]. The common molecular basis of DM1 and DM2 is a toxic RNA transcript containing the expanded repeats. DM is the first disease proven to result from by toxic gain of function of the mutant mRNA and is now recognized as an RNA-mediated disease [4]. The clinical expression of both types of DM is quite similar, including myotonia, progressive muscle weakness, cataracts, insulin

M. Nakamori (✉) • M.P. Takahashi
Department of Neurology, Osaka University Graduate School of Medicine, D-4, 2-2 Yamadaoka, Suita, Osaka 565-0871, Japan
e-mail: mnakamor@neurol.med.osaka-u.ac.jp

S. Takeda et al. (eds.), *Translational Research in Muscular Dystrophy*,
DOI 10.1007/978-4-431-55678-7_3

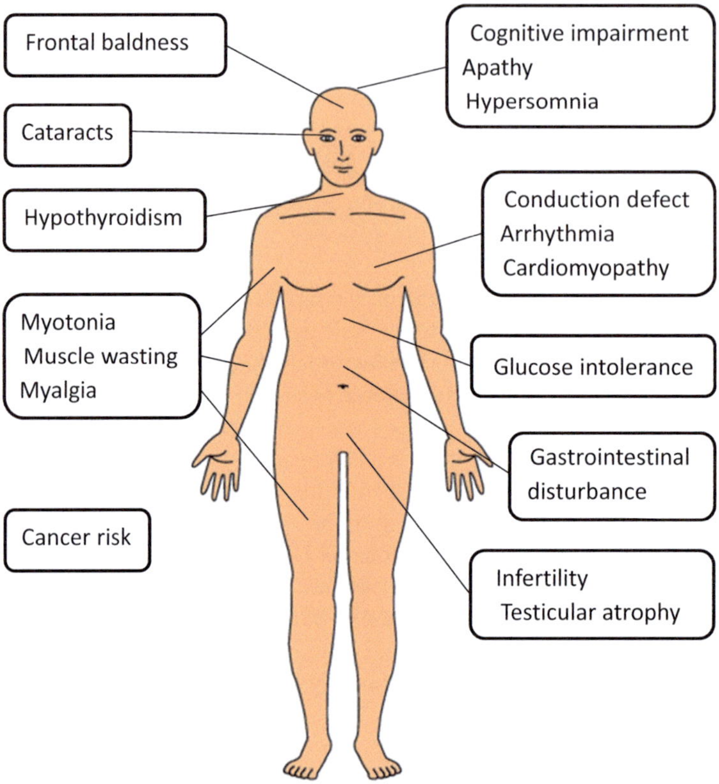

Fig. 3.1 Multisystemic symptoms of DM

resistance, and cardiac conduction defects, although some differences exist between DM1 and DM2 (Fig. 3.1).

3.2 Clinical Features

3.2.1 Adult-Onset DM1

3.2.1.1 Muscle Weakness

The predominant symptom of adult-onset DM1 is facial and distal muscle weakness. Facial weakness is an early feature and atrophy of temporalis and masseter leads to the characteristic facial appearance, so-called hatchet face. Mild ptosis is often seen, but ophthalmoplegia is rare. The neck flexors and sternocleidomastoid muscles are commonly involved. Weakness in the limbs is initially distal, especially finger and wrist flexors and ankle dorsiflexors, leading to difficulty with opening caps and foot drop. Muscle weakness progresses gradually and proximal limb weakness occurs later in the disease course, leading to loss of ambulation. Swallowing and respiratory muscles are often involved in later disease stages, with resultant difficulty in swallowing and breathing.

3.2.1.2 Myotonia

Myotonia, defined as delayed muscle relaxation following voluntary contraction or mechanical percussion, is caused by abnormal muscle fiber membrane activity [5]. Grip myotonia, which is difficulty in relaxing the grip, is often observed in adult-onset DM1. Improvement in myotonia by repeated contractions is termed "warm-up phenomenon." Myotonia can be elicited by percussion of the thenar or tongue. Myotonia can be recorded with electromyography (EMG) as bursts of repetitive muscle fiber discharges, giving a characteristic sound called "dive bomber" or "motorcycle."

3.2.1.3 Cardiac Involvement

Cardiac involvement is the second most frequent cause of death in DM1 [6]. Conduction disturbance is quite common, such as first-degree atrioventricular (AV) block and QRS widening, sometimes progressing to third-degree AV block. Atrial tachyarrhythmia and fatal ventricular tachyarrhythmia can occur. Regular ECG monitoring and early implantation of a pacemaker or cardiac defibrillator are critical for the prevention of sudden unexpected death. In contrast to cardiac arrhythmia, cardiomyopathy is not common, though some DM1 patients suffer from severe dilated cardiomyopathy and heart failure.

3.2.1.4 CNS Involvement

Central nervous system (CNS) involvement is frequently seen in adult-onset DM1. The characteristic neuropsychiatric features are mild cognitive impairment, inertia, apathy, and reduced perception of disease symptoms. Hypersomnia is extremely common even in the absence of respiratory involvement. Polysomnography shows nonobstructive apneas and central hypoventilation. Brain MRI scan frequently shows diffuse white matter lesions, particularly in the frontal or anterior temporal lobes.

3.2.1.5 Endocrine Involvement

Although overt diabetes is not frequent, hyperinsulinemia and insulin resistance are common in adult-onset DM1. Hypothyroidism, dyslipidemia, and male infertility because of testicular atrophy are also seen.

3.2.1.6 Other Multisystemic Symptoms

In addition to striated muscle, smooth muscle is affected in DM1. Gastrointestinal problems, such as diarrhea and constipation, are particularly frequent and may lead to pseudo-obstruction and megacolon. Cholecystitis and gallstones are also common because of increased tone of the gallbladder sphincter. Cataracts (typically iridescent posterior subcapsular forms) develop in most adult-onset DM1 patients and are sometimes the only symptom of very late-onset mild DM1. Early frontal baldness is often seen in male and even in some female DM1 patients. Increased risks of cancers of endometrium, ovary, thyroid, and colon have been reported [7].

3.2.2 Congenital DM1

Congenital DM1 (CDM) is not merely a severe early form of DM1 but rather a distinct clinical phenotype. CDM patients are severely affected at birth with hypotonia and generalized muscle weakness resulting in difficulty of sucking, swallowing, and breathing. Some CDM patients present symptoms even in utero, such as reduced fetal movements and hydramnios in later pregnancy. Talipes and tented upper lip (so-called carp mouth) are also seen in CDM. Despite neonatal intensive support, the mortality from respiratory failure remains high in affected infants. Surviving infants gradually improve in motor function, but nevertheless show delayed motor and mental development. Children with CDM can achieve independent walking, but develop myotonia and progressive muscle weakness in early adulthood. CDM is almost exclusively maternally inherited, even from mothers with mild forms of DM (see Sect. 3.3.2).

3.2.3 DM2

Although DM1 is common in populations of European and Asian descent, most DM2 patients are of northern and eastern European descent. DM2 patients also present myotonia and muscle weakness; however, the weakness typically affects the proximal muscles including the neck, elbow extension, and hip flexors. Significant muscle pain and fatigue are common in DM2. Cardiac conduction defects, cataracts, and insulin resistance are seen, whereas cognitive manifestation is rare in DM2. In contrast to DM1, a severe congenital form of DM2 has not been reported to date.

3.3 Genetics

3.3.1 Repeat Expansion in DM1 and DM2

Short DNA tandem repeats are observed ubiquitously across the human genome [8]. A small fraction of these repetitive elements are prone to become mutable and highly expanded. Such genomic expansions of simple tandem repeats cause various neurogenetic disorders, including DM. DM1 is caused by an expansion of CTG repeats in the 3′ untranslated region (UTR) of the *DMPK* gene [2] (Fig. 3.2). The length of CTG repeats is between 50 and several thousand in DM1, whereas the normal repeat number is between 5 and 37. In general, the length of expanded CTG repeats in blood cells correlates with the age of onset in DM1 [9]. DM2 results from a similar expansion of CCTG repeats in the first intron of the *CNBP/ZNF9* gene [3] (Fig. 3.2). The expanded CCTG repeat in DM2 is much longer than that in DM1, ranging from 75 to over 11,000. Importantly, unlike that seen in DM1, the size of expanded CCTG repeats does not correlate with the age of onset in DM2.

3.3.2 Repeat Instability

The expanded CTG and CCTG repeats in DM are not stable [10]. These mutations exhibit an exceptional degree of genetic instability in germline and somatic cells. For instance, the size of the repeat is prone to change during transmission from one generation to the next. In fact, intergenerational increments in the order of hundreds of repeats are often seen in DM1 (intergenerational instability). These mutations are

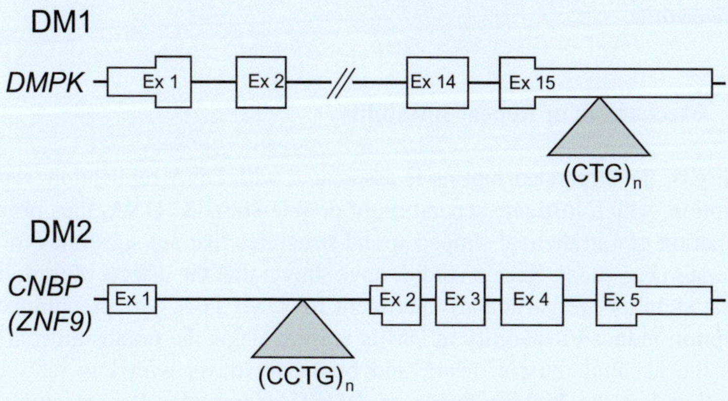

Fig. 3.2 Location of unstable CTG (DM1) or CCTG (DM2) repeats within their respective genes

also unstable in somatic cells, leading to an age-dependent growth of repeat expansion during the life of an individual (somatic instability).

3.3.2.1 Intergenerational Instability

The expanded CTG repeats in DM1 often increase in size when transmitted from parent to offspring, resulting in earlier onset and more severe clinical symptoms in subsequent generations, a phenomenon called "anticipation." A maternal expansion bias is evident in DM1 and cases with CDM are almost exclusively maternal in origin. There are a few cases of repeat contraction through paternal transmission [11]. In contrast to DM1, anticipation is less evident, both clinically and genetically, in DM2.

3.3.2.2 Somatic Instability

The expansion process continues throughout life in somatic cells, at rates that are variable between tissues in DM. This can lead to over tenfold variations of expansion length in different tissues of a DM individual [12]. Progenitor alleles that are estimated in leukocytes in adult-onset DM1 are usually between 100 and 800 CTG repeat, whereas adult biopsy and autopsy samples show typically 2,000–6,000 CTG repeats in the muscle or heart. In DM2, the CCTG expansion length is also considerably longer in the muscle than in leukocytes from the same individual [13]. Since the heterogeneity in fetal tissues is much less extensive, somatic instability causing these highly expanded alleles occurs mainly during postnatal life. The functional significance of somatic instability remains unclear; however, the progression of DM may be depending on the growth of the expanded repeat over time.

3.3.2.3 Mechanism of Repeat Instability

Instability of the expanded repeats is associated with DNA replication, repair, or transcription, which instigate separation of double-stranded DNA, thus promoting the formation of extrahelical slipped strand structures that are substrates for error-prone repair (Fig. 3.3a). Recent studies have shown that the effects of transcription on repeat stability are particularly pertinent for DM1 [14]. The predominance of transcription-induced instability in DM is reasonable as the organs most affected, such as the skeletal muscle, heart, and brain, are those with low rates of cell proliferation but the highest levels of *DMPK* expression. Recent studies also indicate a role for RNA repeats in transcription-induced repeat instability. RNAs comprised of expanded CUG or CCUG repeats bind to the template strand of DNA, then form RNA:DNA hybrids (R-loops) (Fig. 3.3b). The presence of R-loops

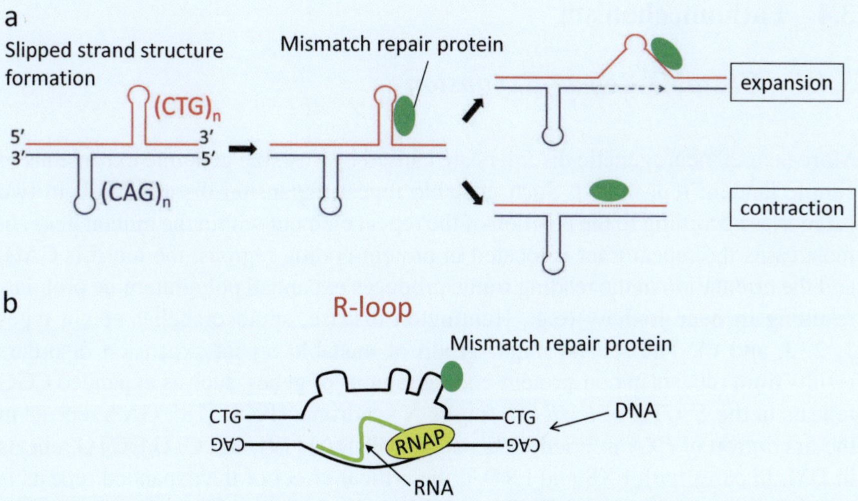

Fig. 3.3 (**a**) Mechanism of repeat instability. Extrahelical slipped strand structures form in (CTG) •(CAG) repeats, resulting in error-prone processing by mismatch repair proteins. (**b**) R-loop formation at the *DMPK* locus. In DM1, expanded CUG RNA binds to the template strand of DNA, then forms RNA:DNA hybrids (R-loops). The presence of R-loops instigates the formation of slipped strand structures on the non-template strand, thereby leading to further repeat instability. RNAP: RNA polymerase

triggers the formation of extrahelical looped-out structures on the non-template strand and thereby stimulates error-prone repair, leading to further expansion or contraction [15].

3.3.3 Genotype-Phenotype Correlation

Although the size of expanded CTG repeats in leukocytes correlates with the age of onset in DM1, there was no correlation between muscle weakness and CTG expansion size in either leukocytes or muscle cells [16]. This suggests that some DM1 patients may tolerate longer expansions better than others and raises the possibility that DM1 severity is modulated by additional factors, such as modifier genes, sequence interruptions in the CTG repeat tract, or epigenetic changes at the *DMPK* locus. The CTG expansion length in the muscle also did not correlate with that in leukocyte from the same subjects [16, 17]. However, the difference in repeat size between leukocytes and muscle is correlated with age, suggesting an age-dependent process of somatic expansion that is more pronounced in the muscle than in leukocytes.

3.4 Pathomechanism

3.4.1 Unstable Repeat Expansion

More than 20 neurogenetic disorders are caused by unstable genomic expansions of simple tandem repeats [8]. Such unstable repeat expansion disorders fall in two categories according to the position of the repeat element within the mutant gene. In most cases the repeat tract is located in protein-coding regions, the motif is CAG, and the orientation in the reading frame produces expanded polyglutamine proteins, resulting in neurotoxicity (e.g., Huntington disease, spinocerebellar ataxia types 1, 2, 3, and 6). The second major group of unstable repeat expansion disorders results from repeats in non-protein-coding regions of genes, such as expanded CGG repeats in the 5′ UTR of *FMR1* in fragile X syndrome (FXS) [18], GAA repeats in the first intron of *FXN* in Friedreich's ataxia (FRDA) [19], and CTG/CCTG repeats in DM. In cases with FXS and FRDA, the critical effect of the expanded repeats is transcriptional silencing of *FMR1* and *FXN*, respectively. However, there is no proven effect on transcription of *DMPK* or *CNBP*/*ZNF9* in DM, indicating that the main pathogenic effect is a deleterious gain of function by the mutant mRNA.

3.4.2 RNA Dominance

Although the mutant mRNA is fully processed in DM1, repeat expansion blocks the nuclear export of mRNA with the expanded repeats of CUG (CUG^{exp}) [20]. Thus, the mRNA containing expanded repeats is retained in the nucleus and accumulates in discrete foci. Since DM1 is an autosomal dominant disease, nuclear retention of the mutant mRNA could theoretically lead to a 50 % reduction in DMPK protein. However, several lines of evidence strongly indicate that symptoms of DM1 result not from haploinsufficiency but from the toxic gain of function by RNA transcripts containing the CUG^{exp}. First, *DMPK* knockout mice, in which DMPK protein can be completely eliminated, show only minor symptoms in the skeletal muscle [21, 22]. Second, muscular features of DM1 can be reproduced by the expression of CUG^{exp} RNA at the 3′ UTR of human skeletal actin transgene in a mouse model [23]. Finally, in DM2, the highly expanded CCUG repeat in *CNBP*/*ZNF9* is fully transcribed, but the intron containing the CCUG expansion is retained and accumulated in nuclear foci similar to that seen in DM1 [3, 24].

3.4.3 RNA-Binding Proteins: MBNL Family and CELF1

The mutant RNA retained in the nucleus affects at least two RNA-binding protein families: the MBNL and CELF. MBNL1, a member of the MBNL family protein, has a strong affinity for CUG^{exp} and CCUG^{exp} [25]. When CUG^{exp} or CCUG^{exp} RNA accumulates in the nucleus, MBNL1 is sequestered in nuclear RNA foci and depleted from the nucleoplasm [26, 27] (Fig. 3.4). Since MBNL1 is a regulator of alternative splicing [28], MBNL1 sequestration in foci leads to the misregulation of alternative splicing of its target exons. One clear example of the functional consequence in DM is the splicing misregulation of *CLCN1* [29, 30]. This gene encodes a chloride ion channel that stabilizes the transmembrane potential in skeletal muscle. When alternative splicing of *CLCN1* is misregulated in response to expression of CUG^{exp} RNA, the channel activity is lost, causing electrical instability of the membrane, which triggers repetitive action potentials and delay of relaxation (myotonia). The loss of MBNL1 has additional effects on gene expression, including transcriptional alterations, mRNA decay, transport of mRNA, and micro-RNA biogenesis [31–33]. *Mbnl1* knockout mice exhibit myotonia and splicing alteration of *Clcn1*, supporting the evidence for MBNL1 dysfunction in DM1 [34]. Two other members of the MBNL family, MBNL2 and MBNL3, may also be involved in DM [34, 35]. Similar to MBNL1, MBNL2 is expressed in the skeletal muscle, heart, and brain, whereas MBNL3 is expressed mainly in the placenta. MBNL2 and MBNL3 are closely related to MBNL1 and can also be sequestered in nuclear foci. These suggest a role for the combinatorial deficiency of all three MBNL family members in DM, depending on the expression of CUG^{exp} or CCUG^{exp} RNA relative to the distinct levels of MBNL proteins in different tissues. Indeed, a recent report showed compound loss of MBNL1 and MBNL2 functions exaggerated cardiac and skeletal muscle symptoms in a mouse model [36].

Expression of CUG^{exp} also causes perturbations in cell signaling via several kinases, including protein kinase C (PKC), Akt kinase, cyclin-dependent kinase 4 (CDK4), and glycogen synthase kinase 3 beta (GSK3B) [37–39]. While the mechanisms of activation of these pathways have not yet been determined, upregulation of PKC enhances the phosphorylation of CELF1, a member of CELF RNA-binding protein family. The phosphorylation of CELF1 extends its half-life, resulting in the upregulation of its steady-state level [37] (Fig. 3.4). Since CELF1 is a multifunctional RNA-binding protein involved in the regulation of alternative splicing and translation, upregulation of CELF1 protein in DM1 results in misregulated alternative splicing of several pre-mRNAs, as well as altered translation or decay of mRNAs that are bound by CELF1 [40–43]. Transgenic mice overexpressing *Celf1* show splicing misregulation and cardiac conduction defect similar to DM1 [44]. As CELF1 plays an important role in developmental splicing switch in the heart, increased CELF1 expression may underlie the cardiac pathology observed in DM1. However, CELF1 upregulation has not been confirmed in DM2 [27, 45].

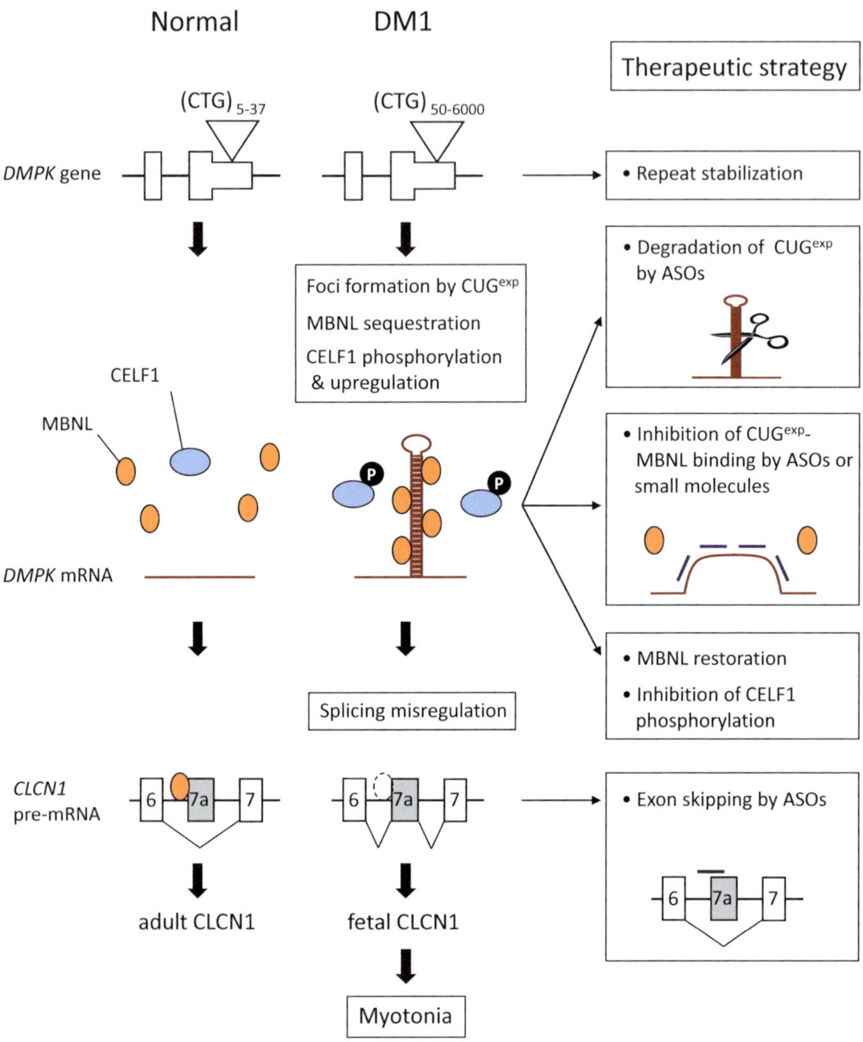

Fig. 3.4 Schematic illustration of the RNA-mediated disease mechanism (*left*) and possible therapeutic strategies (*right*) in DM1. Expanded CUG repeats in the mutant *DMPK* mRNA form hairpin structures and nuclear foci, sequester MBNL1 in the nucleus, and phosphorylate and stabilize CELF1. Loss of functional MBNL1 and upregulation of CELF1 cause misregulation of alternative splicing. Mis-splicing of *CLCN1* exon 7a induces a frameshift and premature termination codon in exon 7, resulting in loss of functional CLCN1 protein on the sarcolemma and myotonia in DM1. Therapeutic strategies are currently being developed for DM, including (1) stabilization of expanded repeats, (2) degradation of the toxic RNA by ASOs, (3) neutralization of CUG^{exp} toxicity by preventing MBNL sequestration with ASOs or small molecules, (4) modulation of MBNL or CELF1, and (5) induction of exon skipping of individual targets (Figure modified from Ref. [82])

3.4.4 Spliceopathy in DM

RNA splicing is the mechanism by which intervening introns are removed, while functional exons are ligated together to form a mature mRNA transcript [46]. There are two types of RNA splicing: constitutive and alternative splicing. Alternative splicing serves to generate a wide variety of unique mRNA transcripts by selecting and pairing discrete exons, resulting in distinct but similar proteins from the same gene (Fig. 3.5).

Although many human genetic disorders have been identified as the consequences of mutations on RNA splicing, in almost all cases, these are cis-acting effects that affect the splicing of a single pre-mRNA. In contrast, DM is caused by a trans-effect of alternative splicing factors on many RNAs and now is recognized as the first example of a human genetic disease resulting from "spliceopathy" [4]. The spliceopathy in DM shares common features in splicing misregulation. First, it does not involve constitutive exons, but selectively affects a group of exons that are subject to alternative splicing. Second, it usually affects alternative exons that normally undergo a developmental splicing switch; therefore, the fetal or neonatal splicing isoforms are expressed in mature muscle fibers in DM1. Third, most target exons in the spliceopathy in DM are regulated by MBNL1, CELF1, or both.

More than 70 mis-splicing events have been reported in DM. Table 3.1 lists the transcripts known to be affected by spliceopathy in DM. In case of *CLCN1*, the

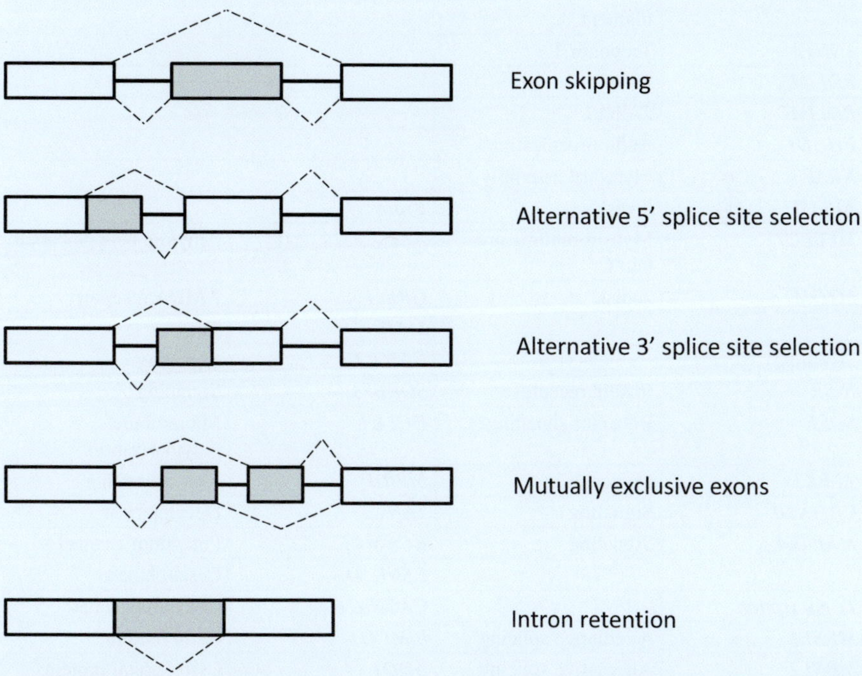

Fig. 3.5 Patterns of alternative splicing. Constitutive exons present in all final mRNAs are indicated by *white* boxes. Alternative RNA segments that may or may not be included in the final mRNA are indicated by *gray* boxes

Table 3.1 Mis-splicing events described in DM

Gene symbol Skeletal muscle	Function of gene product	Gene symbol Heart	Function of gene product
Cl^- ion transport		Cytoskeletal component	
CLCN1	Chloride channel	*TNNT2*	Troponin T
		DMD	Dystrophin
Ca^{2+} homeostasis		*DTNA*	Dystrobrevin
RYR1	Ryanodine receptor	*TTN*	Titin
ATP2A1	Calcium ATPase	*LDB3*	Z-disk
ATP2A2	Calcium ATPase	*PDLIM3*	Z-disk
BIN1	T-Tubule formation	*CAPZB*	Assembly of actin filament
CACNA1S	Calcium channel		
		Ion channel	
Cytoskeletal component		*KCNAB1*	Potassium channel
DMD	Dystrophin	*SCN5A*	Sodium channel
DTNA	Dystrobrevin		
TTN	Titin	*Others*	
LDB3	Z-disk	*MTMR1*	Phosphatase activity
CAPZB	Assembly of actin filament		
TNNT3	Troponin T		
PDLIM3	Z-disk		
PDLIM7	Z-disk		
FHOD1	Actin organization		
NRAP	Myofibril assembly		
ABLIM2	Z-disk	*Brain*	
MYBPC1	Myosin-binding protein C	*APP*	Amyloid beta precursor
MYOM1	Z-disk	*GRIN1*	NMDA receptor
		MAPT	Tau
Signaling		*CAMK2D*	Signaling
INSR	Insulin receptor	*SORBS1*	Signaling
SOS1	Receptor signaling	*DCLK1*	Microtubule polymerization
ALPK3	Myogenesis	*MPRIP*	Rho interacting
CAMK2B	Signaling	*TANC2*	Development
MAP4K4	Signaling	*KCNMA1*	Potassium channel
		CSNK1D	Casein kinase
Transcription		*CACNA1D*	Calcium channel
MBNL1	Alternative splicing	*LIMCH1*	Actin binding
MBNL2	Alternative splicing	*ADD1*	Cytoskeletal protein
NFIX	Transcription factor	*PPP1R12A*	Myosin phosphatase

(continued)

Table 3.1 (continued)

Gene symbol Skeletal muscle	Function of gene product	Gene symbol Heart	Function of gene product
MEF2C	Transcription factor	*CLASP2*	CLIP binding
NCOR2	Transcriptional silencing	*RYR2*	Ryanodine receptor
FXR1	mRNA trafficking		
Others			
GFPT1	Protein glycosylation		
IMPDH2	Nucleotide biosynthesis		
MTMR1	Phosphatase activity		
CAPN3	Intracellular protease		
PHKA1	Glycogenesis		
PHKA2	Glycogenesis		
KIF13A	Endosome positioning		
VPS39	Vesicle trafficking		
ARFGAP2	Vesicle trafficking		
COPZ2	Vesicle trafficking		
TBC1D15	Intracellular trafficking		
ANK2	Membrane targeting		
OPA1	Mitochondrial dynamics		
UBE2D3	Ubiquitination		
USP25	Deubiquitination		
TXNL4A	PQBP1 binding protein		
VEGFA	Angiogenesis		
MAPT	Tau		
MLF1	Oncoprotein		

exon 7a is negatively regulated by MBNL1 [34]. When MBNL1 is depleted in DM muscle, the exon 7a is retained in the mRNA. The inclusion of exon 7a induces a premature termination codon, which causes loss of mature CLCN1 protein in muscle membrane in DM, resulting in myotonia [29]. Misregulated splicing of insulin receptor (*INSR*) is also reported in DM muscle [41]. Alternative splicing of exon 11 is an important factor dictating the function of this receptor. The receptor lacking the exon 11 (non-muscle form) has a higher affinity for insulin than the receptor including the exon (muscle form). Because the inclusion of exon 11 is negatively regulated by CELF1, the non-muscle form lacking exon 11 is increased in DM muscle, leading to insulin resistance. However, whereas numerous mis-splicing events have been identified in DM, the underlying cause of progressive muscle wasting, the main disabling symptom in DM, has not been well defined. One possible candidate is mis-splicing of a group of genes regulating Ca^{2+} homeostasis, such as ryanodine receptor (*RYR1*), sarcoplasmic/endoplasmic reticulum calcium ATPases (*SERCA*s), voltage-dependent Ca^{2+} channel (*CACNA1S*), and T-tubule membrane scaffolding protein (*BIN1*) [47–49]. Because Ca^{2+} concentration is increased in DM1 cells and impaired Ca^{2+} homeostasis triggers muscle damage, misregulated splicing of these transcripts may cause muscle wasting in DM [50]. Another candidate is splicing misregulation of genes encoding cytoskeletal proteins, such as dystrophin (*DMD*), dystrobrevin (*DTNA*), titin (*TTN*), and ZASP (*LDB3*), as mutations or deletions in these genes causes other types of muscular dystrophies and myopathies [27, 51, 52].

The spliceopathy in DM also involves the heart and brain. Although the cause of cardiac symptoms in DM is not well elucidated, mis-splicing of cardiac cytoskeletal proteins (cardiac troponin T, DMD, DTNA, TTN, and LDB3) may contribute to cardiomyopathy [51–54]. In addition, conduction block and arrhythmia in DM may be caused by mis-splicing of cardiac ion channels, such as K^{+} channel beta subunit (*KCNAB1*) and voltage-gated Na^{+} channel (*SCN5A*) [54] (Charlet-Berguerand & Takahashi, manuscript in preparation). In DM1 brain, several splicing misregulations have been reported, including Tau (*MAPT*), *APP*, and *CAMK2D* [26, 55]. However, neither the functional consequences of these mis-splicing events nor the cause of cognitive impairment in DM1 has been determined.

3.4.5 Other Possible Mechanisms

Besides MBNL and CELF1, other RNA-binding proteins, such as hnRNP H and staufen, are implicated in DM pathogenesis [56, 57]. Dysregulation of micro-RNAs and MEF2 transcription factor proteins are also suggested to contribute to cardiac symptoms in DM [33, 58]. Furthermore, repeat-associated non-ATG translation of the *DMPK* antisense transcript was shown to give rise to polyglutamine aggregates [59]. Future studies are needed to elucidate the role of each mechanism in DM pathogenesis.

3.5 Therapeutic Strategies

Although no curative treatment exists in DM at present, recent advances in research and pharmacological approaches provide clues for potential future therapeutic intervention. Along with a better understanding of disease mechanisms such as the spliceopathy because of RNA toxicity, several experimental approaches have been developed and applied to translational research in DM (Fig. 3.4).

3.5.1 Splicing Correction

Since splicing misregulation is the molecular basis of DM, correction of individual mis-splicing events is the most direct way to alleviate the symptoms. Recent advances in technology of antisense oligonucleotides (ASOs) has enabled this strategy. ASOs are short, synthetic, modified nucleic acids that bind complementary RNA and regulate its function [60]. ASOs modulate splicing events by hiding specific sites essential for exon inclusion from the splicing machinery. ASOs blocking target splice sites can skip the target exon(s) and restore normal splicing. This approach has been applied as a treatment for Duchenne muscular dystrophy (DMD). The exon skipping achieved by ASOs restores dystrophin expression in DMD patients and is currently evaluated by clinical trials [61]. In a mouse model of DM1, a morpholino ASO targeting the 3′ splice site of *Clcnl* exon 7a reversed the defect of alternative splicing [62]. The morpholino ASOs repressed the inclusion of exon 7a, restored the normal *Clcnl* mRNA, increased the expression of CLCN1 protein on sarcolemma, stabilized the membrane potential and, thereby, alleviated myotonia. These findings suggest that ASO-induced exon skipping is a powerful tool for correcting mis-splicing in DM. However, there are several hurdles to overcome in the application of this approach in DM patients: (1) alternative splicing of *CLCN1* is more complicated in humans than in mice and (2) mis-splicing events responsible for other symptoms, especially muscle wasting, are not known.

3.5.2 Modulation of Alternative Splicing Factors

In DM, MBNL1 sequestration leads to multiple mis-splicing events, such as *CLCN1* and *ATP2A1* [34]. One therapeutic approach is the restoration of MBNL1 protein in the nucleoplasm. Overexpression of MBNL1 by adeno-associated viral gene delivery in skeletal muscle of mice expressing CUG^{exp} reversed MBNL1-dependent mis-splicing of exons and rescued myotonia [63]. However, the MBNL1 overexpression in a DM1 mouse model did not improve muscle pathology. In addition, *Mbnl1* knockout mice neither reproduce the developmental features of CDM nor display the severe muscle wastings that occur in adult-onset DM1 [34]. Thus, as MBNL1 sequestration does not provide a unifying explanation for the disease process, simultaneous modulation of other splicing factors, such as MBNL2 and CELF1, may be required for successful treatment of DM.

In addition to MBNL1 sequestration, increased steady-state level of CELF1 protein is another important molecular event involved in DM1 pathogenesis [64]. Overexpression of CELF1 in the mouse heart and skeletal muscle causes DM1-associated splicing changes and results in disease phenotypes [44, 65, 66]. Activation of the PKC signaling pathway is suggested to leads to the hyperphosphorylation and stabilization of CELF1 [37]. A recent report showed that PKC inhibitors reduced phosphorylation of CELF1, decreased the steady-state levels, reversed misregulation of splicing events regulated by CELF1, and ameliorated the cardiac conduction defects and contraction abnormalities in a heart-specific DM1 mouse model [67]. Although this approach may be promising for the treatment of cardiac symptoms in DM, there remain important unanswered questions: (1) why is CELF1 not consistently increased in DM2 despite cardiac involvement similar to DM1, and (2) how do CUG^{exp} activate the PKC signaling pathway?

3.5.3 Targeting Toxic RNA

In DM, the mutant RNA exerts a pivotal role in trans-dominant effects on different transcripts and spliceopathy. Thus, interventional strategies against toxic RNA are ideal to accomplish a generalized correction of DM symptoms. Several experimental therapeutic approaches have been attempted to degrade the toxic RNA by small interfering or short hairpin RNA delivered with a retroviral vector and hammerhead ribozyme [68–70]. Although these RNA-based approaches reduced the mutant RNA in DM1 myoblast cells, normal *DMPK* mRNA was simultaneously decreased, raising concerns regarding the loss of endogenous DMPK function. In addition, unmodified nucleic acids are susceptible to cleavage by endogenous nucleases and are rapidly degraded in vivo. From this view point, chemically modified ASOs with high binding affinity and extreme nuclease resistance emerge as a suitable tool for the modulation of toxic RNAs in DM. Depending on the chemistry and sequence, ASO binding can modulate the target RNA metabolism by two distinct mechanisms: neutralization and degradation. Neutralizing ASOs bind to the target RNA and sterically hinder RNA-protein interactions. Therefore, CAG-repeat ASOs can be expected to bind CUG^{exp}, compete with MBNL proteins, and prevent MBNL sequestration in DM1. In fact, recent reports showed that CAG-repeat ASOs with different chemistry (2-*O*-methyl, morpholino, locked nucleic acid) mitigated the RNA toxicity in DM1 model mice [15, 71, 72]. Most strikingly, CAG-morpholino ASOs dispersed nuclear foci of CUG^{exp}, released MBNL1 from foci, corrected mis-splicing events, and eliminated myotonia [72]. One caveat with this approach is the delivery of the ASOs by direct injection into the muscle, followed by electroporation, an approach that is not practical for human patients. However, systemic administration of CAG-ASOs with peptide-linked morpholino (PPMO) modification was reported to improve myotonia in a DM1 mouse model, providing the proof-of-concept for clinical applications given the versatility of CAG-ASOs [73] (see also Sect. 3.5.4). In contrast to these neutralizing ASOs, target-degrading ASOs cleave target RNA by recruiting RNase H to the oligonucleotide-RNA heteroduplex. This degradation capability arises from a characteristic structure called "gapmer" that has chemically modified residues on either side of a stretch of unmodified residues referred to as the gap. The modified wings enhance the binding and stability of the ASOs, and the gap allows for the induction of RNase H activity. Because of the exceptional capability of target degradation, gapmer ASOs are considered as promising for DM treatment and have already been tested in DM1 model mice [15, 74, 75].

In one study, systemic administration of the gapmer ASO with 2-*O*-methyl modification decreased toxic RNA, reduced foci formation, corrected splicing defects, and eliminated myotonia in DM1 mouse model [74]. More importantly, these effects were sustained for up to one year after the discontinuation of treatment. This approach achieved the best therapeutic effects among all strategies in mice so far and led to the development of gapmer ASOs against human *DMPK*. As therapeutic effects were confirmed in a mouse model [74], the gapmer ASOs (ISIS-DMPKRx) will hopefully be applied to a clinical trial soon.

Small molecules are also appropriate tools for targeting mutant RNA. Recent studies have identified numerous small molecules that bind specifically the CUG or CCUG repeats and competitively release the sequestered MBNL1. Several of these molecules were shown to induce the dispersal of RNA foci, redistribution of MBNL1 to the nucleoplasm, and partial reversal of mis-splicing events in mice expressing CUG^{exp} [76–78]. However, toxicity of these compounds in human has not been determined, and none of the candidates achieved a full rescue of mis-splicing of *Clcn1* and myotonia in mice. Pentamidine and related compounds have been recently suggested to inhibit the transcription of CUG^{exp} by binding to the CTG repeat DNA [79, 80]. Indeed, heptamidine, a methylene linker analogue of pentamidine, reversed splicing defects and improved myotonia in the mouse model.

3.5.4 *Stabilization of Expanded Repeats*

Another striking feature of DM is the marked instability of the expanded repeats. The progression of DM1 may depend on the growth of the expanded repeat throughout life. The ongoing repeat expansion also raises a concern that an initial beneficial effect of therapeutic ASOs on the toxic RNA may be lost because of ongoing expansion and increased production of CUG^{exp} RNA. Therefore, stabilization of the repeat is also a potential approach to postpone the onset, slow the progression, or to sustain the effect of therapeutic ASOs. Several compounds that stabilize the repeats in cultured cells have been identified [81]. However, these compounds are DNA intercalators or drugs that affect DNA methylation or replication, evoking concerns about long-term safety. In DM1, the instability of expanded repeats is enhanced by transcription across the repeat and R-loop formation [14, 15]. Because the R-loop is formed with CUG RNA and CAG DNA on the template strand, CAG-ASOs can theoretically prevent its formation. Indeed, a recent report showed that CAG-ASOs suppressed the repeat instability in both a cellular model and a mouse model by reducing the formation of R-loops at the *DMPK* locus [15]. Thus, intervention with CAG-repeat ASOs has the dual benefit of preventing the RNA toxicity and stabilizing the repeat.

3.6 Concluding Remarks

Since the CTG expansion was discovered in DM1, the understanding of the molecular pathomechanisms in DM has been enormously advanced. Promising experimental therapeutic strategies targeting toxic RNA continue to emerge. A recent study showed that several mis-splicing events can be a good biomarker for disease severity and therapeutic response in DM [16]. National and international DM patient registries have already been established in several countries for a clinical trial. Indeed, gapmer-ASOs targeting mutant *DMPK* mRNA for treatment of DM1 is currently being planned for a first-in-human clinical trial. Combination therapy with small molecules is also an attractive option. These developments are opening a new, fascinating, and promissing era for the treatment of DM.

References

1. Harper PS (2001) Myotonic dystrophy. W.B. Saunders Company, London
2. Harley HG, Brook JD, Rundle SA, Crow S, Reardon W, Buckler AJ, Harper PS, Housman DE, Shaw DJ (1992) Expansion of an unstable DNA region and phenotypic variation in myotonic dystrophy. Nature 355(6360):545–546
3. Liquori CL, Ricker K, Moseley ML, Jacobsen JF, Kress W, Naylor SL, Day JW, Ranum LP (2001) Myotonic dystrophy type 2 caused by a CCTG expansion in intron 1 of ZNF9. Science 293(5531):864–867
4. Osborne RJ, Thornton CA (2006) RNA-dominant diseases. Hum Mol Genet 15(2): R162–R169. doi:10.1093/hmg/ddl181
5. Vicart S, Sternberg D, Fontaine B, Meola G (2005) Human skeletal muscle sodium channelopathies. Neurol Sci 26(4):194–202. doi:10.1007/s10072-005-0461-x
6. de Die-Smulders CE, Howeler CJ, Thijs C, Mirandolle JF, Anten HB, Smeets HJ, Chandler KE, Geraedts JP (1998) Age and causes of death in adult-onset myotonic dystrophy. Brain 121(Pt 8):1557–1563
7. Gadalla SM, Lund M, Pfeiffer RM, Gortz S, Mueller CM, Moxley RT 3rd, Kristinsson SY, Bjorkholm M, Shebl FM, Hilbert JE, Landgren O, Wohlfahrt J, Melbye M, Greene MH (2011) Cancer risk among patients with myotonic muscular dystrophy. JAMA 306(22):2480–2486. doi:10.1001/jama.2011.1796
8. Nakamori M, Thornton C (2010) Epigenetic changes and non-coding expanded repeats. Neurobiol Dis 39(1):21–27. doi:10.1016/j.nbd.2010.02.004
9. Harley HG, Rundle SA, MacMillan JC, Myring J, Brook JD, Crow S, Reardon W, Fenton I, Shaw DJ, Harper PS (1993) Size of the unstable CTG repeat sequence in relation to phenotype and parental transmission in myotonic dystrophy. Am J Hum Genet 52(6):1164–1174
10. Lopez Castel A, Cleary JD, Pearson CE (2010) Repeat instability as the basis for human diseases and as a potential target for therapy. Nat Rev Mol Cell Biol 11(3):165–170. doi:10.1038/nrm2854
11. Ashizawa T, Anvret M, Baiget M, Barcelo JM, Brunner H, Cobo AM, Dallapiccola B, Fenwick RG Jr, Grandell U, Harley H (1994) Characteristics of intergenerational contractions of the CTG repeat in myotonic dystrophy. Am J Hum Genet 54(3):414–423
12. Thornton CA, Johnson K, Moxley RT (1994) Myotonic dystrophy patients have larger CTG expansions in skeletal muscle than in leukocytes. Ann Neurol 35:104–107

13. Nakamori M, Sobczak K, Moxley RT 3rd, Thornton CA (2009) Scaled-down genetic analysis of myotonic dystrophy type 1 and type 2. Neuromuscul Disord 19(11):759–762. doi:10.1016/j.nmd.2009.07.012
14. Nakamori M, Pearson CE, Thornton CA (2011) Bidirectional transcription stimulates expansion and contraction of expanded (CTG)•(CAG) repeats. Hum Mol Genet 20(3):580–588. doi:10.1093/hmg/ddq501
15. Nakamori M, Gourdon G, Thornton CA (2011) Stabilization of expanded (CTG)*(CAG) repeats by antisense oligonucleotides. Mol Ther 19(12):2222–2227. doi:10.1038/mt.2011.191
16. Nakamori M, Sobczak K, Puwanant A, Welle S, Eichinger K, Pandya S, Dekdebrun J, Heatwole CR, McDermott MP, Chen T, Cline M, Tawil R, Osborne RJ, Wheeler TM, Swanson MS, Moxley RT 3rd, Thornton CA (2013) Splicing biomarkers of disease severity in myotonic dystrophy. Ann Neurol 74(6):862–872. doi:10.1002/ana.23992
17. Zatz M, Passos-Bueno MR, Cerqueira A, Marie SK, Vainzof M, Pavanello R (1995) Analysis of the CTG repeat in skeletal muscle of young and adult myotonic dystrophy patients: when does the expansion occur? Hum Mol Genet 4(3):401–406
18. Verkerk AJ, Pieretti M, Sutcliffe JS, Fu YH, Kuhl DP, Pizzuti A, Reiner O, Richards S, Victoria MF, Zhang FP et al (1991) Identification of a gene (FMR-1) containing a CGG repeat coincident with a breakpoint cluster region exhibiting length variation in fragile X syndrome. Cell 65(5):905–914. doi:10.1016/0092-8674(91)90397-H
19. Campuzano V, Montermini L, Molto MD, Pianese L, Cossee M, Cavalcanti F, Monros E, Rodius F, Duclos F, Monticelli A, Zara F, Canizares J, Koutnikova H, Bidichandani SI, Gellera C, Brice A, Trouillas P, De Michele G, Filla A, De Frutos R, Palau F, Patel PI, Di Donato S, Mandel JL, Cocozza S, Koenig M, Pandolfo M (1996) Friedreich's ataxia: autosomal recessive disease caused by an intronic GAA triplet repeat expansion. Science 271(5254):1423–1427
20. Miller JW, Urbinati CR, Teng-Umnuay P, Stenberg MG, Byrne BJ, Thornton CA, Swanson MS (2000) Recruitment of human muscleblind proteins to (CUG)(n) expansions associated with myotonic dystrophy. EMBO J 19(17):4439–4448. doi:10.1093/emboj/19.17.4439
21. Jansen G, Groenen PJ, Bachner D, Jap PH, Coerwinkel M, Oerlemans F, van den Broek W, Gohlsch B, Pette D, Plomp JJ, Molenaar PC, Nederhoff MG, van Echteld CJ, Dekker M, Berns A, Hameister H, Wieringa B (1996) Abnormal myotonic dystrophy protein kinase levels produce only mild myopathy in mice. Nat Genet 13(3):316–324. doi:10.1038/ng0796-316
22. Reddy S, Smith DBJ, Rich MM, Leferovich JM, Reilly P, Davis BM, Tran K, Rayburn H, Bronson R, Cros D, Balice-Gordon RJ, Housman D (1996) Mice lacking the myotonic dystrophy protein kinase develop a late onset progressive myopathy. Nat Genet 13:325–334
23. Mankodi A, Logigian E, Callahan L, McClain C, White R, Henderson D, Krym M, Thornton CA (2000) Myotonic dystrophy in transgenic mice expressing an expanded CUG repeat. Science 289(5485):1769–1773
24. Margolis JM, Schoser BG, Moseley ML, Day JW, Ranum LP (2006) DM2 intronic expansions: evidence for CCUG accumulation without flanking sequence or effects on ZNF9 mRNA processing or protein expression. Hum Mol Genet 15(11):1808–1815
25. Kino Y, Mori D, Oma Y, Takeshita Y, Sasagawa N, Ishiura S (2004) Muscleblind protein, MBNL1/EXP, binds specifically to CHHG repeats. Hum Mol Genet 13(5):495–507
26. Jiang H, Mankodi A, Swanson MS, Moxley RT, Thornton CA (2004) Myotonic dystrophy type 1 is associated with nuclear foci of mutant RNA, sequestration of muscleblind proteins and deregulated alternative splicing in neurons. Hum Mol Genet 13(24):3079–3088. doi:10.1093/hmg/ddh327
27. Lin X, Miller JW, Mankodi A, Kanadia RN, Yuan Y, Moxley RT, Swanson MS, Thornton CA (2006) Failure of MBNL1-dependent postnatal splicing transitions in myotonic dystrophy. Hum Mol Genet 15(13):2087–2097
28. Ho TH, Charlet B, Poulos MG, Singh G, Swanson MS, Cooper TA (2004) Muscleblind proteins regulate alternative splicing. EMBO J 23(15):3103–3112

29. Mankodi A, Takahashi MP, Jiang H, Beck CL, Bowers WJ, Moxley RT, Cannon SC, Thornton CA (2002) Expanded CUG repeats trigger aberrant splicing of ClC-1 chloride channel pre-mRNA and hyperexcitability of skeletal muscle in myotonic dystrophy. Mol Cell 10(1): 35–44
30. Charlet-B N, Savkur RS, Singh G, Philips AV, Grice EA, Cooper TA (2002) Loss of the muscle-specific chloride channel in type 1 myotonic dystrophy due to misregulated alternative splicing. Mol Cell 10(1):45–53
31. Osborne RJ, Lin X, Welle S, Sobczak K, O'Rourke JR, Swanson MS, Thornton CA (2009) Transcriptional and post-transcriptional impact of toxic RNA in myotonic dystrophy. Hum Mol Genet 18(8):1471–1481. doi:10.1093/hmg/ddp058
32. Wang ET, Cody NA, Jog S, Biancolella M, Wang TT, Treacy DJ, Luo S, Schroth GP, Housman DE, Reddy S, Lecuyer E, Burge CB (2012) Transcriptome-wide regulation of pre-mRNA splicing and mRNA localization by muscleblind proteins. Cell 150(4):710–724. doi:10.1016/j.cell.2012.06.041
33. Rau F, Freyermuth F, Fugier C, Villemin JP, Fischer MC, Jost B, Dembele D, Gourdon G, Nicole A, Duboc D, Wahbi K, Day JW, Fujimura H, Takahashi MP, Auboeuf D, Dreumont N, Furling D, Charlet-Berguerand N (2011) Misregulation of miR-1 processing is associated with heart defects in myotonic dystrophy. Nat Struct Mol Biol 18(7):840–845. doi:10.1038/nsmb.2067
34. Kanadia RN, Johnstone KA, Mankodi A, Lungu C, Thornton CA, Esson D, Timmers AM, Hauswirth WW, Swanson MS (2003) A muscleblind knockout model for myotonic dystrophy. Science 302(5652):1978–1980
35. Fardaei M, Rogers MT, Thorpe HM, Larkin K, Hamshere MG, Harper PS, Brook JD (2002) Three proteins, MBNL, MBLL and MBXL, co-localize in vivo with nuclear foci of expanded-repeat transcripts in DM1 and DM2 cells. Hum Mol Genet 11(7):805–814
36. Lee KY, Li M, Manchanda M, Batra R, Charizanis K, Mohan A, Warren SA, Chamberlain CM, Finn D, Hong H, Ashraf H, Kasahara H, Ranum LP, Swanson MS (2013) Compound loss of muscleblind-like function in myotonic dystrophy. EMBO Mol Med 5(12):1887–1900. doi:10.1002/emmm.201303275
37. Kuyumcu-Martinez NM, Wang GS, Cooper TA (2007) Increased steady-state levels of CUGBP1 in myotonic dystrophy 1 are due to PKC-mediated hyperphosphorylation. Mol Cell 28(1):68–78. doi:10.1016/j.molcel.2007.07.027
38. Salisbury E, Sakai K, Schoser B, Huichalaf C, Schneider-Gold C, Nguyen H, Wang GL, Albrecht JH, Timchenko LT (2008) Ectopic expression of cyclin D3 corrects differentiation of DM1 myoblasts through activation of RNA CUG-binding protein, CUGBP1. Exp Cell Res 314(11–12):2266–2278. doi:10.1016/j.yexcr.2008.04.018
39. Jones K, Wei C, Iakova P, Bugiardini E, Schneider-Gold C, Meola G, Woodgett J, Killian J, Timchenko NA, Timchenko LT (2012) GSK3beta mediates muscle pathology in myotonic dystrophy. J Clin Invest 122(12):4461–4472. doi:10.1172/JCI64081
40. Charlet BN, Logan P, Singh G, Cooper TA (2002) Dynamic antagonism between ETR-3 and PTB regulates cell type-specific alternative splicing. Mol Cell 9(3):649–658, doi: S1097276502004793 [pii]
41. Savkur RS, Philips AV, Cooper TA (2001) Aberrant regulation of insulin receptor alternative splicing is associated with insulin resistance in myotonic dystrophy. Nat Genet 29(1):40–47
42. Timchenko NA, Cai ZJ, Welm AL, Reddy S, Ashizawa T, Timchenko LT (2001) RNA CUG repeats sequester CUGBP1 and alter protein levels and activity of CUGBP1. J Biol Chem 276(11):7820–7826
43. Vlasova IA, Tahoe NM, Fan D, Larsson O, Rattenbacher B, Sternjohn JR, Vasdewani J, Karypis G, Reilly CS, Bitterman PB, Bohjanen PR (2008) Conserved GU-rich elements mediate mRNA decay by binding to CUG-binding protein 1. Mol Cell 29(2):263–270. doi:10.1016/j.molcel.2007.11.024
44. Koshelev M, Sarma S, Price RE, Wehrens XH, Cooper TA (2010) Heart-specific overexpression of CUGBP1 reproduces functional and molecular abnormalities of myotonic dystrophy type 1. Hum Mol Genet 19(6):1066–1075. doi:10.1093/hmg/ddp570

45. Cardani R, Bugiardini E, Renna LV, Rossi G, Colombo G, Valaperta R, Novelli G, Botta A, Meola G (2013) Overexpression of CUGBP1 in skeletal muscle from adult classic myotonic dystrophy type 1 but not from myotonic dystrophy type 2. PLoS One 8(12):e83777. doi:10.1371/journal.pone.0083777
46. Kornblihtt AR, Schor IE, Allo M, Dujardin G, Petrillo E, Munoz MJ (2013) Alternative splicing: a pivotal step between eukaryotic transcription and translation. Nat Rev Mol Cell Biol 14(3): 153–165. doi:10.1038/nrm3525
47. Kimura T, Nakamori M, Lueck JD, Pouliquin P, Aoike F, Fujimura H, Dirksen RT, Takahashi MP, Dulhunty AF, Sakoda S (2005) Altered mRNA splicing of the skeletal muscle ryanodine receptor and sarcoplasmic/endoplasmic reticulum Ca2+ –ATPase in myotonic dystrophy type 1. Hum Mol Genet 14(15):2189–2200
48. Tang ZZ, Yarotskyy V, Wei L, Sobczak K, Nakamori M, Eichinger K, Moxley RT, Dirksen RT, Thornton CA (2012) Muscle weakness in myotonic dystrophy associated with misregulated splicing and altered gating of CaV1.1 calcium channel. Hum Mol Genet 21(6):1312–1324. doi:10.1093/hmg/ddr568
49. Fugier C, Klein AF, Hammer C, Vassilopoulos S, Ivarsson Y, Toussaint A, Tosch V, Vignaud A, Ferry A, Messaddeq N, Kokunai Y, Tsuburaya R, de la Grange P, Dembele D, Francois V, Precigout G, Boulade-Ladame C, Hummel MC, Lopez de Munain A, Sergeant N, Laquerriere A, Thibault C, Deryckere F, Auboeuf D, Garcia L, Zimmermann P, Udd B, Schoser B, Takahashi MP, Nishino I, Bassez G, Laporte J, Furling D, Charlet-Berguerand N (2011) Misregulated alternative splicing of BIN1 is associated with T tubule alterations and muscle weakness in myotonic dystrophy. Nat Med 17(6):720–725. doi:10.1038/nm.2374
50. Jacobs AE, Benders AA, Oosterhof A, Veerkamp JH, van Mier P, Wevers RA, Joosten EM (1990) The calcium homeostasis and the membrane potential of cultured muscle cells from patients with myotonic dystrophy. Biochim Biophys Acta 1096(1):14–19, doi: 0925-4439(90)90006-B [pii]
51. Nakamori M, Kimura T, Fujimura H, Takahashi MP, Sakoda S (2007) Altered mRNA splicing of dystrophin in type 1 myotonic dystrophy. Muscle Nerve 36(2):251–257. doi:10.1002/mus.20809
52. Nakamori M, Kimura T, Kubota T, Matsumura T, Sumi H, Fujimura H, Takahashi MP, Sakoda S (2008) Aberrantly spliced alpha-dystrobrevin alters alpha-syntrophin binding in myotonic dystrophy type 1. Neurology 70(9):677–685. doi:10.1212/01.wnl.0000302174.08951.cf
53. Philips AV, Timchenko LT, Cooper TA (1998) Disruption of splicing regulated by a CUG-binding protein in myotonic dystrophy. Science 280(5364):737–741
54. Mankodi A, Lin X, Blaxall BC, Swanson MS, Thornton CA (2005) Nuclear RNA foci in the heart in myotonic dystrophy. Circ Res 97(11):1152–1155
55. Suenaga K, Lee KY, Nakamori M, Tatsumi Y, Takahashi MP, Fujimura H, Jinnai K, Yoshikawa H, Du H, Ares M Jr, Swanson MS, Kimura T (2012) Muscleblind-like 1 knockout mice reveal novel splicing defects in the myotonic dystrophy brain. PLoS One 7(3):e33218. doi:10.1371/journal.pone.0033218
56. Paul S, Dansithong W, Kim D, Rossi J, Webster NJ, Comai L, Reddy S (2006) Interaction of muscleblind, CUG-BP1 and hnRNP H proteins in DM1-associated aberrant IR splicing. EMBO J 25(18):4271–4283
57. Ravel-Chapuis A, Belanger G, Yadava RS, Mahadevan MS, DesGroseillers L, Cote J, Jasmin BJ (2012) The RNA-binding protein Staufen1 is increased in DM1 skeletal muscle and promotes alternative pre-mRNA splicing. J Cell Biol 196(6):699–712. doi:10.1083/jcb.201108113
58. Kalsotra A, Singh RK, Gurha P, Ward AJ, Creighton CJ, Cooper TA (2014) The Mef2 transcription network is disrupted in myotonic dystrophy heart tissue, dramatically altering miRNA and mRNA expression. Cell Rep 6(2):336–345. doi:10.1016/j.celrep.2013.12.025
59. Zu T, Gibbens B, Doty NS, Gomes-Pereira M, Huguet A, Stone MD, Margolis J, Peterson M, Markowski TW, Ingram MA, Nan Z, Forster C, Low WC, Schoser B, Somia NV, Clark HB, Schmechel S, Bitterman PB, Gourdon G, Swanson MS, Moseley M, Ranum LP (2011) Non-

ATG-initiated translation directed by microsatellite expansions. Proc Natl Acad Sci U S A 108(1):260–265. doi:10.1073/pnas.1013343108
60. Southwell AL, Skotte NH, Bennett CF, Hayden MR (2012) Antisense oligonucleotide therapeutics for inherited neurodegenerative diseases. Trends Mol Med 18(11):634–643. doi:10.1016/j.molmed.2012.09.001
61. Koo T, Wood MJ (2013) Clinical trials using antisense oligonucleotides in Duchenne muscular dystrophy. Hum Gene Ther 24(5):479–488. doi:10.1089/hum.2012.234
62. Wheeler TM, Lueck JD, Swanson MS, Dirksen RT, Thornton CA (2007) Correction of ClC-1 splicing eliminates chloride channelopathy and myotonia in mouse models of myotonic dystrophy. J Clin Invest 117(12):3952–3957. doi:10.1172/JCI33355
63. Kanadia RN, Shin J, Yuan Y, Beattie SG, Wheeler TM, Thornton CA, Swanson MS (2006) Reversal of RNA missplicing and myotonia after muscleblind overexpression in a mouse poly (CUG) model for myotonic dystrophy. Proc Natl Acad Sci U S A 103(31):11748–11753
64. Roberts R, Timchenko NA, Miller JW, Reddy S, Caskey CT, Swanson MS, Timchenko LT (1997) Altered phosphorylation and intracellular distribution of a (CUG)n triplet repeat RNA-binding protein in patients with myotonic dystrophy and in myotonin protein kinase knockout mice. Proc Natl Acad Sci U S A 94(24):13221–13226
65. Ho TH, Bundman D, Armstrong DL, Cooper TA (2005) Transgenic mice expressing CUG-BP1 reproduce splicing mis-regulation observed in myotonic dystrophy. Hum Mol Genet 14(11): 1539–1547
66. Ward AJ, Rimer M, Killian JM, Dowling JJ, Cooper TA (2010) CUGBP1 overexpression in mouse skeletal muscle reproduces features of myotonic dystrophy type 1. Hum Mol Genet 19(18):3614–3622. doi:10.1093/hmg/ddq277
67. Wang GS, Kuyumcu-Martinez MN, Sarma S, Mathur N, Wehrens XH, Cooper TA (2009) PKC inhibition ameliorates the cardiac phenotype in a mouse model of myotonic dystrophy type 1. J Clin Invest 119(12):3797–3806. doi:10.1172/JCI37976
68. Furling D, Doucet G, Langlois MA, Timchenko L, Belanger E, Cossette L, Puymirat J (2003) Viral vector producing antisense RNA restores myotonic dystrophy myoblast functions. Gene Ther 10(9):795–802. doi:10.1038/sj.gt.3301955
69. Langlois MA, Boniface C, Wang G, Alluin J, Salvaterra PM, Puymirat J, Rossi JJ, Lee NS (2005) Cytoplasmic and nuclear retained DMPK mRNAs are targets for RNA interference in myotonic dystrophy cells. J Biol Chem 280(17):16949–16954. doi:10.1074/jbc.M501591200
70. Langlois MA, Lee NS, Rossi JJ, Puymirat J (2003) Hammerhead ribozyme-mediated destruction of nuclear foci in myotonic dystrophy myoblasts. Mol Ther 7(5 Pt 1):670–680, doi: S1525001603000686 [pii]
71. Mulders SA, van den Broek WJ, Wheeler TM, Croes HJ, van Kuik-Romeijn P, de Kimpe SJ, Furling D, Platenburg GJ, Gourdon G, Thornton CA, Wieringa B, Wansink DG (2009) Triplet-repeat oligonucleotide-mediated reversal of RNA toxicity in myotonic dystrophy. Proc Natl Acad Sci U S A 106(33):13915–13920. doi:10.1073/pnas.0905780106
72. Wheeler TM, Sobczak K, Lueck JD, Osborne RJ, Lin X, Dirksen RT, Thornton CA (2009) Reversal of RNA dominance by displacement of protein sequestered on triplet repeat RNA. Science 325(5938):336–339. doi:10.1126/science.1173110
73. Leger AJ, Mosquea LM, Clayton NP, Wu IH, Weeden T, Nelson CA, Phillips L, Roberts E, Piepenhagen PA, Cheng SH, Wentworth BM (2013) Systemic delivery of a Peptide-linked morpholino oligonucleotide neutralizes mutant RNA toxicity in a mouse model of myotonic dystrophy. Nucleic Acid Ther 23(2):109–117. doi:10.1089/nat.2012.0404
74. Wheeler TM, Leger AJ, Pandey SK, MacLeod AR, Nakamori M, Cheng SH, Wentworth BM, Bennett CF, Thornton CA (2012) Targeting nuclear RNA for in vivo correction of myotonic dystrophy. Nature 488(7409):111–115. doi:10.1038/nature11362
75. Lee JE, Bennett CF, Cooper TA (2012) RNase H-mediated degradation of toxic RNA in myotonic dystrophy type 1. Proc Natl Acad Sci U S A 109(11):4221–4226. doi:10.1073/pnas.1117019109

76. Parkesh R, Childs-Disney JL, Nakamori M, Kumar A, Wang E, Wang T, Hoskins J, Tran T, Housman D, Thornton CA, Disney MD (2012) Design of a bioactive small molecule that targets the myotonic dystrophy type 1 RNA via an RNA motif-ligand database and chemical similarity searching. J Am Chem Soc 134(10):4731–4742. doi:10.1021/ja210088v
77. Childs-Disney JL, Parkesh R, Nakamori M, Thornton CA, Disney MD (2012) Rational design of bioactive, modularly assembled aminoglycosides targeting the RNA that causes myotonic dystrophy type 1. ACS Chem Biol 7(12):1984–1993. doi:10.1021/cb3001606
78. Ofori LO, Hoskins J, Nakamori M, Thornton CA, Miller BL (2012) From dynamic combinatorial 'hit' to lead: in vitro and in vivo activity of compounds targeting the pathogenic RNAs that cause myotonic dystrophy. Nucleic Acids Res 40(13):6380–6390. doi:10.1093/nar/gks298
79. Warf MB, Nakamori M, Matthys CM, Thornton CA, Berglund JA (2009) Pentamidine reverses the splicing defects associated with myotonic dystrophy. Proc Natl Acad Sci U S A 106(44):18551–18556. doi:10.1073/pnas.0903234106
80. Coonrod LA, Nakamori M, Wang W, Carrell S, Hilton CL, Bodner MJ, Siboni RB, Docter AG, Haley MM, Thornton CA, Berglund JA (2013) Reducing levels of toxic RNA with small molecules. ACS Chem Biol 8(11):2528–2537. doi:10.1021/cb400431f
81. Gomes-Pereira M, Monckton DG (2006) Chemical modifiers of unstable expanded simple sequence repeats: what goes up, could come down. Mutat Res 598(1–2):15–34. doi:10.1016/j.mrfmmm.2006.01.011
82. Nakamori M, Takahashi MP (2011) Myotonic dystrophy: therapeutic approaches to RNA toxicity. Brain Nerve 63(11):1161–1168, doi: 1416101048 [pii]

Chapter 4
Molecular Pathogenesis and Therapeutic Strategy in GNE Myopathy

Hiroaki Nishimura and Satoru Noguchi

Abstract GNE myopathy is an autosomal recessive disease, which is characterized by gradually progressive muscle atrophy and weakness, and preferentially involves the distal muscles of lower extremities, especially the *tibialis anterior* muscle. GNE myopathy is caused by mutations in the UDP-N-acetylglucosamine 2-epimerase/N-acetylmannosamine kinase (*GNE*) gene which encodes the bifunctional enzyme catalyzing the rate-limiting step in sialic acid biosynthesis. GNE myopathy model mouse, in which *Gne* is knocked out with human GNE transgene with D176V, recaptured the symptoms of human GNE myopathy. The supplementation of ManNAc, NeuAc, and sialyllactose prevented the onset of the disorder and also recovered the muscle function from symptomatic status, suggesting hyposialylation is one of key factors in the pathogenesis of this disorder. Based on the studies with GNE myopathy model, the clinical trials are conducted at the three places in the world (USA, Japan, and Israel). Expectedly GNE myopathy will be treatable in the near future.

Keywords GNE myopathy • *GNE* gene • Sialic acid • Clinical trial

4.1 Introduction

GNE myopathy is an autosomal recessive myopathy, which was initially identified by its unique pathological characters, the presence of rimmed vacuoles and cytosolic inclusions in myofibers in 1981 [1]. Then this disease was characterized clinically by progressive atrophy and weakness of preferentially distal muscles of lower extremities, especially the tibialis anterior muscles as "distal myopathy with rimmed vacuoles," and by the unique finding of quadriceps sparing even in the advanced stages as "quadriceps sparing rimmed vacuolar myopathy" [2]. In 2001, the identification of causative gene and gene mutations in the patients made an initial breakthrough on a research on this disease [3]. After this finding, the researches on this disorder were accelerated remarkably; more than 100 genetic

H. Nishimura • S. Noguchi (✉)
Department of Neuromuscular Research, National Institute of Neuroscience, National Center of Neurology and Psychiatry, 4-1-1 Ogawahigashi-cho, Kodaira, Tokyo 187-8502, Japan
e-mail: noguchi@ncnp.go.jp

S. Takeda et al. (eds.), *Translational Research in Muscular Dystrophy*,
DOI 10.1007/978-4-431-55678-7_4

mutations were listed up [4, 5], phenotypes of the identified patients were documented in detail, and the impacts of the identified mutations and natures of the affected muscles were evaluated on cell culture experiments. Most importantly, the efficacy of treatment with sugar metabolites on the patients' cells served a strong possibility for the therapy for this disorder [6]. The second breakthrough on the research was the development of the animal models mimicking patients' phenotypes which enable to make up a detailed strategy for the therapeutic application. The success of the preclinical studies on the animal model by sugar compound supplementation further encouraged the researchers, clinicians, as well as the patients to have a reality of the therapy, as considering that GNE myopathy is a treatable disorder. Now the clinical trials for this disease are conducted at three places. GNE myopathy might be a special case with successful research progression just taking for only 10 years from starting research to clinical trials. What makes it possible for such a shorter time? In this chapter, we will give an outline of the GNE myopathy and explain the researches using animal models. In the last part, we will also introduce the ongoing clinical trials and discuss the further perspectives in therapy for the GNE myopathy.

4.2 Nomenclature of the Disease and Causative Gene

As described in "Introduction," GNE myopathy has been reported as "Nonaka distal myopathy" [1]. Later this disorder was commonly referred to as "distal myopathy with rimmed vacuoles" in Japan. Argov et al. independently identified this disorder in Iranian-Jewish families and termed as "vacuolar myopathy sparing the quadriceps" [2] and later it was commonly referred to as "inclusion body myopathy 2" or "hereditary inclusion body myopathy" in Western countries. Genetic analyses by mapping of the causative gene to 9p1-9q1 on chromosome 9 and identification of mutations in the *GNE* gene in all cohorts clarified that these disorders are the same condition [7]. These multiple names to one disorder make confusing for clinicians, researchers, and patients. An international consortium has recently proposed to rename this disorder as "GNE myopathy" and recommended only to use this term [8].

In 2001, *GNE* gene had been identified as a causative gene for GNE myopathy. After this finding, the several kinds of transcripts from *GNE* gene were identified. According to the rule of mutation nomenclature of HGVS, the longest transcript (hGNE2: NM_001128227) and protein (NP_001121699) should be used to describe mutations. The protein and transcript originally used are hGNE1 (NP_005467) and variant 2(NM_005476), respectively, in GenBank. The protein isoform hGNE1 covers 722 amino acids which is 31 amino acids shorter than hGNE2. So, amino acid numbering of previously reported *GNE* mutations should be supplemented with 31 amino acids to adhere to the current nomenclature guidelines [8]. However, several previous studies have used the shorter protein, hGNE1, and old nomenclature based on hGNE1. To express the information, for avoiding confusion, it was also recommended to describe the *GNE* mutation position with the name of corresponding transcript or protein, if the research used the specific isoform.

4.3 Clinical Features and Pathological Findings of GNE Myopathy

The onset age of GNE myopathy is from 15 to 40 years, with the average onset of 26 years. Patients become wheelchair bound for an average of 12 years after the onset. Serum creatine kinase level is normal to mildly elevated.

Though GNE myopathy is a mildly progressive disease, annual reduction in summed manual muscle testing, grip power, percent force vital capacity, 6 min walk test scores, and gross motor function measurement were observed. Among all the muscles examined, shoulder extension and abduction and knee flexion showed significant annual decrement [9]. Respiratory dysfunction had rarely been reported in GNE myopathy patients. In 2012, some of GNE myopathy patients were reported to have mild but progressive respiratory loss, and some of them experienced recurrent pneumonia due to reduced airway clearance [10].

In muscle pathology, the most characteristic feature in GNE myopathy is the presence of rimmed vacuoles (RVs) in myofibers (Fig. 4.1). Some of these RVs include congophilic materials which have immunoreactivity to amyloid proteins [11], phosphorylated tau, ubiquitin, and various proteins. Scattered atrophic fibers are also seen. Necrotic and regenerating fibers or inflammatory cell infiltration is not common but occasionally can be observed. In ultrastructural observation, accumulated autophagic vacuoles with amorphous inclusions are seen in the center of the myofibers making "autophagy buildup" as described in Pompe disease [12, 13], and the myofibrils neighbor to the autophagy buildup were well

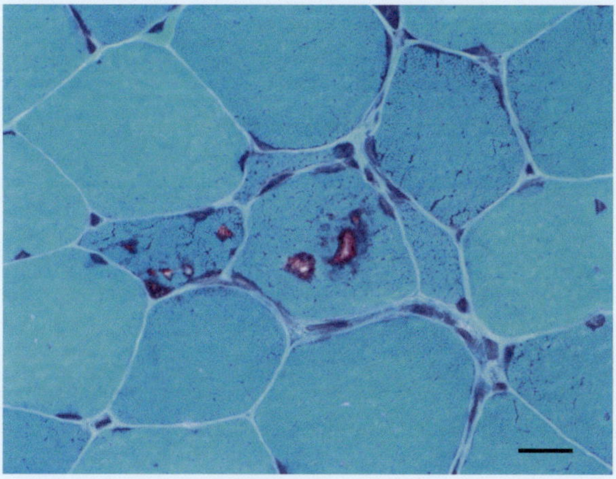

Fig. 4.1 RV in GNE myopathy muscle. Bar 20 μm

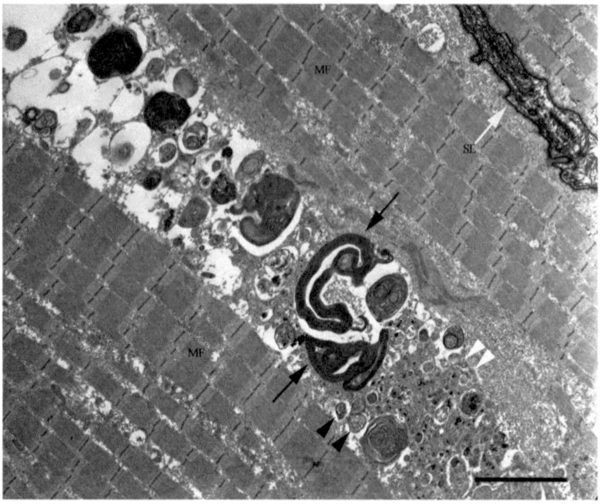

Fig. 4.2 Electron microscopic findings of GNE myopathy muscle. Autophagic vacuoles (*black arrow head*) are seen in the regions with various cellular debris and protein deposit (*white arrow head*). Multilamellar bodies (*black arrow*) are also formed. Myofibrils (MF) themselves are maintained to be almost normal. Sarcolemma (*white arrow*) is intact. Bar 5 μm

maintained (Fig. 4.2). Filamentous inclusions with 18–20 nm in diameter are also seen in the cytoplasm and the nucleus.

4.4 Genetic Cause and Proposed Molecular Mechanism of GNE Myopathy

More than 100 mutations in the *GNE* gene have been reported so far [4, 5]. It is known that different mutations lead to different ranges of severity in symptoms [4, 5, 14]. For example, the patients with homozygous p.V572L mutations exhibit earlier onset age and the time from disease onset to wheelchair use is shorter. On the other hand, the patients with p.D176V mutations show later onset age and most of them are ambulatory at the older ages.

GNE gene encodes a bifunctional enzyme working on the rate-limiting step in sialic acid biosynthesis in higher vertebrates. GNE protein catalyzes the epimerization of UDP-GlcNAc to ManNAc and the phosphorylation of ManNAc to ManNAc-6-P. The phosphorylated ManNAc eventually is converted to NeuAc and then CMP-NeuAc. The final product CMP-NeuAc is used as a sialic acid donor for sialylation of gangliosides or sialoglycoproteins in Golgi (Fig. 4.3). Sialic acid production is regulated by a negative feedback inhibition of the GNE activity by CMP-NeuAc. *GNE* mutations have been reported to lead to decreased GNE activities, subsequently resulting in the reduction in sialic acid production in cells.

Although decreased sialic acid production in GNE myopathy has been controversial [15], we have demonstrated the hyposialylation in primary culture cells and muscles in GNE myopathy patients [7]. Importantly, the hyposialylation in culture

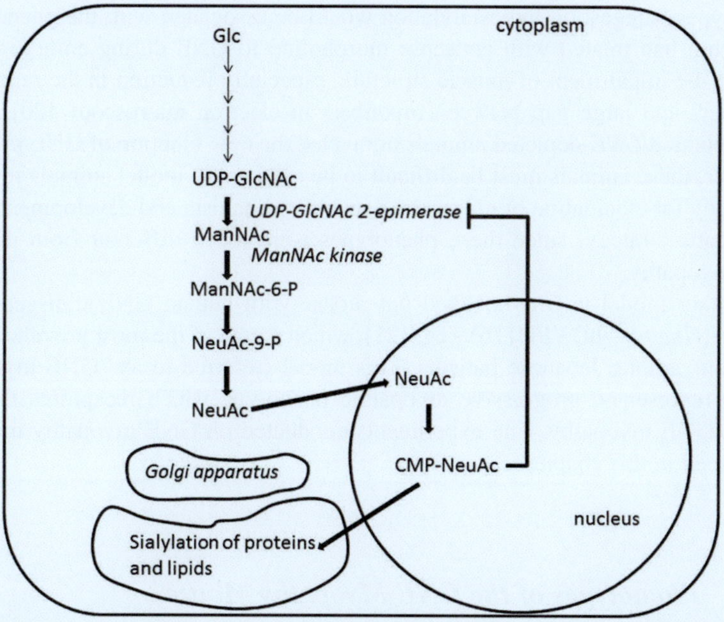

Fig. 4.3 Sialic acid biosynthetic pathway. The initial step in sialic acid biosynthesis is started by a bifunctional enzyme encoded by the *GNE* gene: UDP-GlcNAc 2-epimerase which epimerizes UDP-GlcNAc into ManNAc and ManNAc kinase which catalyzes the phosphorylation of ManNAc into ManNAc-6-P. The next two steps in the pathway eventually convert ManNAc-6-P into NeuAc. Activation of free NeuAc into CMP-NeuAc occurs in the nucleus. CMP-NeuAc is later transported to the Golgi apparatus and used for sialylation of oligosaccharide chains of gangliosides or sialoglycoproteins in Golgi. CMP-NeuAc regulates UDP-GlcNAc 2-epimerase activity by negative feedback to determine sialic acid biosynthesis in cells

cells was recovered to normal level with NeuAc and ManNAc supplementation [6]. However, no overall hyposialylation in the myoblasts and lymphoblastoid cell line from GNE myopathy patients had been also reported in other papers [16, 17].

4.5 GNE Myopathy Model Animals

Model animals are essential to elucidate the pathomechanism of diseases and to develop therapeutic methods. Three kinds of *Gne* gene-modified mice and *gne*-knocked down zebra fish with antisense oligonucleotides have been reported. Two mice strains with the recessive mutations of M712T and V572L (mutation nomenclature is based on GenBank NP_005467) represented the severe glomerular proteinuria without myopathic phenotype [18, 19]. Both mice displayed quite similar renal phenotypes, enlarged glomerulosclerosis, and podocyte foot process abnormalities in the kidney. ManNAc administration to M712T homozygotes and NeuAc administration to V572L homozygotes could prevent the nephrotic-like phenotypes, suggesting hyposialylation would be associated with the phenotypes. The zebra fish treated with antisense morpholino to GNE during embryogenesis showed the impairment of muscle structure, especially reduction in the number of myofibers and large gap between myofibers in electron microscopy [20]. These *GNE*-mutated/*GNE*-depleted animals unraveled the new function of GNE proteins; however, these animals must be difficult to be used as the model animals for GNE myopathy for elucidation of myopathy-causing mechanism and development of the therapeutic strategy, since these phenotypes were much different from those in GNE myopathy.

Another model is *Gne*-knocked out mouse with human GNE transgene with D176V (*Gne*−/−•h*GNE*D176V-Tg) [21], which is one of the most prevalent *GNE* mutations among Japanese patients. This model (referred to as "GNE myopathy mice") represented progressive myopathic phenotype which recaptures those in human GNE myopathy. The experiments conducted on GNE myopathy mice are introduced in this chapter.

4.5.1 Phenotypes of the GNE Myopathy Mouse

The *Gne*−/−•h*GNE*D176V-Tg mice can be littered in Mendelian rate and no apparent phenotype at birth. The cellular sialic acid levels in various organs other than the brain were remarkably reduced. The weights of the GNE myopathy mice were lighter than control littermates, and this difference in weight becomes more remarkable with age [22]. The motor performance and exercise endurance of the model mice were worse than their littermates, and the impairment of the motor performance became evident from the age of 21 weeks and displayed remarkable disease progression after 31 weeks of age.

In isolated gastrocnemius muscles, peak isometric twitch and maximum tetanic force showed gradual decrements with age: decrease to 90 % by 10 weeks, 80 % by 21 weeks, 70 % by 31 weeks, and 50 % by 41 weeks. The tetanic force was markedly reduced after 41 weeks of age, so the twitch-tetanic ratio is significantly higher in GNE myopathy mice compared with control mice. The gastrocnemius muscles of the GNE myopathy mice were smaller as compared with those of control mice, even in younger age. Furthermore, the muscles demonstrated a steadily decreasing muscle mass of at least 10–20 % from 31 weeks of age and decreasing more remarkably from 41 weeks of age. Cross-sectional area-normalized twitch and tetanic forces showed similar temporal pattern of force reduction in GNE myopathy mice, but interestingly significant differences between GNE myopathy and control mice were only seen from the age of 31 weeks, indicating the only atrophy but not muscle degeneration attributes to muscle weakness in younger age by 30 weeks, and symptomatic muscle degeneration, which would cause the remarkable reduction of tetanic force, begins from 31 weeks of age and results in the severe muscle weakness after 41 weeks.

4.5.2 *Atrophic Change Proceeds Development of Pathological Hallmarks in Muscles of GNE Myopathy Mice*

No remarkable change in morphological appearance on light microscopy was seen in the muscles from the GNE myopathy mice from 10 to 20 weeks of age, except for minimal variation in fiber size in the gastrocnemius, TA, and QF muscles. The number of small size fibers increased from 21 to 30 weeks of age in gastrocnemius and TA muscles, which contribute to the increasing variation in fiber size. From 31 to 40 weeks of age, a few intracellular inclusions, which were Congo red positive and immunoreactive to various antibodies to amyloid, were observed. The appearance of RVs delayed from 42 weeks (Fig. 4.4). In electron microscopy, the protein inclusions were observed between the bundles of myofibrils in 30 weeks of age, and both the protein inclusions and autophagic vacuoles were accumulated in the center

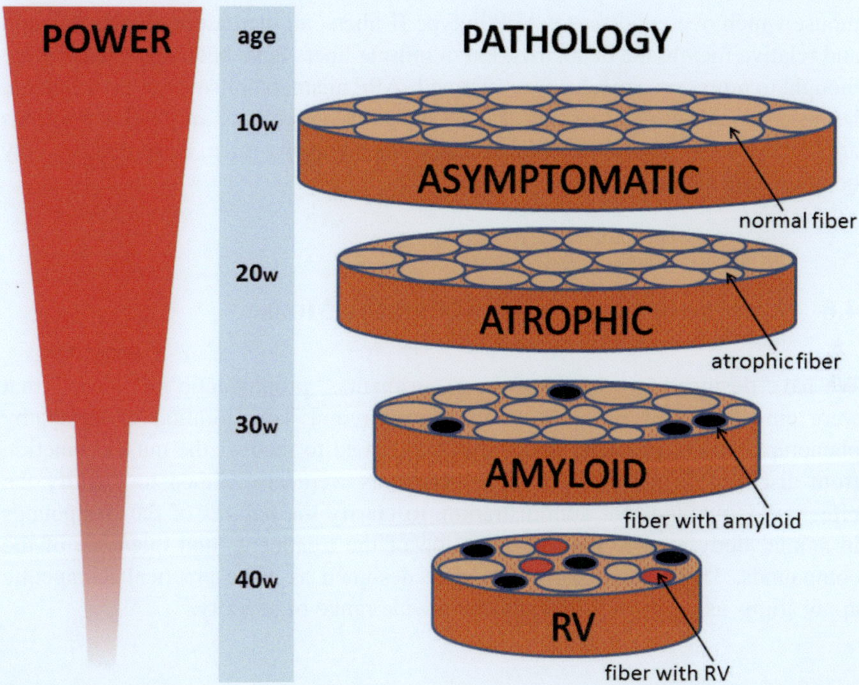

Fig. 4.4 The course of muscle changes in GNE myopathy mouse. No remarkable changes in morphological appearance, but slight weakness in muscle power is seen from 10 to 20 weeks of age. The myofiber atrophy is evident from 21 to 30 weeks of age, which contributes to the increasing variation in fiber size. From 31 to 40 weeks of age, fiber size variation is enhanced and amyloid protein positive – intracellular inclusions are observed. RVs are seen after 40 weeks

of myofibers apart from the myofibrils after 41 weeks as observed in human GNE patients' muscles. This accumulation would be results of active cellular response to intracellular inclusion proteins, gathering them into central region by intracellular transport system and inducing macroautophagy process for proteolysis of them.

Fiber-type selective atrophy was not observed at least in gastrocnemius, TA, and QF muscle. However, surprisingly, almost all fibers that had either RVs or intracellular depositions were type II fibers. In other murine models of muscular dystrophy and myopathies, the predominant involvement of type II muscle fibers [23] has been estimated to be due to the increased susceptibility of these muscles to eccentric contraction-induced damage [24, 25]. In the GNE myopathy mice, this is interesting since the mechanism underlying the disease is remarkably different from these other types of murine myopathy models. Interestingly, in a transgenic mouse overexpressing β-amyloid precursor protein (β-APP), intracellular amyloid deposition has been reported predominantly in type II fibers [26]. This could suggest that the involvement of type II fibers may be secondary to susceptibility to oxidative stress and/or calcium dysregulation attributed to type II fibers. Moreover, in a mouse which overexpresses β-APP in type II fibers, an increase in resting calcium and relative membrane depolarization in muscle fibers have been observed and are thought to represent a mechanism relating β-APP mismetabolism to altered calcium homeostasis and clinical weakness [27]. Because intracellular amyloid depositions are key events in muscle degeneration of GNE myopathy mice, these findings may be of interest for future investigations.

4.6 Treatment of the GNE Myopathy Mouse

We have designed two kinds of the experiments: "prophylactic treatments" that were aimed to prevent onset of the disorder and "amelioration of myopathy phenotypes in symptomatic mice" that was aimed to recover the muscle function from diseased status. The former experiments were also aimed to identify the effective compounds for administration, to clarify the natures of the compounds in animal body, and to get the limitation of the treatments and tolerance of the compounds. The latter experiments were designed as more practical therapeutic applications using weaker animals and a wide range of severity.

4.6.1 Prophylactic Treatment with Sialic Acid Metabolites

ManNAc was effective in preventing the myopathic symptoms of the GNE myopathy mice, equally with low dose (20 mg per kg bodyweight per day), medium dose (200 mg per kg bodyweight per day), and high dose (2000 mg per kg bodyweight per day) [28]. The serum creatine kinase concentration was lowered and motor performance, body weight, and muscle mass were increased after treatment. The number of rimmed vacuoles was significantly lower than the mice who received control treatment. Treatment also increased muscle cross-sectional area and force production and substantially diminished congophilic, amyloid-positive, or tau-positive inclusions. There was no apparent dose effect of ManNAc supplementation in preventing the myopathic symptoms of the GNE myopathy mice. NeuAc and sialyllactose were also effective for the prevention of disease with lower dose at 20 mg per kg bodyweight per day.

To aim for the enhancement of cellular uptake of the administered sialic acid metabolites in mice, we used peracetylated ManNAc for prophylactic treatment of the GNE myopathy mice [29]. Peracetylated ManNAc showed similar recovery of cellular sialylation at less than 1/10 concentration of regular ManNAc in culture medium. As expected, cellular sialic acid levels were highly increased to control levels in all organs including serum, and all aspects in muscle phenotypes, such as muscle power, size, and pathology, were well recovered to those in control mice.

These results provided us important insights: the properties of supplemented compounds, timing of treatment and measurement outcomes, for treatment of GNE myopathy. For the prevention of the disorder, small amounts of metabolites must be enough. More importantly, since NeuAc and ManNAc are rapidly excreted after oral administration, the repeated administration and modification of the compounds for increment of cellular uptake or for sustained release preparation must be necessary.

4.6.2 *Amelioration of Myopathy in Symptomatic Model Mice by Treatment with Sialyllactose*

6′-Sialyllactose showed slower excretion into urine than free sialic acid compounds. Treatment with 6′-sialyllactose led to marked amelioration of hyposialylation in muscle and consequently to improvement in the muscle size, contractile parameters, and pathology as compared to NeuAc [30]. These results suggest that GNE myopathy is treatable even at a progressive stage and 6-′-sialyllactose has more remarkable advantage than free sialic acid. These facts also provided an evidence of concept in the use of slowly metabolized sialic acid in the clinical trial of patients with GNE myopathy. Much amounts of sialic acid must be needed to rescue myopathic phenotypes. There are several points that we have to consider to achieve efficient increase in sialic acid level in peripheral tissues, including the variation of the recovery effects among the individual mice and the pharmacological advantages of the less metabolized compounds such as 6′-sialyllactose.

4.7 Clinical Trials by Sialic Acid-Related Compounds

After the success of preclinical studies on GNE myopathy model mice with supplementation of sialic acid metabolites, the clinical trials were carried on in three places in the world (NIH, Japan, and Ultragenyx) [31]. In this chapter, the design and the present status of the clinical trial in each place are explained.

4.7.1 Registration of GNE Myopathy Patients

In NCNP, Japan, the patients of GNE myopathy are registered with Remudy, Registry of Muscular Dystrophy. Remudy of GNE myopathy started in June 2012 and 155 patients were registered by July 2014.

4.7.2 ManNAc

In 2012–2013, a phase 1a study (ClinicalTrials.gov NCT01634750; IND No.78 091) with ManNAc was conducted at the NIH. This was the randomized, placebo-controlled, double-blind, single-dose study. The aim of this study was to evaluate the safety, pharmacokinetics, and pharmacodynamics of ManNAc in patients with GNE myopathy. A total of 22 patients were recruited in three cohorts. The dose levels investigated were 3, 6, and 10 g in each cohort. ManNAc was safe and well tolerated in all participants in this study. A multiple-dose study as a phase 1b study and an efficacy study of ManNAc in participants with GNE myopathy as a phase 2 study are being planned.

4.7.3 NeuAc

From November 2010 to June 2011, phase 1 clinical trial was performed at Tohoku University in Japan (ClinicalTrials.gov: NCT01236898). Three genetically confirmed patients were enrolled and were given 800 mg of NeuAc 3 times a day up to 5 consecutive days. No significant side effects were observed.

Because free sialic acid is rapidly excreted after administration, a slow release product (sialic acid extended release: SA-ER) was developed by Ultragenyx, a company involved in developing metabolic treatments for rare diseases. The trial was started in 2012 by Ultragenyx (ClinicalTrials.gov: NCT01517880). The 46 patients were enrolled and this new drug was orally supplemented. The trial design was double-blind administration of 2 doses (3 or 6 g per day) of SA-ER and a placebo control for 24 weeks. This was followed by continued administration of either the high or the low dose for an additional 24 weeks. Results of the first phase of the trial gave a modest improvement in the upper limb functional measurements, compared with deterioration in the placebo group. Patients with better walking ability at baseline had a better effect, which suggests that the degree of advancement of this disease may be a factor in the observed response. The serum sialic acid levels rose significantly as expected. There were no serious adverse events, and minimal side effects were not dose related.

4.7.4 Intravenous Immunoglobulin G Trial (IVIG)

Immunoglobulin G is a glycoprotein that contains 8 μ moles of NeuAc per gram. In 2005, IVIG was conducted in four patients with GNE myopathy at the NIH (ClinicalTrials.gov: NCT00195637) [32]. IVIG was infused as a loading dose of 1 g per kg on 2 continuous days followed by 3 doses of 400 mg per kg at weekly intervals, providing a total of 1.8 mmol (0.55 g) of NeuAc for an average participant weighing 70 kg, that is, approximately equal to 6 days normal production of NeuAc (0.3 mmol/24 h). The objective measurements of muscle strength were improved by IVIG administration (35 % in the quadriceps and 46 % in the shoulders). About 2 weeks after finishing IVIG administration, patients lost the benefit of IVIG. Distinct histological changes were not observed, possibly because such changes need longer-term treatment or muscle regeneration. Although the improvements of muscle strength after IVIG treatments suggest that supplementation of sialic acid has therapeutic promise, the therapeutic advantages in the use of IVIG, such as target organs of IVIG and the metabolism pathway of immunoglobulin G to produce sialic acids, should be considered.

4.8 Conclusion

Sialic acid deficiency might be a critical factor for the pathogenesis of GNE myopathy. Treatments for GNE model mouse by the supplementation of sialic acid-related compounds have been successfully conducted. Clinical trials using sialic acid compounds are in progress.

References

1. Nonaka I, Sunohara N, Ishiura S et al (1981) Familial distal myopathy with rimmed vacuole and lamellar (myeloid) body formation. J Neurol Sci 51:141–155
2. Argov Z, Yarom R (1984) "Rimmed vacuole myopathy" sparing the quadriceps. A unique disorder in Iranian Jews. J Neurol Sci 64:33–43

3. Eisenberg I, Avidan N, Potikha T et al (2001) The UDP-N-acetylglucosamine 2-epimerase/N-acetylmannosamine kinase gene is mutated in recessive hereditary inclusion body myopathy. Nat Genet 29:83–87
4. Cho A, Hayashi YK, Monma K (2013) Mutation profile of the GNE gene in Japanese patients with distal myopathy with rimmed vacuoles (GNE myopathy). J Neurol Neurosurg Psychiatry. doi:10.1136/jnnp-2013-305587
5. Celeste FV, Vilboux T, Ciccone C et al (2014) Mutation update for GNE gene variants associated with GNE myopathy. Hum Mutat 35:915–926
6. Noguchi S, Keira Y, Murayama K et al (2004) Reduction of UDP-N-acetylglucosamine 2-epimerase/N-acetylmannosamine kinase activity and sialylation in distal myopathy with rimmed vacuoles. J Biol Chem 279:11402–11407
7. Nishino I, Noguchi S, Murayama K (2002) Distal myopathy with rimmed vacuoles is allelic to hereditary inclusion body myopathy. Neurology 59:1689–1693
8. Huizing M, Carrillo-Carrasco N, Malicdan MC et al (2014) GNE myopathy: new name and new mutation nomenclature. Neuromuscul Disord 24:387–389
9. Mori-Yoshimura M, Oya Y, Yajima H (2014) GNE myopathy: a prospective natural history study of disease progression. Neuromuscul Disord 24:380–386
10. Mori-Yoshimura M, Oya Y, Hayashi YK (2013) Respiratory dysfunction in patients severely affected by GNE myopathy (distal myopathy with rimmed vacuoles). Neuromuscul Disord 23:84–88
11. Malicdan MC, Noguchi S, Nishino I (2007) Autophagy in a mouse model of distal myopathy with rimmed vacuoles or hereditary inclusion body myopathy. Autophagy 3:396–398
12. Shea L, Raben N (2009) Autophagy in skeletal muscle: implications for Pompe disease. Int J Clin Pharmacol Ther 47(Suppl 1):S42–S47
13. Malicdan MC, Noguchi S, Nonaka I et al (2008) Lysosomal myopathies: an excessive build-up in autophagosomes is too much to handle. Neuromuscul Disord 18:521–529
14. Mori-Yoshimura M, Monma K, Suzuki N et al (2012) Heterozygous UDP-GlcNAc 2-epimerase and N-acetylmannosamine kinase domain mutations in the GNE gene result in a less severe GNE myopathy phenotype compared to homozygous N-acetylmannosamine kinase domain mutations. J Neurol Sci 318:100–105
15. Malicdan MC, Noguchi S, Nishino I (2010) A preclinical trial of sialic acid metabolites on distal myopathy with rimmed vacuoles/hereditary inclusion body myopathy, a sugar-deficient myopathy: a review. Ther Adv Neurol Disord 3:127–135
16. Salama I, Hinderlich S, Shlomai Z et al (2005) No overall hyposialylation in hereditary inclusion body myopathy myoblasts carrying the homozygous M712T GNE mutation. Biochem Biophys Res Commun 328:221–226
17. Hinderlich S, Salama I, Eisenberg I (2004) The homozygous M712T mutation of UDP-N-acetylglucosamine 2-epimerase/N-acetylmannosamine kinase results in reduced enzyme activities but not in altered overall cellular sialylation in hereditary inclusion body myopathy. FEBS Lett 566:105–109
18. Kakani S, Yardeni T, Poling J et al (2012) The Gne M712T mouse as a model for human glomerulopathy. Am J Pathol 180:1431–1440
19. Ito M, Sugihara K, Asaka T (2012) Glycoprotein hyposialylation gives rise to a nephrotic-like syndrome that is prevented by sialic acid administration in GNE V572L point-mutant mice. PLoS One 7:e29873
20. Daya A, Vatine GD, Becker-Cohen M et al (2014) Gne depletion during zebrafish development impairs skeletal muscle structure and function. Hum Mol Genet 23:3349–3361
21. Malicdan MC, Noguchi S, Nonaka I et al (2007) A Gne knockout mouse expressing human GNE D176V mutation develops features similar to distal myopathy with rimmed vacuoles or hereditary inclusion body myopathy. Hum Mol Genet 16:2669–2682
22. Malicdan MC, Noguchi S, Hayashi YK (2008) Muscle weakness correlates with muscle atrophy and precedes the development of inclusion body or rimmed vacuoles in the mouse model of DMRV/hIBM. Physiol Genomics 35:106–115

23. North KN, Laing NG, Wallgren-Pettersson C (1997) Nemaline myopathy: current concepts. The ENMC International Consortium and Nemaline Myopathy. J Med Genet 34:705–713
24. D'Antona G, Brocca L, Pansarasa O et al (2007) Structural and functional alterations of muscle fibres in the novel mouse model of facioscapulohumeral muscular dystrophy. J Physiol 584:997–1009
25. Yeung EW, Head SI, Allen DG (2003) Gadolinium reduces short-term stretch-induced muscle damage in isolated mdx mouse muscle fibres. J Physiol 552:449–458
26. Sugarman MC, Kitazawa M, Baker M (2006) Pathogenic accumulation of APP in fast twitch muscle of IBM patients and a transgenic model. Neurobiol Aging 27:423–432
27. Schwarzkopf M, Knobeloch KP, Rohde E et al (2002) Sialylation is essential for early development in mice. Proc Natl Acad Sci U S A 99:5267–5270
28. Malicdan MC, Noguchi S, Hayashi YK et al (2009) Prophylactic treatment with sialic acid metabolites precludes the development of the myopathic phenotype in the DMRV-hIBM mouse model. Nat Med 15:690–695
29. Malicdan MC, Noguchi S, Tokutomi T (2012) Peracetylated N-acetylmannosamine, a synthetic sugar molecule, efficiently rescues muscle phenotype and biochemical defects in mouse model of sialic acid-deficient myopathy. J Biol Chem 287:2689–2705
30. Yonekawa T, Malicdan MC, Cho A et al (2014) Sialyllactose ameliorates myopathic phenotypes in symptomatic GNE myopathy model mice. Brain 137:2670–2679
31. Nishino I, Carrillo-Carrasco N, Argov Z (2014) GNE myopathy: current update and future therapy. J Neurol Neurosurg Psychiatry 86:385–392
32. Sparks S, Rakocevic G, Joe G (2007) Intravenous immune globulin in hereditary inclusion body myopathy: a pilot study. BMC Neurol 29(7):3

Chapter 5
Targeting the Type I TGF-β Receptor for Treating Caveolin-3-Deficient Autosomal Dominant Limb-Girdle Muscular Dystrophy Type 1C and Muscle Wasting Disorders

Yutaka Ohsawa, Shin-ichiro Nishimatsu, Masahiro Fujino, and Yoshihide Sunada

Abstract Caveolin-3, the principal scaffold protein in sarcolemmal caveolae, regulates signal transduction and vesicular trafficking. Dominant-negative mutations in the caveolin-3 gene (CAV3) cause autosomal dominant limb-girdle muscular dystrophy 1C (LGMD1C) and autosomal dominant rippling muscle disease (AD-RMD). Myostatin, a member of the muscle-specific transforming growth factor (TGF)-β family, negatively regulates muscle growth and volume. We recently showed that wild-type caveolin-3 binds to and inhibits TGF-β type I receptor (TβRI), thereby suppressing intracellular TGF-β signaling. In contrast, LGMD1C-causing mutant caveolin-3 activates TβRI, resulting in muscle atrophy. Recently, small-molecule compounds suppressing activation of TβRI, also known as activin receptor-like kinase 5 (ALK5), have been developed as anticancer agents. Oral administration of a TβRI inhibitor, Ki26894, ameliorates muscle atrophy and weakness in a caveolin-3-deficient LGMD1C mouse model. The therapeutic effect of Ki26894 is associated with a reduction in TGF-β signaling and an increase in the number of muscle precursor satellite cells. This suggests that the caveolin-3/TβRI signaling pathway plays an important role in the pathogenesis of LGMD1C and that it regulates skeletal muscle size by controlling the number of muscle precursor cells. Consequently, drugs that target the TGF-β pathway may have therapeutic potential for diseases characterized by muscle atrophy.

Keywords Caveolin-3 • LGMD1C • AD-RMD • ALK5 • TβRI inhibitors

Y. Ohsawa (✉) • Y. Sunada
Department of Neurology, Kawasaki Medical School, 577 Matsushima, Kurashiki, Okayama 701-0192, Japan
e-mail: yosawa@med.kawasaki-m.ac.jp

S.-i. Nishimatsu
Molecular and Developmental Biology, Kawasaki Medical School, Okayama, Japan

M. Fujino
Department of Health and Sports Science, Faculty of Health Science and Technology, Kawasaki University of Medical Welfare, Okayama, Japan

S. Takeda et al. (eds.), *Translational Research in Muscular Dystrophy*,
DOI 10.1007/978-4-431-55678-7_5

5.1 Mutations in the Caveolin-3 Gene Cause Autosomal Dominant Limb-Girdle Muscular Dystrophy 1C and Autosomal Dominant Rippling Muscle Disease

Caveolins, 18–24-kDa integral membrane proteins, play a crucial role in the formation of caveolae, flask-shaped pits in the plasma membrane, in terminally differentiated cells, such as adipocytes, endothelial cells, and skeletal muscle cells [1, 2]. Caveolin-1 and caveolin-2 are co-expressed and form hetero-oligomers in non-muscle cells, whereas caveolin-3 forms homo-oligomers in muscle cells [3, 4]. De novo synthesized caveolins assemble to form ~350-kDa oligomers in the endoplasmic reticulum (ER) and are subsequently targeted to the plasma membrane via the trans-Golgi network. Caveolins participate in diverse cellular processes, including vesicular trafficking, lipid metabolism, and signal transduction [1–4]. They bind to and regulate specific lipid and lipid-modified signaling proteins, including cholesterol, G-proteins, G-protein-coupled receptors, Src family kinases, Ha-Ras, and nitric oxide synthases [3, 4]. The interaction between caveolins and these molecules is mediated by a caveolin-binding motif on the target protein and a scaffolding domain in caveolins [5]. Numerous recent in vitro studies have demonstrated an important role of caveolins in regulating signaling by these various effectors. However, very few studies have examined the role of caveolins in signal transduction pathways in vivo [2, 3].

Mutations in the caveolin-3 gene (*CAV3*) have been identified in autosomal dominant limb-girdle muscular dystrophy 1C (LGMD1C) and autosomal dominant rippling muscle disease (AD-RMD) [6]. These mutations cause a significant reduction in sarcolemmal caveolin-3 protein levels and, to a lesser extent, mistargeting of the mutant protein to the Golgi complex from the sarcolemma [6–8]. The loss of caveolin-3 by mutations in *CAV3* in LGMD1C/AD-RMD patients may also impact the function of caveolin-3-binding molecules. Indeed, we and another group have shown that the enzymatic activity of neuronal nitric oxide synthase, which is suppressed by caveolin-3 in vitro, is elevated in skeletal muscles in a transgenic mouse model of LGMD1C and in LGMD1C/AD-RMD patients [7, 8]. Cytokine-induced nitric oxide production is increased in C2C12 myoblast cells transfected with LGMD1C/AD-RMD-causing mutant caveolin-3, compared with cells transfected with wild-type caveolin-3 [8]. Src, a membrane tyrosine kinase that regulates the balance between cell survival and cell death, is highly activated and accumulates in the perinuclear region, instead of the plasma membrane, in cells transfected with mutant LGMD1C/AD-RMD-causing caveolin-3 [9]. Furthermore, muscle-specific phosphofructokinase, a glycolytic enzyme, is significantly reduced in cells transfected with LDMD1C/AD-RMD-causing mutant caveolin-3, likely because of enhanced ubiquitin-mediated proteasomal degradation [10]. Of note, dysferlin, a protein involved in skeletal muscle repair, is deficient in LGMD2B/Miyoshi myopathy and is mistargeted to the cytoplasm in skeletal muscle of LGMD1C/AD-RMD patients, probably due to misdelivery of mutant caveolin-3 to the trans-Golgi network [11]. We previously showed that the ER stress molecule

GRP78 is upregulated in parallel with the gene dosage of mutant caveolin-3 ($CAV3^{P104L}$) in skeletal muscle in a rodent model of LGMD1C [12]. Despite the recent insight into the function of wild-type and mutant caveolin-3, the pathogenetic mechanisms underlying LGMD1C/AD-RMD remain fully understood.

5.2 Myostatin is a Promising Therapeutic Target for Muscle Wasting Disorders

Myostatin, a muscle-specific TGF-β family member, was discovered as a negative regulator of muscle growth and muscle volume. Overexpression of myostatin causes severe muscle atrophy, whereas targeted disruption of the myostatin gene increases skeletal muscle mass in mice [13, 14]. Like most other TGF-β family members, myostatin is synthesized as a precursor that undergoes proteolytic processing to generate a peptide with an N-terminal prodomain and a biologically active C-terminal disulfide-linked dimer [15, 16] (Fig. 5.1a). In the circulating inactive state, the N-terminal prodomain suppresses the biological activity of the C-terminal dimer [17, 18]. Once the prodomain is cleaved by BMP-1/tolloid-like proteases in the extracellular matrix, the C-terminal active dimer binds to and phosphorylates the activin receptor IIB/IIA (ActRIIB/IIA), a receptor type II serine/threonine kinase [18, 19]. This, in turn, recruits and phosphorylates activin receptor-like kinase 4/5 (ALK4/5), a receptor type I serine/threonine kinase, at the plasma membrane [16, 18–20]. The activation of a heteromeric complex of receptor type II and type I serine/threonine kinases results in the phosphorylation of intracellular effectors, including the receptor-regulated Smads (R-Smads), such as Smad2/3 [16, 21]. Phosphorylated R-Smads translocate to the nucleus from the cytoplasm, where they regulate the transcription of specific target genes leading to skeletal muscle atrophy [16]. In 2002, Khurana's group reported that administration of a neutralizing antibody against myostatin ameliorated symptoms in dystrophin-deficient *mdx* mice, including muscle atrophy, muscle weakness, and dystrophic changes [22]. However, a clinical trial using a humanized neutralizing antibody against myostatin showed no significant improvement in muscle strength in patients with Becker-type muscular dystrophy (BMD), facioscapulohumeral muscular dystrophy (FSHD), or LGMD [23]. Recently, highly potent myostatin signal blockers have been developed for clinical application in patients with muscle wasting disorders. A clinical trial of an antibody against the receptor type II serine/threonine kinase is currently ongoing in patients with sporadic inclusion body myositis (sIBM). This antibody, named bimagrumab, was designated as a breakthrough therapy by the US Food and Drug Administration (FDA) in 2013 [24, 25].

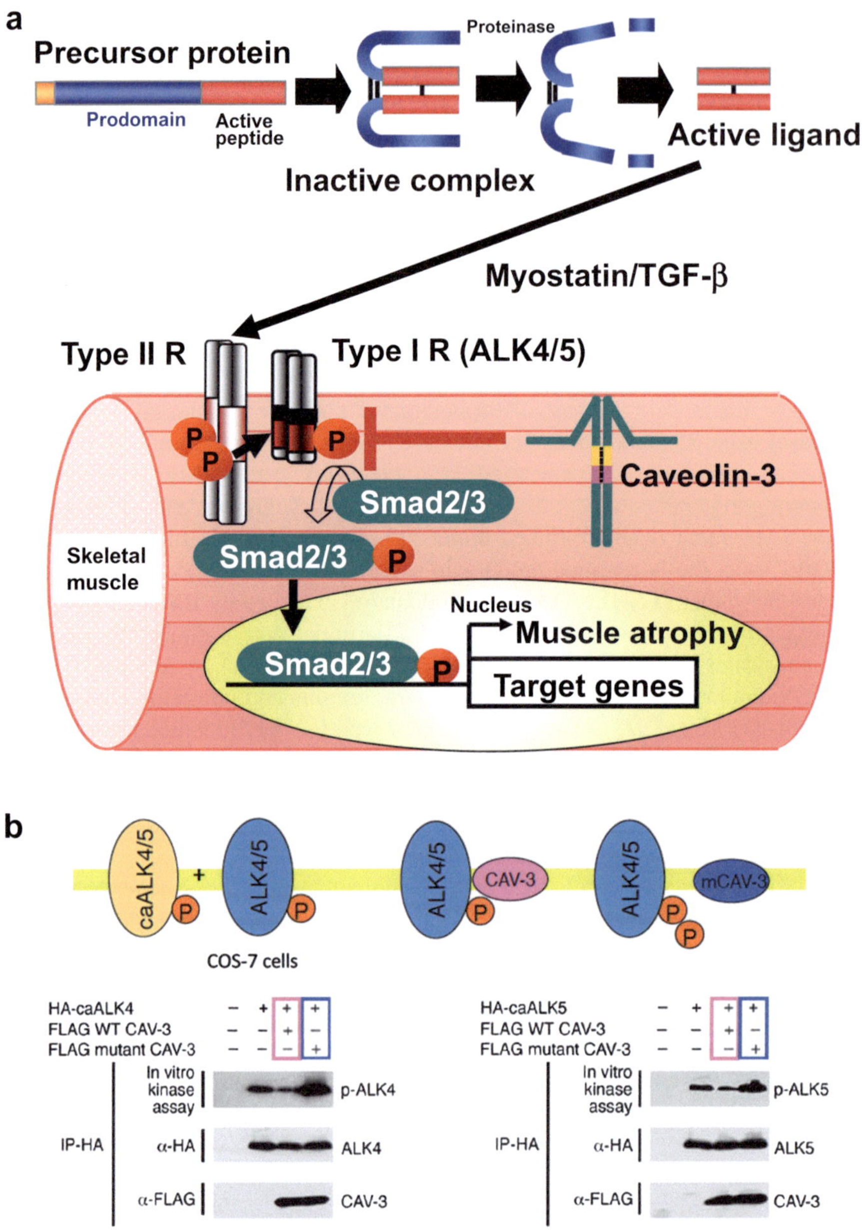

Fig. 5.1 Caveolins regulate myostatin and related TGF-β signaling at the type I receptor level. (**a**) Schematic representation of myostatin and related TGF-β signaling and caveolin-3. Type I serine/threonine receptor (R) controls intramuscular signaling by activating R-Smad (Smad2/3). Caveolin-3 suppresses the type I receptor. (**b**) In vitro autophosphorylation of constitutively active type I TGF-β receptors, ALK4 and ALK5. Cell lysates from COS-7 cells cotransfected with FLAG-tagged wild-type or mutant caveolin-3 ($CAV3^{P104L}$) and HA-tagged constitutively active ALK4 (HA-caALK4) or ALK5 (HA-caALK5) were immunoprecipitated with anti-HA agarose. The in vitro kinase reaction was initiated by the addition of kinase reaction buffer and [γ-^{32}P] ATP.

5.3 Caveolin-3 Suppresses the Type I TGF-β Receptor: Relationship to the Pathogenesis of Caveolin-3-Deficient LGMD1C

Recently, caveolin-1 has drawn considerable attention as a critical regulator of TGF-β signaling. Caveolin-1 binds to and suppresses activation of the TGF-β1 receptor type I serine/threonine kinase (TβRI), which induces growth arrest in non-muscle cells [26]. Caveolin-1 facilitates ligand-bound TβRI internalization and ubiquitin-mediated degradation [27]. In addition, caveolin-1 interacts with type II and type I receptors for bone morphogenic proteins (BMPs) in vivo [28]. These findings indicate that caveolin-1 regulates TGF-β signaling at the receptor level.

Based on the role of caveolin-1 in non-muscle cells, we postulated that caveolin-3 likely inhibits myostatin and TGF-β signaling in muscle cells. Indeed, we found several caveolin-3 binding motifs in the cytoplasmic kinase domain of the TβRI [29]. We cotransfected caveolin-3 and a constitutively active TβRI in COS-7 monkey kidney cells (Fig. 5.1b). We found that caveolin-3 colocalized and co-immunoprecipitated with the TβRI. Furthermore, phosphorylation of the TβRI was decreased by wild-type caveolin-3 and, conversely, increased by the P104L disease-causing mutant caveolin-3 in vitro [3]. These results indicate that wild-type caveolin-3 inhibits activation of the TβRI, whereas mutant caveolin-3 enhances activation. Genetic introduction of the myostatin prodomain or administration of type II decoy receptor (ActRIIB-Fc) drastically rescues muscle atrophy in a LGMD1C mouse model ($CAV3^{P104L}$). This therapeutic effect is associated with a decrease in TGF-β signaling, which is elevated in mutant mouse muscle [29]. Thus, caveolin-3 normally suppresses myostatin and TGF-β signaling at the type I receptor level, thereby preventing muscular atrophy. These findings suggest that excessive TGF-β signaling, triggered by caveolin-3 deficiency, could participate in the pathogenesis of muscular atrophy in LGMD1C.

5.4 TβRI Inhibitors Potentially Suppress Multiple TGF-β Signaling Pathways

Small-molecule compounds antagonizing TGF-β signaling at type I receptors (TβRIs) have recently been developed as targeted drugs for advanced cancer [30]. Tumor cells in advanced stages become refractory to TGF-β-induced growth

Fig. 5.1 (continued) Phosphorylated caALK4 and caALK5 were detected by autoradiography. Immunoprecipitated caALK4, caALK5, and caveolin-3 were analyzed by immunoblotting with anti-HA (α-HA) or anti-FLAG (α-FLAG) mAb. Bands corresponding to phosphorylated type I receptor (in vitro kinase assay), total type I receptor (α-HA), and caveolin-3 (α-FLAG) are shown

arrest, but often overexpress TGF-β1, TGF-β2, and TGF-β3 [31]. TGF-β family members promote the epithelial–mesenchymal transition, immunosuppression, and angiogenesis, resulting in tumor growth and metastasis [31]. Each member of the TGF-β family binds to the type II receptor, which, in turn, recruits a TβRI. Seven different TβRIs—activin receptor-like kinases 1–7 (ALK1–7)—determine the intracellular signaling specificity of the 33 members of the TGF-β family. Small-molecule TβRI inhibitors were originally developed to compete with the binding of adenosine triphosphate (ATP) to the kinase domain of ALK5, the TβRI for TGF-β1–3 [15, 16]. TβRI inhibitors have been found to suppress tumor enlargement and metastasis in the advanced stages of cancer in animals [32, 33]. Notably, these inhibitors also suppress a similar kinase domain in ALK4, the type I receptor for activin, and potentially block ALK4/5, the type I receptor for myostatin [30]. However, the effects of TβRI inhibitors on activin, myostatin, and TGF-β1–3 signaling in muscle remain unclear.

5.5 A TβRI Inhibitor Ameliorates Muscle Atrophy and Weakness in a Rodent Model of Caveolin-3-Deficient LGMD1C by Impacting Muscle Precursor Cells

Myostatin suppresses the differentiation of C2C12 myoblasts exposed to low-serum conditions [34]. Using an efficient retrovirus-mediated gene transfer system [35], we assessed the effect of a TβRI inhibitor, Ki26894 [33], on the differentiation of C2C12 myoblasts expressing TGF-β1 or activin A, as well as myostatin (Fig. 5.2a) [36]. Transferring C2C12 myoblasts expressing an empty vector from high-serum (growth) to low-serum (differentiation) media caused them to fuse and form multinucleated myotubes. We then stained the cells with antibodies against myosin heavy chain (MyHC). Adding Ki26894 to the culture media enhanced myoblast fusion and myotube formation (Fig. 5.2a, green). In comparison, myotube formation was impaired in C2C12 myoblasts expressing myostatin, activin A, or TGF-β1 (Fig. 5.2a, blue), compared with controls harboring an empty vector. Notably, Ki26894 alleviated the impairment in myotube formation induced by the TGF-β family members (Fig. 5.2a, red). TβRI inhibitors enhance myoblast differentiation in vitro by suppressing the activity of several members of the anti-myogenic TGF-β family, including activin, TGF-β1, and myostatin. Ki26894 also prevented the impairment in myotube formation induced by LGMD-causing mutant caveolin-3 [36].

We orally administered Ki26894 to a rodent model of caveolin-3-deficient LGMD ($CAV3^{P104L}$) from 6 to 16 weeks of age. Muscle atrophy was reduced in Ki26894-treated animals compared with untreated mice (Fig. 5.2b). Ki26894 increased muscle weight, muscle strength, and myofiber size, as well as centrally nucleated regenerative myofiber number in the mouse [36]. Furthermore, Ki26894

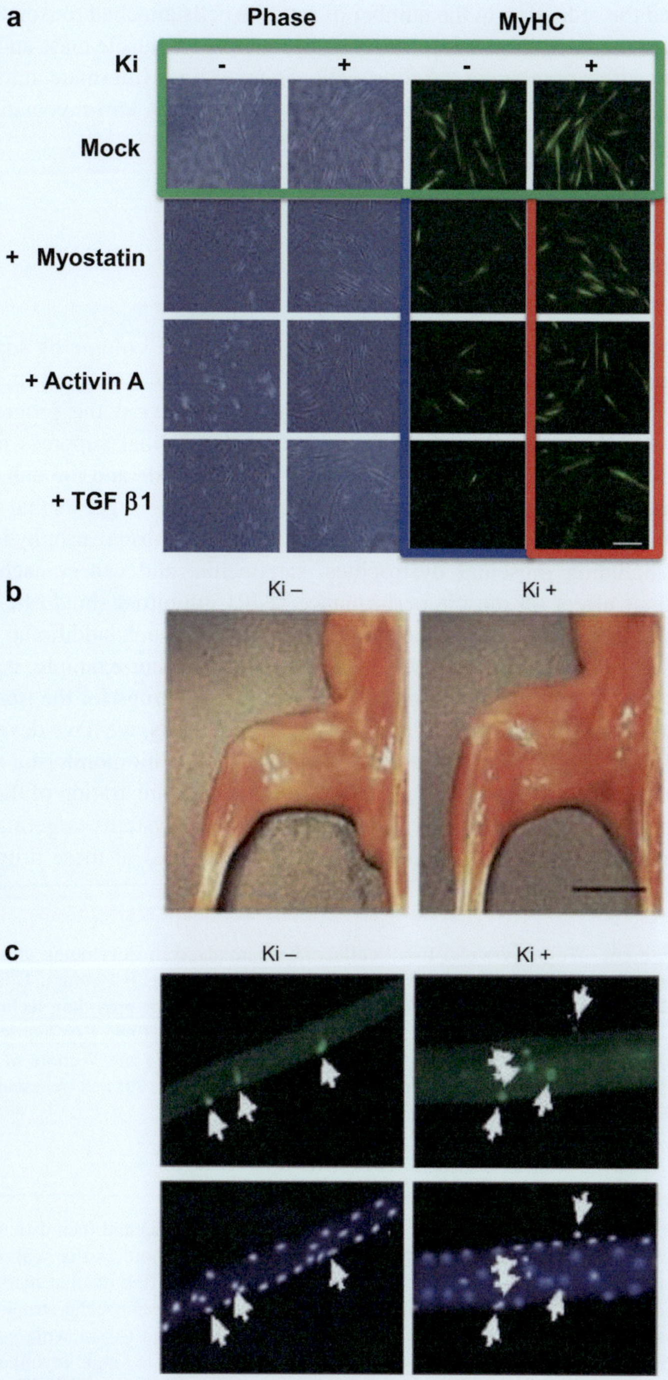

Fig. 5.2 TβRI inhibitor Ki26894 (Ki) prevents muscular atrophy in a caveolin-3-deficient LGMD1C mouse model. (**a**) Ki26894 suppresses the impairment in myogenesis produced by myostatin, activin A, and TGF-β1. C2C12 myoblasts expressing an empty vector were grown in

ameliorated the reduction in the number of satellite cells attached to isolated single myofibers in the mice (Fig. 5.2c). Ki26894 also increased muscle mass and strength and elevated the number of satellite cells, in wild-type littermate mice. These findings indicate that TβRI inhibitors strongly antagonize anti-myogenic TGF-β signaling and alleviate muscle atrophy.

5.6 Future Directions

As mentioned above, caveolin-3 regulates skeletal muscle volume by suppressing multiple anti-myogenic TGF-β signaling pathways. Pharmacological intervention strategies based on TβRI inhibitors are expected to prevent the progression of muscle weakness better than those based on inhibitors that suppress myostatin signaling alone. An increase in the number of satellite cells and the enhancement of myoblast differentiation induced by this type of inhibitor suggests that they may hold substantial therapeutic potential for the treatment of muscle atrophy in various diseases, including muscular dystrophies, sarcopenia, and cancer cachexia. To evaluate their effect on muscle performance, TβRI inhibitors should be tested in large-animal models of muscular atrophy. However, much additional study is required before clinical application of these compounds. For example, it is necessary to define the optimal, but nontoxic, dosage of these drugs for the treatment of individual patients with muscular atrophy. To facilitate this, we have developed an ex vivo myostatin activity assay as a convenient real-time biomonitoring system to determine how myostatin signaling is affected by the administration of these drugs in individual patients [36]. Furthermore, novel delivery systems targeting skeletal muscles also require development before the full potential of these drugs can be realized.

Acknowledgment We are grateful to all collaborators involved in developing anti-myostatin therapeutics and to T. Kenmotsu, N. Naoe, M Harada, M. Kimura, F Uemura, E Sugita, and K. Tanda (Department of Neurology, Kawasaki Medical School) for providing technical assistance. This work was supported by a research grant for Neurological and Psychiatric Disorders from the National Center of Neurology and Psychiatry (23–5, 26–8) and Welfare of Japan and from the Japan Society for the Promotion of Science (JST, AS24212769) and by research project grants from Kawasaki Medical School (23-T1, 26-T1).

Fig. 5.2 (continued) DMEM containing 10 % FBS (growth medium) and then differentiated in DMEM containing 2 % horse serum (differentiation medium), without (−) or with (+) 10 nM Ki26894 for 6 days. The cells were then stained with the muscle differentiation marker myosin heavy chain (MyHC). (**b**) Oral administration of Ki26894 ameliorates muscular atrophy. Appearance of de-skinned hind limb from 16-week-old mice treated without (−) or with (+) Ki26894. Scale bar, 5 mm. (**c**) Fluorescence images of satellite cells attached to single myofibers isolated from the EDL muscles of a rodent model of caveolin-3-deficient LGMD ($CAV3^{P104L}$) at 16 weeks of age. The white arrow indicates caveolin-1-positive satellite cells

References

1. Parton RG (2003) Caveolae-from ultrastructure to molecular mechanisms. Nat Rev Mol Cell Biol 4:162–167
2. Parton RG, Simons K (2007) The multiple faces of caveolae. Nat Rev Mol Cell Biol 8:185–194
3. Razani B, Schlegel A, Lisanti MP (2000) Caveolin proteins in signaling, oncogenic transformation and muscular dystrophy. J Cell Sci 113:2103–2109
4. Galbiati F, Razani B, Lisanti MP (2001) Emerging themes in lipid rafts and caveolae. Cell 106:403–411
5. Couet J, Li S, Okamoto T, Ikezu T et al (1997) Identification of peptide and protein ligands for the caveolin-scaffolding domain. Implications for the interaction of caveolin with caveolae-associated proteins. J Biol Chem 272:6525–6533
6. Minetti C, Sotgia F, Bruno C et al (1998) Mutations in the caveolin-3 gene cause autosomal dominant limb-girdle muscular dystrophy. Nat Genet 18:365–368
7. Sunada Y, Ohi H, Hase A et al (2001) Transgenic mice expressing mutant caveolin-3 show severe myopathy associated with increased nNOS activity. Hum Mol Genet 10:173–178
8. Kubisch C, Schoser BG, von Düring M et al (2003) Homozygous mutations in caveolin-3 cause a severe form of rippling muscle disease. Ann Neurol 53:512–520
9. Smythe GM, Eby JC, Disatnik MH et al (2003) A caveolin-3 mutant that causes limb girdle muscular dystrophy type lC disrupts Src localization and activity and induces apoptosis in skeletal myotubes. J Cell Sci 116:4739–4749
10. Sotgia F, Bonuccelli G, Minetti C et al (2003) Phosphofructokinase muscle-specific isoform requires caveolin-3 expression for plasma membrane recruitment and caveolar targeting: implications for the pathogenesis of caveolin-related muscle diseases. Am J Pathol 163:2619–2634
11. Matsuda C, Hayashi YK, Ogawa M et al (2001) The sarcolemmal proteins dysferlin and caveolin-3 interact in skeletal muscle. Hum Mol Genet 10:1761–1766
12. Kuga A, Ohsawa Y, Okada T et al (2011) Endoplasmic reticulum stress response in P104L mutant caveolin-3 transgenic mice. Hum Mol Genet 20:2975–2983
13. Zimmers TA, Davies MV, Koniaris LG et al (2002) Induction of cachexia in mice by systemically administered myostatin. Science 296:1486–1488
14. McPherron AC, Lawler AM, Lee SJ (1997) Regulation of skeletal muscle mass in mice by a new TGF-beta superfamily member. Nature 387:83–90
15. Massagué J (1998) TGF-beta signal transduction. Annu Rev Biochem 67:753–791
16. Tsuchida K (2004) Activins, myostatin and related TGF-beta family members as novel therapeutic targets for endocrine, metabolic and immune disorders. Curr Drug Targets Immune Endocr Metabol Disord 4:157–166
17. Hill JJ, Davies MV, Pearson AA et al (2002) The myostatin propeptide and the follistatin-related gene are inhibitory binding proteins of myostatin in normal serum. J Biol Chem 277:40735–40741
18. Lee SJ, McPherron AC (2001) Regulation of myostatin activity and muscle growth. Proc Natl Acad Sci U S A 98:9306–9311
19. Wolfman NM, McPherron AC, Pappano WN et al (2003) Activation of latent myostatin by the BMP-1/tolloid family of metalloproteinases. Proc Natl Acad Sci U S A 100:15842–15846
20. Rebbapragada A, Benchabane H, Wrana JL et al (2003) Myostatin signals through a transforming growth factor beta-like signaling pathway to block adipogenesis. Mol Cell Biol 23:7230–7242
21. Moustakas A, Souchelnytskyi S, Heldin CH (2001) Smad regulation in TGF-beta signal transduction. J Cell Sci 114:4359–4369
22. Bogdanovich S, Krag TO, Barton ER et al (2002) Functional improvement of dystrophic muscle by myostatin blockade. Nature 420:418–421

23. Wagner KR, Fleckenstein JL, Amato AA et al (2008) A phase I/II trial of MYO-029 in adult subjects with muscular dystrophy. Ann Neurol 63:561–571
24. Lach-Trifilieff E, Minetti GC, Sheppard K et al (2014) An antibody blocking activin type II receptors induces strong skeletal muscle hypertrophy and protects from atrophy. Mol Cell Biol 34:606–618
25. http://clinicaltrials.gov/show/NCT0192520.
26. Razani B, Zhang XL, Bitzer M et al (2001) Caveolin-1 regulates transforming growth factor (TGF) -beta/SMAD signaling through an interaction with the TGF-beta type I receptor. J Biol Chem 276:6727–6738
27. Le Roy C, Wrana JL (2005) Clathrin- and non-clathrin-mediated endocytic regulation of cell signaling. Nat Rev Mol Cell Biol 6:112–126
28. Nohe A, Keating E, Underhill TM et al (2005) Dynamics and interaction of caveolin-l isoforms with BMP-receptors. J Cell Sci 118:643–650
29. Ohsawa Y, Hagiwara H, Nakatani M et al (2006) Muscular atrophy of caveolin-3-deficient mice is rescued by myostatin inhibition. J Clin Invest 116:2924–2934
30. Yingling JM, Blanchard KL, Sawyer JS (2004) Development of TGF-beta signalling inhibitors for cancer therapy. Nat Rev Drug Discov 3:1011–1022
31. Derynck R, Akhurst RJ, Balmain A (2001) TGF-beta signaling in tumor suppression and cancer progression. Nat Genet 29:117–129
32. Uhl M, Aulwurm S, Wischhusen J et al (2004) SD-208, a novel transforming growth factor beta receptor I kinase inhibitor, inhibits growth and invasiveness and enhances immunogenicity of murine and human glioma cells in vitro and in vivo. Cancer Res 64:7954–7961
33. Kano MR, Bae Y, Iwata C et al (2007) Improvement of cancer-targeting therapy, using nanocarriers for intractable solid tumors by inhibition of TGF-beta signaling. Proc Natl Acad Sci U S A 104:3460–3465
34. Rios R, Fernández-Nocelos S, Carneiro I et al (2004) Differential response to exogenous and endogenous myostatin in myoblasts suggests that myostatin acts as an autocrine factor in vivo. Endocrinology 145:2795–2803
35. Kitamura T, Koshino Y, Shibata F et al (2003) Retrovirus-mediated gene transfer and expression cloning: powerful tools in functional genomics. Exp Hematol 31:1007–1014
36. Ohsawa Y, Okada T, Nishimatsu S et al (2012) An inhibitor of transforming growth factor beta type I receptor ameliorates muscle atrophy in a mouse model of caveolin 3-deficient muscular dystrophy. Lab Invest 92:1100–1114

Chapter 6
Translational Research in Nucleic Acid Therapies for Muscular Dystrophies

Joshua J.A. Lee and Toshifumi Yokota

Abstract Nucleic acid therapies have gained significant traction in recent years as a promising new approach to treating various genetic diseases. Such therapies employ synthetic, small molecules called antisense oligonucleotides (AOs) which are capable of modulating the transfer of genetic information from nucleic acid to protein through various mechanisms, including the augmentation of pre-mRNA splicing and downregulation of expression. Thus, AOs can prevent the incorporation of genetic mutations causing disease into final protein transcripts as well as reduce levels of mutant transcripts, potentially ameliorating disease phenotype. This process, also known as antisense therapy, has recently been the subject of several preclinical and clinical trials aimed at treating muscular dystrophies. Thanks to recent advancements in antisense drug chemistries, numerous studies have demonstrated the safety, tolerability, and efficacy of AOs administered to patients with Duchenne muscular dystrophy, the most common form of muscular dystrophy. In the wake of promising clinical trial data, it may well be that the first federally approved marketable antisense drug for treating muscular dystrophy could be on the horizon.

Keywords Antisense oligonucleotides • Muscular dystrophy • Exon skipping

6.1 Introduction

A potential therapeutic strategy for the treatment of the muscular dystrophies which has gained significant momentum in the last several years is antisense therapy. Antisense therapy involves the use of short, synthetic, nucleic acid-like molecules known as antisense oligonucleotides (AOs). AOs are designed to bind in a

J.J.A. Lee
Department of Medical Genetics, University of Alberta Faculty of Medicine and Dentistry, 8812-112 Street, Edmonton, AB T6G 2H7, Canada

T. Yokota (✉)
Department of Medical Genetics, University of Alberta Faculty of Medicine and Dentistry, 8812-112 Street, Edmonton, AB T6G 2H7, Canada

Muscular Dystrophy Canada Research Chair, Edmonton, AB, Canada
e-mail: toshifumi.yokota@ualberta.ca

S. Takeda et al. (eds.), *Translational Research in Muscular Dystrophy*,
DOI 10.1007/978-4-431-55678-7_6

sequence-specific manner to target regions on pre-mRNA, whereupon they can modulate splicing or inhibit protein synthesis through various mechanisms, such as translational arrest and RNase-mediated degradation of target RNA [1, 2]. By modulating the transfer of information from transcription to translation, antisense therapy could provide therapeutic treatment for a wide range of diseases, including muscular dystrophy, by preventing the incorporation of deleterious disease-causing mutations found in patients' genetic information from inclusion in the final protein product or by silencing the expression of a given mutant protein [3]. This chapter focuses on antisense oligonucleotides and their use as a therapeutic agent for the treatment of muscular dystrophies.

6.2 AO History and Early Challenges

The regulatory role of antisense RNA was first alluded to in studies involving transcription in Phage lambda [4] but was later defined through the study of *E. coli* plasmid ColE1, wherein plasmid replication is negatively controlled by antisense RNAs that modulate the formation of a replication-initiating primer [5–8]. Several other prokaryotic antisense systems were later described [5, 7, 9–11]. Antisense-mediated regulation of gene expression through the application of AOs was first reported by Zamecnik and Stephenson [12] who demonstrated the inhibition of Rous sarcoma virus (RSV) replication in chick embryo fibroblasts through the addition of a 13-mer oligonucleotide complementary to the 3′- and 5′-redundant terminal sequences of the RSV 35S RNA. Subsequent studies supporting the feasibility of antisense-mediated regulation of gene expression in eukaryotic systems were conducted using mouse β-actin, chicken thymidine kinase, and *Drosophila* hsp26, to name just a few [13, 14]. These early studies helped prepare the way for translational research utilizing AOs to target specific nucleic acid sequences to treat human diseases.

As the potential applications for AOs became apparent, so did the challenges and limitations of early antisense technology. These challenges have, in part, been responsible for the slow progress of antisense therapeutics into clinical application, but they have also propelled the breakthroughs that have brought nucleic acid therapies to where they are today; a few such early challenges will be discussed briefly as follows.

Initially, the method of AO delivery presented a major problem. The effectiveness of early AO chemistries was greatly hindered by their inefficiency at crossing the cell membrane, thus being unable to reach their intracellular targets at therapeutically beneficial quantities [15–18]. Off-target toxic effects caused by the immunostimulatory nature of traditional nucleic acids were another challenge faced by early AOs. Toll-like receptors, key players in the body's immune response, can be activated by the hybridization of DNA or RNA and can even recognize some AO chemistries [19]. Another challenge of AO-based therapies lies in the fact that depending on the nature of the disease or mutation, a very large proportion of nucleic acid targets (possibly greater than 90 %) must be specifically silenced through direct base-pairing with an AO in order to prove therapeutically beneficial [20]. Determining biochemically effective concentrations of AOs can therefore prove quite challenging when compounded with other challenges such as toxicity. A final challenge to consider in nucleic acid therapy is the intracellular sequestration of AOs. Administered AOs can sometimes be taken up and sequestered in phagolysosomes, oligo-protein complexes, and the reticuloendothelial system [20]. To overcome all of these challenges, AOs have undergone extensive changes in their chemistries since their initial discovery and development. These chemical modifications have produced several classes of AOs that exhibit increased stability and greater effectiveness at reaching and hybridizing with their transcript targets.

6.3 Comparative AO Chemistries

To counter the many opposing barriers which have impeded the development of effective nucleic acid therapies, many unique chemical modifications have been developed. These "next-generation" antisense chemistries exhibit improved target specificity, biological stability, intracellular delivery, and reduced off-target toxic effects. Some of these AO modifications will be discussed presently.

A widely popular antisense chemistry is the phosphorodiamidate morpholino oligomer (PMO, morpholino) [21]. Unlike DNA or RNA, base pairs within the PMO chemistry are bound to morpholine rings rather than the traditional deoxyribose/ribose rings. Additionally, PMOs differ from classical nucleic acid structures in the design of their backbone which is comprised of phosphorodiamidate linkages as opposed to phosphodiester linkages [22]. PMO antisense oligos exhibit high nuclease stability as well as binding affinity for their mRNA targets. PMOs are also well tolerated and do not activate toll-like receptors, the interferon system, or the NF-κB-mediated inflammatory response [23]. The encouraging toxicokinetic profile of PMO-based antisense drugs has helped catapult them to the forefront of clinical research, and there have been several clinical trials employing them as a potential therapeutic agent for treating neuromuscular disorders. A phase II trial for Duchenne muscular dystrophy has already been concluded and has yielded very promising results [24].

Another AO chemistry which has also been the focus of several clinical investigations is the 2'O-methyl phosphorothioate-modified (2'OMePS) antisense oligo [25]. The increased stability and cellular uptake of this particular AO come from a 2′-ribose ring modification and the substitution of sulfur for oxygen groups along its backbone, creating a phosphorothioate linkage. As mentioned, this AO has demonstrated its safety and effectiveness through several preclinical and clinical investigations for a host of diseases and is also currently being studied as a potential therapeutic agent for the treatment of Duchenne muscular dystrophy [26].

While not all AO chemistries have advanced to the clinical trial phase, many have demonstrated great potential through extensive in vitro and in vivo investigations. For example, vivo-morpholinos (vPMOs) are morpholino AOs conjugated to a cell-penetrating octa-guanidine moiety. These have been shown to effectively modulate splicing of the *FCMD* gene for the potential treatment of Fukuyama congenital muscular dystrophy, as well as facilitate multiple exon skipping of exons 45–55 and 6–8 in mice and dogs, respectively [27–29].

2’-methoxyethoxy (2’-MOE)-modified oligonucleotides contain 2’-O-alkyl-substitutions and function as antisense gapmers, supporting RNase-H-mediated cleavage of target RNAs [30–32]. Preclinical studies involving 2’-MOE AOs to treat spinal muscular atrophy (SMA) in the mouse model have shown the ability of this AO to ameliorate disease pathology in severely affected mice [33]. This antisense chemistry has been employed by Isis Pharmaceuticals in human clinical trials for SMA. Isis Pharmaceuticals’ lead candidate drug, ISIS-SMN$_{Rx}$, is designed to target a splice enhancer region of the *survival of motor neuron 2* (*SMN2*) gene, facilitating inclusion of exon 7 and producing full-length SMN protein. Current phase II clinical trials involving children with infantile-onset (type I) as well as type II and type III SMA have demonstrated the safety and tolerability of ISIS-SMN$_{Rx}$ (clinical trials ID: NCT01703988, NCT01839656).

6.4 Antisense Therapy and Muscular Dystrophy

As newer and more effective AO chemistries have been developed, their potential to treat a wide range of genetic diseases has been vigorously investigated. One promising group of genetic diseases for which antisense therapy holds great promise is the muscular dystrophies. Despite there being more than 30 different types of muscular dystrophy, with new sub-types being added regularly, only a relative few have found their way to the forefront of antisense therapy-based investigations.

6.4.1 Duchenne Muscular Dystrophy

Of all the muscular dystrophies, Duchenne muscular dystrophy is the most prevalent and, not surprisingly, it is also the foremost muscular dystrophy under investigation as a target for antisense therapy – specifically, exon skipping therapy (Fig. 6.1). Antisense-mediated exon skipping is a process that employs AOs to restore the open reading frame by either removing in-frame mutation-carrying exons or by removing exons flanking deletions [3, 34]. Numerous in vitro and in vivo studies have demonstrated the feasibility of exon skipping in the *DMD* gene [35–38]. The first successful *DMD* exon skipping in vitro was demonstrated in lymphoblastoid cells. In that study, researchers achieved successful skipping of exon 19 using a 2′O-methyl AO targeted to an exon recognition site and delivered via cationic lipid transfection [39]. The first demonstration of *DMD* exon skipping in vivo was shown in *mdx* mice using a 2′O-methyl AO designed to catalyze the

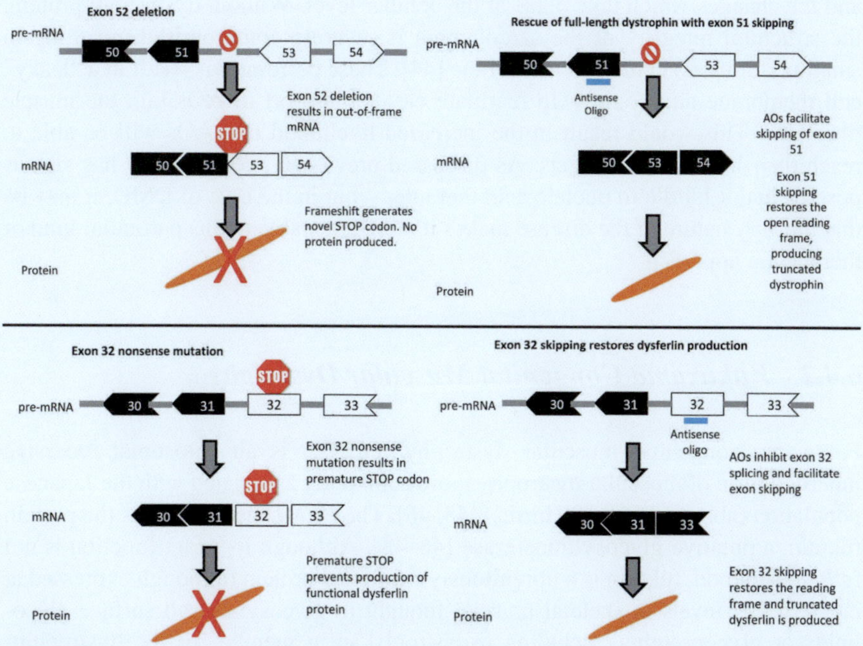

Fig. 6.1 Mechanism of exon skipping therapy in *DMD* and *DYSF*. The deletion of exon 52 in the *DMD* gene results in an out-of-frame transcript that does not produce functional protein (*upper left*). Antisense oligonucleotides are able to bind in a sequence-specific manner to regions of pre-mRNA and modulate splicing through interference with the spliceosome, resulting in the in-frame skipping of exon 51 and restoration of the reading frame (*upper right*). A nonsense mutation in exon 32 of the *DYSF* gene generates a novel stop codon, disrupting the reading frame and preventing the production of functional protein (*bottom left*). Antisense oligonucleotides can bind to a region of exon 32 and prevent incorporation of the exonic sequence into the final mRNA transcript, restoring the reading frame and producing a truncated protein that may retain some functionality (*bottom right*). Phasing or "framed-ness" of each exon is denoted by the shape of the ends of the exon – ends that fit together are in-frame

removal of exon 23 [40]. Lu et al. conducted the first systemic study of AO-mediated exon skipping in mice and were able to achieve bodywide dystrophin expression in all skeletal muscles using a 2′O-methyl AO chemistry [41]. Systemic administration of PMOs and local injection of 2′O-methyl AOs were able to restore dystrophin expression in the canine X-linked muscular dystrophy (*CXMD*) dog model; furthermore, this was the first successful demonstration of multiple exon skipping, wherein researchers used a cocktail of multiple AOs to achieve bodywide skipping of exons 6 and 8 [42, 43]. These discoveries have paved the way for AO clinical trials, and several have been conducted, with others ongoing or planned in the near future. The current status of nucleic acid therapies in clinical trials will be discussed in the section below.

One possible explanation for the remarkable success in antisense-based therapies for the treatment of DMD lies in understanding the pathology of the disease and the changes which take place at the cellular level. Without dystrophin protein, the structural integrity of the sarcolemma is severely compromised, resulting in small perforations in the cell membrane [44]. These perforations result in a "leaky" cell membrane and could help facilitate easier transport of AOs into the muscle fiber [18]. This would result in the increased likelihood that AOs will be able to reach their intracellular targets. As discussed previously, cell delivery has always posed a major hurdle to nucleic acid therapies – but in the case of DMD, it may be that the very nature of the disease makes it more amenable to this particular kind of therapeutic approach.

6.4.2 Fukuyama Congenital Muscular Dystrophy

Fukuyama congenital muscular dystrophy (FCMD) is an autosomal recessive inherited form of muscular dystrophy more commonly associated with the Japanese population (about 1 in 10,000 births) [45, 46]. The *FCMD* gene encodes the protein fukutin, a putative glycosyltransferase [46–48]. Although its exact function is not fully understood, fukutin is a ubiquitously expressed protein (although expressed at much higher levels in skeletal muscle) thought to glycosylate cell-surface glycolipids or glycoproteins, including α-dystroglycan, a member of the dystrophin-associated glycoprotein complex (DGC) [47]. Patients with FCMD harbor a 3-kb retrotransposon insertion in the 3′-untranslated region (UTR) of the gene, which introduces a splicing error that causes premature truncation of exon 10 [28]. Researchers have successfully utilized a cocktail of multiple vPMOs targeting intronic and exonic splice enhancers to restore normal fukutin expression and protein levels both in a mouse model and in human patient cells (Fig. 6.2) [28]. Although initially promising, there have yet to be any further investigations into the antisense-mediated treatment of FCMD.

6.4.3 Dysferlinopathy

Mutations in the *dysferlin* (*DYSF*) gene are associated with three autosomal recessive inherited muscular dystrophies – limb-girdle muscular dystrophy type 2B (LGMD2B), Miyoshi myopathy (MM), and distal myopathy with anterior tibial onset (DMAT) – and are collectively referred to as the dysferlinopathies [49–56]. The clinical symptoms of dysferlinopathy present across a wide pathological spectrum which narrows with disease progression until each subtype becomes practically indistinguishable. The protein product of *DYSF*, dysferlin, is a ubiquitously expressed transmembrane protein found at higher levels in skeletal and cardiac muscles where it plays an essential role in vesicle trafficking and plasma membrane resealing [54]. Providing "natural" proof of principle evidence that exon skipping could be amenable to treating dysferlinopathies, a female patient was

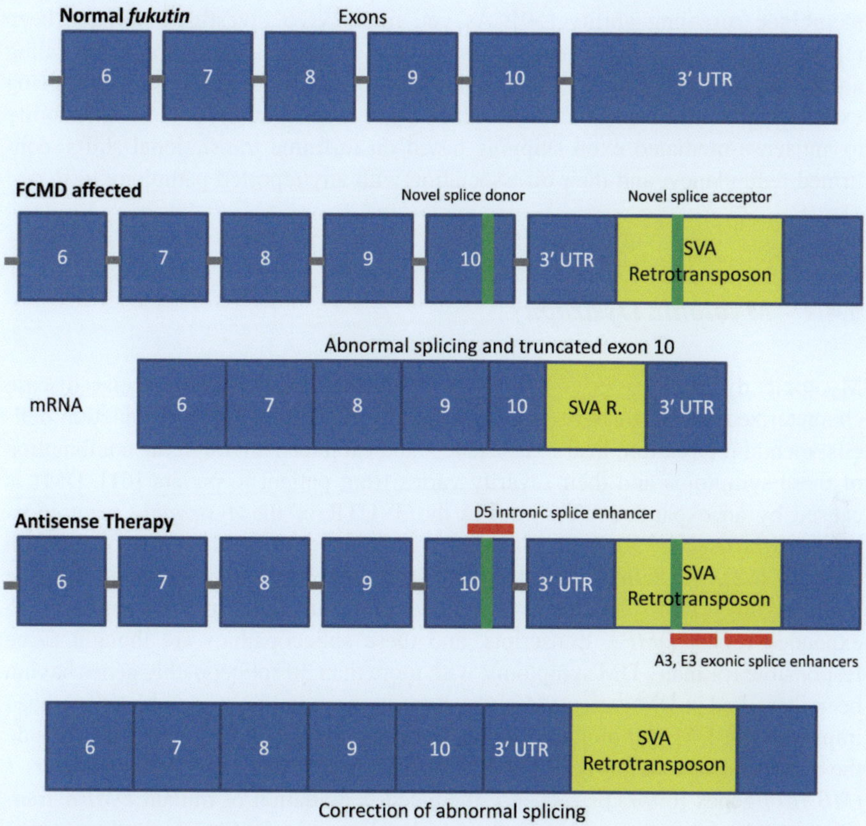

Fig. 6.2 Mechanism of antisense therapy in treating FCMD. The addition of a retrotransposal unit into the 3′ UTR of the *fukutin* gene generates novel splice acceptor and donor sites, resulting in aberrant splicing and truncation of exon 10. A cocktail of three antisense oligos targeting splice enhancer regions is able to correct splicing abnormalities and restore protein expression

previously reported as having a *DYSF* mutation causing the in-frame skipping of exon 32. Although the patient had two daughters with homozygous null mutations and severe LGMD2B, the patient herself presented with only mild symptoms, a phenotype attributed to the action of truncated DYSF protein caused by her mutation [57]. These observations drove subsequent investigations into the feasibility of *DYSF* exon skipping in vitro. One group utilized myoblasts generated from dysferlinopathy patients to test the effectiveness of 2′-O-methyl AOs targeting exonic splice enhancer/silencer sites and was able to achieve efficient exon skipping of exon 32 (Fig. 6.1) [58]. Another natural observation supporting the potential therapeutic action of truncated dysferlin comes from the report of a male dysferlinopathy patient who, despite proximodistal muscle weakness, was still ambulant unassisted at 41 years [59]. Intramuscular injections of a viral vector containing a *DYSF* construct corresponding to the patient's mutation were administered to *DYSF*-null mice and resulted in significant protein expression and restoration of membrane resealing ability [59]. As yet, no in vivo investigations have been reported that assess the effectiveness of AOs in restoring membrane resealing ability and ameliorating dysferlinopathy phenotype, although several promising exonic targets have been identified and are under investigation for their amenability to antisense-mediated exon skipping based on in-frame translational shifts, confirmed redundancy, and their disassociation with any reported pathology [60].

6.4.4 Myotonic Dystrophy

Myotonic dystrophy type 1 (DM1) is a multisystemic neuromuscular disease characterized by progressive muscle wasting, myotonia, cardiac conduction deficits, mental retardation, insulin resistance, and cataracts, although the combination of these symptoms and their severity varies from patient to patient [61]. DM1 is caused by an expanded CTG tract in the 3′ UTR of the *dystrophia myotonica-protein kinase* (*DMPK*) gene, which is believed to result in RNA-gain-of-function toxicity [62]. A hallmark feature of DM pathogenesis is aberrant splicing (spliceopathy). DM spliceopathy is believed to occur due to protein binding with expanded repeat *DMPK* transcripts, and these spliceopathies are thought to be responsible for many DM symptoms, with more than 30 spliceopathic genes having been identified in DM patients [63–68]. Some spliceopathic genes which have been implicated in DM pathology, specifically in the progression of myotonia, include the *chloride channel 1* (*CLCN1*) and *muscleblind-like splicing regulator 1* (*MBNL1*) genes [69–71]. Antisense-mediated degradation of mutant *DMPK* transcripts and/or the correction of abnormal splicing in DM-related spliceopathic genes through nucleic acid-based therapy are, therefore, promising avenues for treating DM1 (Fig. 6.3). Using 2′-O-methyl AOs, a novel DM1 myoblast-myotube cell model, and a well-characterized DM mouse model (HSA^{LR}), Mulders et al. achieved efficient silencing of mutant *DMPK* transcripts in vitro and in vivo, a reduction in the amount of RNA nuclear foci, and normalization of spliceopathy in several affected genes [72]. In human cells, expanded CUG transcripts were significantly reduced following the addition of AOs, and in DM300-328-XXL mice harboring a 45-kb human genomic fragment containing human *DMPK* with an expanded CTG repeat, there were reduced levels of mutant transcripts following AO injection into skeletal muscles [73]. In another study, systemically administered 2’-MOE AOs were effective in reducing expanded CUG repeats and nuclear foci and achieved transcriptome normalization and normalization of splicing in four genes: sarcoplasmic/endoplasmic reticulum calcium ATPase 1 (ATP2A1 or SERCA1), titin (TTN), LIM domain binding 3 (LDB3 or ZASP), and chloride channel 1 (CLCN1) with no signs of toxicity [74]. In the same study, persistent AO activity was detected up to 1 year following initial treatment and was accompanied by the sustained amelioration of several myopathic features including reduced numbers of centrally nucleated fibers and increased muscle fiber diameter [74].

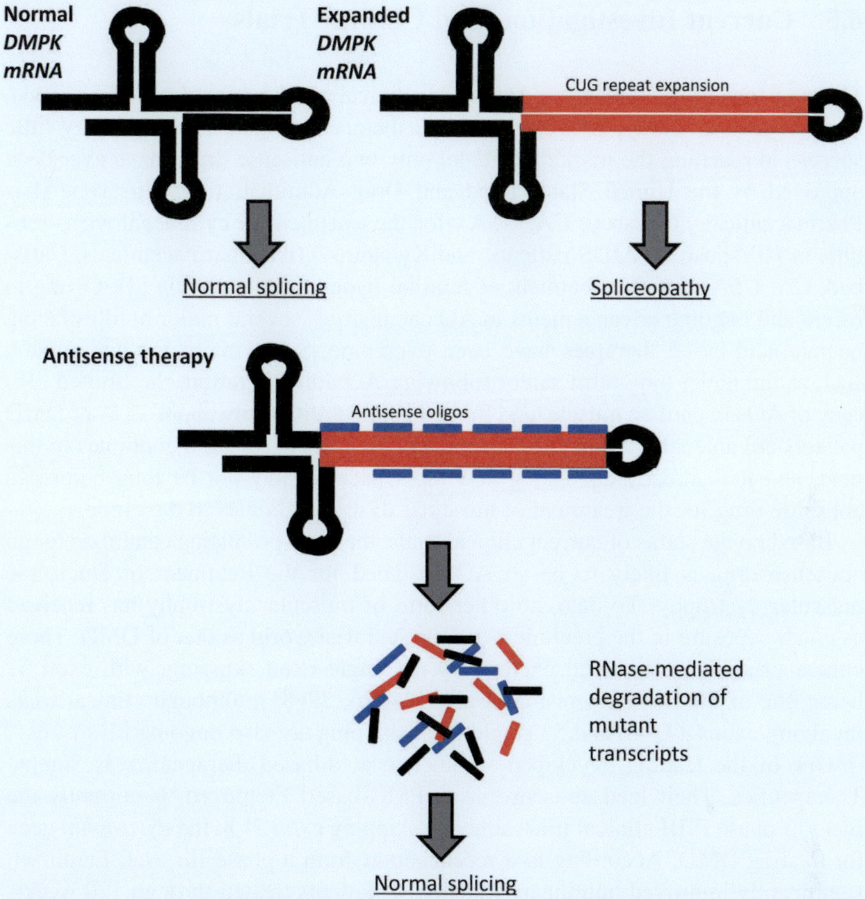

Fig. 6.3 Antisense-mediated degradation of toxic DMPK expanded repeat transcripts. DM1 is caused by a CUG repeat expansion in the *DMPK* gene, which results in spliceopathy in several other genes. Expression of mutant DMPK transcripts can be silenced through the use of antisense oligos which catalyze RNase-mediated degradation

Focusing on the correction of splicing in CLCN1, researchers employed PMOs to prevent incorporation of frame-shift-causing exon 7a and were able to suppress exon 7a inclusion, restore CLCN1 protein expression, rescue channel function, and reverse myotonia using two different DM mouse models [75]. Another group achieved amelioration of myotonia in mice who received PMOs delivered via bubble liposome-ultrasound, highlighting an effective method of AO administration and further demonstrating the feasibility of AO-based therapies for the treatment of DM [64].

6.5 Current Investigations and Clinical Trials

The road toward implementing AOs in the clinical arena has not been an easy one. Despite years of study, AOs as a licensed therapeutic agent have had very little success in reaching the market. To date, only two antisense drugs have ever been approved by the United States Food and Drug Administration: Vitravene (Isis Pharmaceuticals, Carlsbad, CA, USA), for the treatment of cytomegalovirus retinitis in HIV-positive AIDS patients, and Kynamro® (Isis Pharmaceuticals, Carlsbad, CA, USA), for the treatment of familial hypercholesterolemia [3]. Owing to recent and ongoing advancements in AO chemistries, several major hurdles facing nucleic acid-based therapies have been overcome. Some major hurdles remain, such as unknown long-term safety following AO administration, the limited efficacy of AOs in cardiac muscle, and limited applicability (only about 13 % of DMD patients are amenable to exon 51 skipping) [76, 77]. As research continues in this field, and it is already advancing at a rapid pace, it may not be long before an antisense drug for the treatment of muscular dystrophy comes to the clinic.

Based on the status of current clinical trials, the most promising candidate for an antisense drug is likely to be an AO designed for the treatment of Duchenne muscular dystrophy. To date, no other form of muscular dystrophy has received as much exposure in the preclinical and clinical trial world as that of DMD. These clinical trials have centered exclusively on single exon skipping, with exon 51 being one of the most promising targets [24, 26, 78–81], although clinical trials involving exons 44, 45, and 53 single exon skipping are also ongoing [2].

One of the leading developers of nucleic acid-based therapeutics is Sarepta Therapeutics. Their lead antisense drug, PMO-based Eteplirsen, is currently the focus of phase II/III clinical trials aimed at skipping exon 51 in the *dystrophin* gene for treating DMD. According to a recent report from a phase IIb trial, Eteplirsen significantly improved pulmonary function in patients treated through 120 weeks. This finding comes in the wake of preceding data from a 120-week study which found a significant improvement in walking ability in treated patients, as demonstrated by the 6-min walk test. No clinically significant negative effects due to Eteplirsen treatment have been reported. Another DMD exon 51-targeting drug, the 2′OMePS oligo Drisapersen, was developed jointly by GlaxoSmithKline (GSK) and Prosensa, and previous phase II clinical trial data demonstrated the safety, tolerability, and effectiveness of the drug at improving walking distance after 12 weeks of treatment. Unfortunately, Drisapersen did not demonstrate significant improvement in the 6-min walk test in a more recent phase III clinical trial. As a result, GSK is no longer involved in pursuing further clinical trials with Drisapersen, although Prosensa continues to be involved with the drug's development. There are plenty of lessons we can learn from this failure as recently pointed out [3]. For example, the doses of injections in this trial (up to 6 mg/kg) were much lower than the effective dose in *mdx* mice (2 mg/mouse; approximately 75–100 mg/kg) [41]. A very recent development in DMD clinical trials involves the joint efforts of Nippon Shinyaku Co., Ltd. and the National Center of Neurology and Psychiatry

(NCNP, Kodaira City, Japan), which have been developing a PMO-based antisense drug that facilitates exon 53 skipping in DMD patients. The first clinical trial involving their lead candidate drug NS-065/NCNP-01 is underway in 2014. This marks the first ever nucleic acid-based clinical trial in Japan and the first DMD exon 53-targeting clinical trial in the world.

While single exon skipping may be a focus of current clinical trials, future investigations involving multiple exon skipping could widen the door of applicability for AOs in treating muscular dystrophies, especially DMD. The majority of DMD patients (about 63 %) with deletion mutations harbor a mutation between the region of exons 45–55 in the *DMD* gene, a region known as the "mutation hot spot" [27, 37]. The development of a novel antisense approach to skipping exons 45–55 in the human *DMD* gene could overcome the enormous clinical heterogeneity observed in DMD by providing a single therapeutic tactic to treating a large proportion of patients. Furthermore, naturally occurring exons 45–55 deletions in patients are associated with an exceptionally mild, even asymptomatic phenotype [27, 35]. Bodywide exon skipping of exons 45–55 has been accomplished in a mouse model of DMD but has yet to be reported in human cells [27].

With successes in recent clinical trials, ongoing translational research using both in vitro and in vivo models, and continual advancements in AO chemistries, nucleic acid therapies for muscular dystrophies have become one of the most rapidly improving therapeutic strategies in medical research and may soon cease to be a technology exclusive to just the lab bench or to clinical trial cohorts.

Acknowledgments This work was supported by the University of Alberta Faculty of Medicine and Dentistry, Parent Project Muscular Dystrophy (USA), The Friends of Garrett Cumming Research Funds, HM Toupin Neurological Science Research Funds, Muscular Dystrophy Canada, Canada Foundation for Innovation, Alberta Enterprise and Advanced Education, Jesse's Journey, Slipchuk SMA Research Funds, the Women and Children's Health Research Institute, and Canadian Institutes of Health Research.

References

1. Helene C, Toulme JJ (1990) Specific regulation of gene expression by antisense, sense and antigene nucleic acids. Biochim Biophys Acta 1049(2):99–125
2. Lee J, Yokota T (2013) Antisense therapy in neurology. J Pers Med 3(3):144–176. doi:10.3390/jpm3030144#sthash.EzKjmG9w.dpuf
3. Touznik A, Lee JJ, Yokota T (2014) New developments in exon skipping and splice modulation therapies for neuromuscular diseases. Expert Opin Biol Ther 14(6):809–819. doi:10.1517/14712598.2014.896335
4. Spiegelman WG, Reichardt LF, Yaniv M, Heinemann SF, Kaiser AD, Eisen H (1972) Bidirectional transcription and the regulation of Phage lambda repressor synthesis. Proc Natl Acad Sci U S A 69(11):3156–3160
5. Green PJ, Pines O, Inouye M (1986) The role of antisense RNA in gene regulation. Annu Rev Biochem 55:569–597. doi:10.1146/annurev.bi.55.070186.003033
6. Itoh T, Tomizawa J (1980) Formation of an RNA primer for initiation of replication of ColE1 DNA by ribonuclease H. Proc Natl Acad Sci U S A 77(5):2450–2454

7. Simons RW, Kleckner N (1988) Biological regulation by antisense RNA in prokaryotes. Annu Rev Genet 22:567–600. doi:10.1146/annurev.ge.22.120188.003031
8. Tomizawa J, Itoh T, Selzer G, Som T (1981) Inhibition of ColE1 RNA primer formation by a plasmid-specified small RNA. Proc Natl Acad Sci U S A 78(3):1421–1425
9. Light J, Molin S (1983) Post-transcriptional control of expression of the repA gene of plasmid R1 mediated by a small RNA molecule. EMBO J 2(1):93–98
10. Mizuno T, Chou MY, Inouye M (1984) A unique mechanism regulating gene expression: translational inhibition by a complementary RNA transcript (microRNA). Proc Natl Acad Sci U S A 81(7):1966–1970
11. Simons RW, Kleckner N (1983) Translational control of IS10 transposition. Cell 34(2): 683–691
12. Zamecnik PC, Stephenson ML (1978) Inhibition of Rous sarcoma virus replication and cell transformation by a specific oligodeoxynucleotide. Proc Natl Acad Sci U S A 75(1):280–284
13. Izant JG, Weintraub H (1985) Constitutive and conditional suppression of exogenous and endogenous genes by anti-sense RNA. Science 229(4711):345–352
14. McGarry TJ, Lindquist S (1986) Inhibition of heat shock protein synthesis by heat-inducible antisense RNA. Proc Natl Acad Sci U S A 83(2):399–403
15. Yokota T, Takeda S, Lu QL, Partridge TA, Nakamura A, Hoffman EP (2009) A renaissance for antisense oligonucleotide drugs in neurology: exon skipping breaks new ground. Arch Neurol 66(1):32–38
16. Miller PS, Braiterman LT, Ts'o PO (1977) Effects of a trinucleotide ethyl phosphotriester, Gmp(Et)Gmp(Et)U, on mammalian cells in culture. Biochemistry 16(9):1988–1996
17. Bendifallah N, Rasmussen FW, Zachar V, Ebbesen P, Nielsen PE, Koppelhus U (2006) Evaluation of cell-penetrating peptides (CPPs) as vehicles for intracellular delivery of antisense peptide nucleic acid (PNA). Bioconjug Chem 17(3):750–758. doi:10.1021/bc050283q
18. Hoffman EP, Bronson A, Levin AA, Takeda S, Yokota T, Baudy AR, Connor EM (2011) Restoring dystrophin expression in Duchenne muscular dystrophy muscle progress in exon skipping and stop codon read through. Am J Pathol 179(1):12–22. doi:10.1016/j.ajpath.2011.03.050
19. Iwasaki A, Medzhitov R (2004) Toll-like receptor control of the adaptive immune responses. Nat Immunol 5(10):987–995. doi:10.1038/ni1112
20. Juliano R, Bauman J, Kang H, Ming X (2009) Biological barriers to therapy with antisense and siRNA oligonucleotides. Mol Pharm 6(3):686–695. doi:10.1021/mp900093r
21. Lu QL, Yokota T, Takeda S, Garcia L, Muntoni F, Partridge T (2011) The status of exon skipping as a therapeutic approach to Duchenne muscular dystrophy. Mol Ther 19(1):9–15. doi:10.1038/mt.2010.219
22. Moulton JD, Jiang S (2009) Gene knockdowns in adult animals: PPMOs and vivo-morpholinos. Molecules 14(3):1304–1323. doi:10.3390/molecules14031304
23. Sazani P, Ness KP, Weller DL, Poage D, Nelson K, Shrewsbury AS (2011) Chemical and mechanistic toxicology evaluation of exon skipping phosphorodiamidate morpholino oligomers in mdx mice. Int J Toxicol 30(3):322–333. doi:10.1177/1091581811403504
24. Cirak S, Arechavala-Gomeza V, Guglieri M, Feng L, Torelli S, Anthony K, Abbs S, Garralda ME, Bourke J, Wells DJ, Dickson G, Wood MJ, Wilton SD, Straub V, Kole R, Shrewsbury SB, Sewry C, Morgan JE, Bushby K, Muntoni F (2011) Exon skipping and dystrophin restoration in patients with Duchenne muscular dystrophy after systemic phosphorodiamidate morpholino oligomer treatment: an open-label, phase 2, dose-escalation study. Lancet 378(9791):595–605. doi:10.1016/S0140-6736(11)60756-3
25. Heemskerk H, de Winter C, van Kuik P, Heuvelmans N, Sabatelli P, Rimessi P, Braghetta P, van Ommen GJ, de Kimpe S, Ferlini A, Aartsma-Rus A, van Deutekom JC (2010) Preclinical PK and PD studies on 2′-O-methyl-phosphorothioate RNA antisense oligonucleotides in the mdx mouse model. Mol Ther 18(6):1210–1217. doi:10.1038/mt.2010.72
26. Goemans NM, Tulinius M, van den Akker JT, Burm BE, Ekhart PF, Heuvelmans N, Holling T, Janson AA, Platenburg GJ, Sipkens JA, Sitsen JM, Aartsma-Rus A, van Ommen GJ, Buyse G,

Darin N, Verschuuren JJ, Campion GV, de Kimpe SJ, van Deutekom JC (2011) Systemic administration of PRO051 in Duchenne's muscular dystrophy. N Engl J Med 364(16): 1513–1522. doi:10.1056/NEJMoa1011367

27. Aoki Y, Yokota T, Nagata T, Nakamura A, Tanihata J, Saito T, Duguez SM, Nagaraju K, Hoffman EP, Partridge T, Takeda S (2012) Bodywide skipping of exons 45-55 in dystrophic mdx52 mice by systemic antisense delivery. Proc Natl Acad Sci U S A 109(34):13763–13768. doi:10.1073/pnas.1204638109
28. Taniguchi-Ikeda M, Kobayashi K, Kanagawa M, Yu CC, Mori K, Oda T, Kuga A, Kurahashi H, Akman HO, DiMauro S, Kaji R, Yokota T, Takeda S, Toda T (2011) Pathogenic exon-trapping by SVA retrotransposon and rescue in Fukuyama muscular dystrophy. Nature 478(7367): 127–131. doi:10.1038/nature10456
29. Yokota T, Nakamura A, Nagata T, Saito T, Kobayashi M, Aoki Y, Echigoya Y, Partridge T, Hoffman EP, Takeda S (2012) Extensive and prolonged restoration of dystrophin expression with vivo-morpholino-mediated multiple exon skipping in dystrophic dogs. Nucleic Acid Ther 22(5):306–315. doi:10.1089/nat.2012.0368
30. Prakash TP, Bhat B (2007) 2′-Modified oligonucleotides for antisense therapeutics. Curr Top Med Chem 7(7):641–649
31. Altmann KH, Fabbro D, Dean NM, Geiger T, Monia BP, Muller M, Nicklin P (1996) Second-generation antisense oligonucleotides: structure-activity relationships and the design of improved signal-transduction inhibitors. Biochem Soc Trans 24(3):630–637
32. Monia BP, Lesnik EA, Gonzalez C, Lima WF, McGee D, Guinosso CJ, Kawasaki AM, Cook PD, Freier SM (1993) Evaluation of 2′-modified oligonucleotides containing 2′-deoxy gaps as antisense inhibitors of gene expression. J Biol Chem 268(19):14514–14522
33. Hua Y, Sahashi K, Rigo F, Hung G, Horev G, Bennett CF, Krainer AR (2011) Peripheral SMN restoration is essential for long-term rescue of a severe spinal muscular atrophy mouse model. Nature 478(7367):123–126. doi:10.1038/nature10485
34. Aartsma-Rus A, Bremmer-Bout M, Janson AA, den Dunnen JT, van Ommen GJ, van Deutekom JC (2002) Targeted exon skipping as a potential gene correction therapy for Duchenne muscular dystrophy. Neuromuscul Disord 12(Suppl 1):S71–77
35. Echigoya Y, Yokota T (2014) Skipping multiple exons of dystrophin transcripts using cocktail antisense oligonucleotides. Nucleic Acid Ther 24(1):57–68. doi:10.1089/nat.2013.0451
36. Yokota T, Duddy W, Echigoya Y, Kolski H (2012) Exon skipping for nonsense mutations in Duchenne muscular dystrophy: too many mutations, too few patients? Expert Opin Biol Ther 12(9):1141–1152. doi:10.1517/14712598.2012.693469
37. Aoki Y, Yokota T, Wood MJ (2013) Development of multiexon skipping antisense oligonucleotide therapy for Duchenne muscular dystrophy. Biomed Res Int 2013:402369. doi:10.1155/2013/402369
38. Yokota T, Duddy W, Partridge T (2007) Optimizing exon skipping therapies for DMD. Acta Myol 26(3):179–184
39. Pramono ZA, Takeshima Y, Alimsardjono H, Ishii A, Takeda S, Matsuo M (1996) Induction of exon skipping of the dystrophin transcript in lymphoblastoid cells by transfecting an antisense oligodeoxynucleotide complementary to an exon recognition sequence. Biochem Biophys Res Commun 226(2):445–449
40. Mann CJ, Honeyman K, Cheng AJ, Ly T, Lloyd F, Fletcher S, Morgan JE, Partridge TA, Wilton SD (2001) Antisense-induced exon skipping and synthesis of dystrophin in the mdx mouse. Proc Natl Acad Sci U S A 98(1):42–47
41. Lu QL, Rabinowitz A, Chen YC, Yokota T, Yin H, Alter J, Jadoon A, Bou-Gharios G, Partridge T (2005) Systemic delivery of antisense oligoribonucleotide restores dystrophin expression in body-wide skeletal muscles. Proc Natl Acad Sci U S A 102(1):198–203
42. Yokota T, Lu QL, Partridge T, Kobayashi M, Nakamura A, Takeda S, Hoffman E (2009) Efficacy of systemic morpholino exon-skipping in Duchenne dystrophy dogs. Ann Neurol 65(6):667–676. doi:10.1002/ana.21627

43. Yokota T, Hoffman E, Takeda S (2011) Antisense oligo-mediated multiple exon skipping in a dog model of Duchenne muscular dystrophy. Methods Mol Biol 709:299–312. doi:10.1007/978-1-61737-982-6_20
44. McCarter GC, Steinhardt RA (2000) Increased activity of calcium leak channels caused by proteolysis near sarcolemmal ruptures. J Membr Biol 176(2):169–174
45. Kamoshita S, Konishi Y, Segawa M, Fukuyama Y (1976) Congenital muscular dystrophy as a disease of the central nervous system. Arch Neurol 33(7):513–516
46. Kobayashi K, Nakahori Y, Miyake M, Matsumura K, Kondo-Iida E, Nomura Y, Segawa M, Yoshioka M, Saito K, Osawa M, Hamano K, Sakakihara Y, Nonaka I, Nakagome Y, Kanazawa I, Nakamura Y, Tokunaga K, Toda T (1998) An ancient retrotransposal insertion causes Fukuyama-type congenital muscular dystrophy. Nature 394(6691):388–392. doi:10.1038/28653
47. Hayashi YK, Ogawa M, Tagawa K, Noguchi S, Ishihara T, Nonaka I, Arahata K (2001) Selective deficiency of alpha-dystroglycan in Fukuyama-type congenital muscular dystrophy. Neurology 57(1):115–121
48. Michele DE, Barresi R, Kanagawa M, Saito F, Cohn RD, Satz JS, Dollar J, Nishino I, Kelley RI, Somer H, Straub V, Mathews KD, Moore SA, Campbell KP (2002) Post-translational disruption of dystroglycan-ligand interactions in congenital muscular dystrophies. Nature 418(6896): 417–422. doi:10.1038/nature00837
49. Guglieri M, Bushby K (2008) How to go about diagnosing and managing the limb-girdle muscular dystrophies. Neurol India 56(3):271–280
50. Illa I, Serrano-Munuera C, Gallardo E, Lasa A, Rojas-Garcia R, Palmer J, Gallano P, Baiget M, Matsuda C, Brown RH (2001) Distal anterior compartment myopathy: a dysferlin mutation causing a new muscular dystrophy phenotype. Ann Neurol 49(1):130–134
51. Liu J, Aoki M, Illa I, Wu C, Fardeau M, Angelini C, Serrano C, Urtizberea JA, Hentati F, Hamida MB, Bohlega S, Culper EJ, Amato AA, Bossie K, Oeltjen J, Bejaoui K, McKenna-Yasek D, Hosler BA, Schurr E, Arahata K, de Jong PJ, Brown RH Jr (1998) Dysferlin, a novel skeletal muscle gene, is mutated in Miyoshi myopathy and limb girdle muscular dystrophy. Nat Genet 20(1):31–36. doi:10.1038/1682
52. Matsuda C, Aoki M, Hayashi YK, Ho MF, Arahata K, Brown RH Jr (1999) Dysferlin is a surface membrane-associated protein that is absent in Miyoshi myopathy. Neurology 53(5): 1119–1122
53. Argov Z, Sadeh M, Mazor K, Soffer D, Kahana E, Eisenberg I, Mitrani-Rosenbaum S, Richard I, Beckmann J, Keers S, Bashir R, Bushby K, Rosenmann H (2000) Muscular dystrophy due to dysferlin deficiency in Libyan Jews. Clinical and genetic features. Brain 123(Pt 6):1229–1237
54. Bansal D, Miyake K, Vogel SS, Groh S, Chen CC, Williamson R, McNeil PL, Campbell KP (2003) Defective membrane repair in dysferlin-deficient muscular dystrophy. Nature 423(6936):168–172
55. Anderson LV, Davison K, Moss JA, Young C, Cullen MJ, Walsh J, Johnson MA, Bashir R, Britton S, Keers S, Argov Z, Mahjneh I, Fougerousse F, Beckmann JS, Bushby KM (1999) Dysferlin is a plasma membrane protein and is expressed early in human development. Hum Mol Genet 8(5):855–861
56. Aoki M, Liu J, Richard I, Bashir R, Britton S, Keers SM, Oeltjen J, Brown HE, Marchand S, Bourg N, Beley C, McKenna-Yasek D, Arahata K, Bohlega S, Cupler E, Illa I, Majneh I, Barohn RJ, Urtizberea JA, Fardeau M, Amato A, Angelini C, Bushby K, Beckmann JS, Brown RH Jr (2001) Genomic organization of the dysferlin gene and novel mutations in Miyoshi myopathy. Neurology 57(2):271–278
57. Sinnreich M, Therrien C, Karpati G (2006) Lariat branch point mutation in the dysferlin gene with mild limb-girdle muscular dystrophy. Neurology 66(7):1114–1116. doi:10.1212/01.wnl.0000204358.89303.81
58. Wein N, Avril A, Bartoli M, Beley C, Chaouch S, Laforet P, Behin A, Butler-Browne G, Mouly V, Krahn M, Garcia L, Levy N (2010) Efficient bypass of mutations in dysferlin deficient patient cells by antisense-induced exon skipping. Hum Mutat 31(2):136–142. doi:10.1002/humu.21160

59. Krahn MWN, Nguyen K, Vial C, Courrier S, Lostal W, Bartoli M, Labelle V, Leturcq F, Cau P, Richard I, Levy N (2007) Functional evaluation of a putative mini-dysferlin identified in a patient with moderate Miyoshi myopathy phenotype. Neuromuscul Disord 17(9):790–790. doi:10.1016/j.nmd.2007.06.102
60. Aartsma-Rus A, Singh KH, Fokkema IF, Ginjaar IB, van Ommen GJ, den Dunnen JT, van der Maarel SM (2010) Therapeutic exon skipping for dysferlinopathies? Eur J Hum Genet 18(8): 889–894. doi:10.1038/ejhg.2010.4
61. Harper P (2001) Myotonic dystrophy, 3rd edition: major problems in neurology series, No 37. W B Saunders, London
62. Harley HG, Brook JD, Rundle SA, Crow S, Reardon W, Buckler AJ, Harper PS, Housman DE, Shaw DJ (1992) Expansion of an unstable DNA region and phenotypic variation in myotonic dystrophy. Nature 355(6360):545–546. doi:10.1038/355545a0
63. Fugier C, Klein AF, Hammer C, Vassilopoulos S, Ivarsson Y, Toussaint A, Tosch V, Vignaud A, Ferry A, Messaddeq N, Kokunai Y, Tsuburaya R, de la Grange P, Dembele D, Francois V, Precigout G, Boulade-Ladame C, Hummel MC, Lopez de Munain A, Sergeant N, Laquerriere A, Thibault C, Deryckere F, Auboeuf D, Garcia L, Zimmermann P, Udd B, Schoser B, Takahashi MP, Nishino I, Bassez G, Laporte J, Furling D, Charlet-Berguerand N (2011) Misregulated alternative splicing of BIN1 is associated with T tubule alterations and muscle weakness in myotonic dystrophy. Nat Med 17(6):720–725. doi:10.1038/nm.2374
64. Koebis M, Ohsawa N, Kino Y, Sasagawa N, Nishino I, Ishiura S (2011) Alternative splicing of myomesin 1 gene is aberrantly regulated in myotonic dystrophy type 1. Genes Cells 16(9): 961–972. doi:10.1111/j.1365-2443.2011.01542.x
65. Ohsawa N, Koebis M, Suo S, Nishino I, Ishiura S (2011) Alternative splicing of PDLIM3/ALP, for alpha-actinin-associated LIM protein 3, is aberrant in persons with myotonic dystrophy. Biochem Biophys Res Commun 409(1):64–69. doi:10.1016/j.bbrc.2011.04.106
66. Philips AV, Timchenko LT, Cooper TA (1998) Disruption of splicing regulated by a CUG-binding protein in myotonic dystrophy. Science 280(5364):737–741
67. Ranum LP, Cooper TA (2006) RNA-mediated neuromuscular disorders. Annu Rev Neurosci 29:259–277. doi:10.1146/annurev.neuro.29.051605.113014
68. Savkur RS, Philips AV, Cooper TA (2001) Aberrant regulation of insulin receptor alternative splicing is associated with insulin resistance in myotonic dystrophy. Nat Genet 29(1):40–47. doi:10.1038/ng704
69. Charlet BN, Savkur RS, Singh G, Philips AV, Grice EA, Cooper TA (2002) Loss of the muscle-specific chloride channel in type 1 myotonic dystrophy due to misregulated alternative splicing. Mol Cell 10(1):45–53
70. Kanadia RN, Johnstone KA, Mankodi A, Lungu C, Thornton CA, Esson D, Timmers AM, Hauswirth WW, Swanson MS (2003) A muscleblind knockout model for myotonic dystrophy. Science 302(5652):1978–1980. doi:10.1126/science.1088583
71. Mankodi A, Takahashi MP, Jiang H, Beck CL, Bowers WJ, Moxley RT, Cannon SC, Thornton CA (2002) Expanded CUG repeats trigger aberrant splicing of ClC-1 chloride channel pre-mRNA and hyperexcitability of skeletal muscle in myotonic dystrophy. Mol Cell 10(1): 35–44
72. Mulders SA, van den Broek WJ, Wheeler TM, Croes HJ, van Kuik-Romeijn P, de Kimpe SJ, Furling D, Platenburg GJ, Gourdon G, Thornton CA, Wieringa B, Wansink DG (2009) Triplet-repeat oligonucleotide-mediated reversal of RNA toxicity in myotonic dystrophy. Proc Natl Acad Sci U S A 106(33):13915–13920. doi:10.1073/pnas.0905780106
73. Nakamori M, Gourdon G, Thornton CA (2011) Stabilization of expanded (CTG)*(CAG) repeats by antisense oligonucleotides. Mol Ther 19(12):2222–2227. doi:10.1038/mt.2011.191
74. Wheeler TM, Leger AJ, Pandey SK, MacLeod AR, Nakamori M, Cheng SH, Wentworth BM, Bennett CF, Thornton CA (2012) Targeting nuclear RNA for in vivo correction of myotonic dystrophy. Nature 488(7409):111–115. doi:10.1038/nature11362

75. Wheeler TM, Lueck JD, Swanson MS, Dirksen RT, Thornton CA (2007) Correction of ClC-1 splicing eliminates chloride channelopathy and myotonia in mouse models of myotonic dystrophy. J Clin Invest 117(12):3952–3957
76. Aartsma-Rus A, Fokkema I, Verschuuren J, Ginjaar I, van Deutekom J, van Ommen GJ, den Dunnen JT (2009) Theoretic applicability of antisense-mediated exon skipping for Duchenne muscular dystrophy mutations. Hum Mutat 30(3):293–299
77. Yokota T, Pistilli E, Duddy W, Nagaraju K (2007) Potential of oligonucleotide-mediated exon-skipping therapy for Duchenne muscular dystrophy. Expert Opin Biol Ther 7(6):831–842
78. Aartsma-Rus A, van Ommen GJ (2009) Less is more: therapeutic exon skipping for Duchenne muscular dystrophy. Lancet Neurol 8(10):873–875. doi:10.1016/S1474-4422(09)70229-7
79. Cirak S, Feng L, Anthony K, Arechavala-Gomeza V, Torelli S, Sewry C, Morgan JE, Muntoni F (2012) Restoration of the dystrophin-associated glycoprotein complex after exon skipping therapy in Duchenne muscular dystrophy. Mol Ther 20(2):462–467. doi:10.1038/mt.2011.248
80. Kinali M, Arechavala-Gomeza V, Feng L, Cirak S, Hunt D, Adkin C, Guglieri M, Ashton E, Abbs S, Nihoyannopoulos P, Garralda ME, Rutherford M, McCulley C, Popplewell L, Graham IR, Dickson G, Wood MJ, Wells DJ, Wilton SD, Kole R, Straub V, Bushby K, Sewry C, Morgan JE, Muntoni F (2009) Local restoration of dystrophin expression with the morpholino oligomer AVI-4658 in Duchenne muscular dystrophy: a single-blind, placebo-controlled, dose-escalation, proof-of-concept study. Lancet Neurol 8(10):918–928
81. Muntoni F, Bushby K, van Ommen G (2005) 128th ENMC international workshop on 'pre-clinical optimization and phase I/II clinical trials using antisense oligonucleotides in Duchenne muscular dystrophy' 22–24 October 2004, Naarden, The Netherlands. Neuromuscul Disord 15(6):450–457

Chapter 7
Toward Regenerative Medicine for Muscular Dystrophies

Lessons from Regeneration Processes

Akiyoshi Uezumi and So-ichiro Fukada

Abstract The US National Institutes of Health defines regenerative medicine as "the process of creating living, functional tissues to repair or replace tissue or organ function lost due to age, disease, damage, or congenital defects." In many cases, physiological regenerative processes give us multiple clues for creating new therapeutic methodologies. In skeletal muscle fields, the first attempt at regenerative medicine was transplantation of myoblasts into Duchenne muscular (DMD) patients in the early 1990s, but the clinical trials were not successful. At that time, not much was known about the regenerative process in skeletal muscle. However, due to the efforts of scientists and progress in technologies, many important discoveries have emerged. One is the study of muscle stem cells, named satellite cells, and another is identification of muscle-resident mesenchymal progenitors. In this chapter, we focus on satellite cells and mesenchymal progenitors and discuss the newest information concerning them to realize regenerative medicine.

Keywords Muscle satellite cell • Muscle-resident mesenchymal progenitors • Cell transplantation

7.1 Introduction

Skeletal muscle has great regenerative ability, which depends on muscle stem cells, also known as muscle satellite cells, and skeletal muscle differentiation is one of the best models for the study of cellular differentiation. Establishment of myogenic cell lines, discovery of myogenic transcription factors, and studies of developmental

A. Uezumi
Division for Therapies Against Intractable Diseases, Institute for Comprehensive Medical Science, Fujita Health University, Aichi, Japan

S.-i. Fukada (✉)
Laboratory of Molecular and Cellular Physiology, Graduate School of Pharmaceutical Sciences, Osaka University, 1-6 Yamada-oka, 565-0871 Suita, Osaka, Japan
e-mail: fukada@phs.osaka-u.ac.jp

S. Takeda et al. (eds.), *Translational Research in Muscular Dystrophy*,
DOI 10.1007/978-4-431-55678-7_7

myogenesis allow us to understand the outline of regenerative and myogenic differentiation processes. However, some fundamental issues remain to be elucidated. Among them, molecular regulation of satellite cells in both a steady homeostatic state and during regeneration is of great interest. In addition, in order to exploit the efficient regenerative potential of satellite cells, the contributions of non-myogenic cells are also considered essential. The representative type of non-myogenic cell is the hematopoietic cell, especially the macrophage, because a lack of macrophages results in a decreased number of proliferating myogenic cells and eventually leads to impaired regeneration with fibrosis [1]. In addition to macrophages, recent studies have shown the contribution of regulatory T cells to muscle regeneration [2]. Skeletal muscle-resident mesenchymal progenitors, which were originally identified as a source of both fibrosis and fat accumulation in muscle [3, 4], have attracted great attention for their vital roles in both undamaged muscle and muscle regeneration. Similarly, new factors in maintaining the homeostasis of skeletal muscle have been proposed recently, and a deeper understanding of them will lead to the development of new therapeutic approaches. We introduce satellite cell and mesenchymal progenitors on the basis of new findings that are closely related to the progression of muscular disorders, including muscular dystrophies, and the establishment of regenerative medicine for skeletal muscle.

7.2 Cellular Components of Skeletal Muscle

Well-recognized cellular components of skeletal muscle are myofibers, endothelial cells, nerve cells, hematopoietic cells, and satellite cells. The myofiber is multinuclear and the largest cell in the body, surrounded by the basal lamina and connected to bone via tendons. Except for myofibers, all other cells are mononuclear. When mononuclear cells derived from uninjured skeletal muscle are analyzed by FACS, endothelial cells account for 60–70 % of them. Endothelial cells are positive for both CD31 (PECAM-1) and Sca-1, but negative for CD45. Nerve cells innervate myofibers via neuromuscular junctions and are essential in skeletal muscle for locomotion. In uninjured muscle, only a few hematopoietic cells exist, but when muscles are damaged, abundant neutrophils appear and then infiltration by macrophages follows them [1]. Besides these myeloid lineage cells, the importance of lymphoid cells in the regeneration process is also reported. Recent studies showed that a special population of regulatory T ($CD4^+Foxp3^+$) cells controls muscle inflammation and promotes skeletal muscle repair [2].

The most indispensable type of mononuclear cell for muscle regeneration is the satellite cell, which is known as the physiological stem cell of skeletal muscle [5, 6]. Only satellite cells are found between the basal lamina and plasma membrane of myofibers [7]. Pax7, M-cadherin, calcitonin receptor, Syndecan4, HeyL, and Odz4/Ten-m4 are specifically expressed in satellite cells in skeletal muscle [8–14]. Besides satellite cells, many studies have reported other myogenic stems/progenitors, for example, bone marrow cells, side population (SP) cells, and muscle-resident interstitial cells, that can participate in generating myofibers [15–24]. However, their potentials for generating myofibers are limited. Therefore, they seem inadequate as cell sources for regenerative medicine. When Pax7-expressing cells (satellite cells) are conditionally depleted utilizing a CreER^{T2}-DTA (diphtheria toxin) system, skeletal muscle regeneration is almost completely inhibited [25, 26]. Therefore, these two studies confirmed the essential roles of satellite cells during skeletal muscle regeneration. On the other hand, an early response in muscle hypertrophy does not depend on satellite cells in a compensatory hypertrophy model mice [27], although satellite cells had been thought to be required for muscle hypertrophy based on the "myonuclear domain theory." This study implied that satellite cells do not contribute to an acute change of myofiber size. On the other hand, there is a decrease in myofiber size during the lifelong process known as sarcopenia, the age-related loss of muscle mass. Although the contribution of the loss of the satellite cell pool to the onset of sarcopenia remains to be elucidated, many investigations have demonstrated a decreased number of satellite cells and impaired muscle regeneration in aged animals [28, 29]. In order to reveal the mechanism of the decline in the satellite cell pool, we need to reveal the molecular mechanism for maintaining the satellite cell pool. Fortunately, recent studies are starting to uncover the mechanism, which is expected to lead to the development of an ideal cell source for regenerative medicine [30–32].

Several types of stem cells or progenitors in the interstitial space of muscle are reported. Among them, the mesenchymal progenitor was recently identified as the origin of fibrosis and adipogenesis [3, 4, 33]. Mesenchymal progenitors are positive for both PDGFRα and Sca-1 and negative for CD31, CD45, and satellite cell markers. In addition, they do not have myogenic potential; therefore, mesenchymal progenitors are a completely distinct population of satellite cells. Notably, although mesenchymal progenitors were originally identified as a cell contributing to a pathogenic condition, they likely promote successful regeneration as well [34]. The physiological roles of mesenchymal progenitors are largely unknown, but an elegant in vivo study implied that mesenchymal progenitors play potent roles in muscle repair [35]. Utilizing Tcf4-CreER^{T2} knock-in and DTA mice, Mathew et al. ablated Tcf4^{+} cells and found impaired muscle regeneration with premature satellite cell differentiation, depletion of the early pool of satellite cells, and smaller regenerated myofibers. The direct relationship between mesenchymal progenitors and Tcf4^{+} fibroblasts is not fully understood, but Tcf4^{+} fibroblasts express PDGFRα. Therefore, we can speculate that the roles of mesenchymal progenitors overlap with those of Tcf4^{+} fibroblasts in many aspects. In addition to their roles in the regenerative process, a supportive effect of mesenchymal progenitors on myofibers has been proposed, even in a steady condition [36]. Taken together, the mesenchymal progenitor, like the satellite cell, is becoming recognized as an essential type of cell in skeletal muscle. In order to utilize the full potential of muscle regeneration for the treatment of muscle disorders, we have to understand their roles in skeletal muscle biology. Below, we introduce recent research on both satellite cells and mesenchymal progenitors and discuss their functions in muscular dystrophies, sarcopenia, and cancer-induced loss of muscle mass (cancer cachexia).

7.2.1 Satellite Cells

There is no doubt that prior research on embryonic stem (ES) cells enabled the generation of iPS cells. If there were no established methodology for maintaining ES cells in an undifferentiated state, it would be impossible to generate iPS cells. In the same way, in order to expand satellite cells in vitro while maintaining their original ability, we have to elucidate the maintenance and self-renewal mechanisms of satellite cells in physiological events. In this part, we introduce a brief history of satellite cells and the key molecules for maintaining satellite cells.

7.2.1.1 Brief History of Satellite Cells

In 1961, Dr. Alexander Mauro first reported the existence of satellite cells in frog muscle [7]. Subsequently, satellite cells were discovered in mammalian skeletal muscle. The name is derived from its specific location. One side of a satellite cell is directly attached to a myofiber via cell-cell adhesion molecules such as M-cadherin, and the other side is attached to the basal lamina; therefore, satellite cells are located between the myofiber and basal lamina. Other types of cells are never found in this position. Before the satellite cell-expressing molecules were identified, electron microscopy was the only means to identify and observe satellite cells. However, identifying the proteins expressed in satellite cells and establishing methodologies (FACS analysis, single-myofiber culture, and so on) allow us to observe satellite cells more easily [11, 37–39].

A stem cell is defined as a cell having both differentiation and self-renewal potentials. In 2008, Sacco et al. transplanted a single satellite cell and demonstrated that the satellite cell has both potentials [6]. Although there are many reports indicating the existence of muscle stem cells besides satellite cells, as described above, many recent studies leave no doubt that the satellite cell is a physiological stem cell having both differentiation and self-renewal potentials [5, 25, 26, 40].

7.2.1.2 Maintenance Mechanism of Satellite Cells

Like other stem cells, satellite cells are maintained in an undifferentiated and quiescent state [41]. This state is considered essential for maintaining a satellite cell pool. In general, each tissue stem cell can be found in a specific location, called its niche, composed of certain types of cellular and extracellular matrix proteins. The satellite cell locates beneath the basal lamina and attaches to a myofiber; therefore, both of them together are thought to create the niche for satellite cells. In addition, Christov et al. reported that satellite cells exist in close proximity to endothelial cells [42]. Therefore, endothelial cells might also be a niche cell for maintaining satellite cells, like hematopoietic, neural, and spermatogonic stem cells [42–44].

Recent studies are starting to reveal the molecular mechanism for keeping satellite cells in an undifferentiated and quiescent state [31]. A report by Seale and colleagues was the first that showed a decreased number of satellite cells in genetically modified animals. They found expression of Pax7 in myogenic cells and discovered the loss of the satellite cell pool in Pax7 knockout mice [12]. Because Pax7 is specifically expressed in satellite cells in skeletal muscle, Pax7 has been the best molecule for identifying satellite cells in skeletal muscle. Importantly, the expression of Pax7 has been also confirmed in across species (human, rodent, avian). Although Lepper et al. had reported that the role of Pax7 in adult satellite cells was dispensable [45], two independent groups demonstrated that it was essential even in adult satellite cells [46, 47]. The discrepancy is likely due to the construct of Pax7-floxed mice [46].

What is the role of Pax7 in satellite cells? Taking the abovementioned studies together, Pax7 is involved in both the generation and maintenance of satellite cells. Originally Seale et al. proposed the specification of muscle satellite cells by Pax7 [48]. Relaix et al. showed the antiapoptotic roles of Pax7 in satellite cells [49]. In addition to those roles, McKinnell et al. indicated that Pax7 directly regulates Myf5 expression by association with the Wdr5-Ash2L-MLL2 histone methyltransferase complex that causes methylation of histone H3 lysine 4 [50]. The phenotype of Myf5-null mice [51] is much milder than that of Pax7-null mice; therefore, other targets of Pax7 might be also important for the specification and/or survival of satellite cells. Significantly, Pax7 was used for generating satellite cell-like cells from human iPS cells [52], demonstrating that Pax7 is one of the important discoveries in satellite cell biology that promotes the achievement of cell therapy.

Another molecule essential for regulating satellite cells in adult skeletal muscle is the Notch signaling pathway, which is an evolutionarily conserved intracellular signaling system. When Notch signaling is activated by its ligand (Dll1, Dll3, Dll4, Jag1, or Jag2), the intracellular domain of Notch is cleaved by a protease like γ-secretase and transported to the nucleus [53]. Then, the target genes are transcribed through interaction with Rbpj. Rbpj-dependent Notch signaling is known as canonical Notch signaling, and the representative target genes of canonical Notch signaling are the Hes (Hairy and enhancer of split) and Hesr (Hes related, also known as Hey/Herp/Hrt/Ghf/Gridlock) families of bHLH transcriptional repressor genes [54]. Using conditional ablation of Rbpj in Pax7-CreER^{T2} mice, two independent groups have indicated the essential roles of Rbpj for maintaining adult satellite cells in an undifferentiated and quiescent state [55, 56]. Intriguingly, when satellite cells in adult skeletal muscle lack Rbpj, they start to show precocious myogenic differentiation following protein expressions of MyoD and myogenin. They eventually fuse with myofibers and the satellite cell pool is diminished. When C2C12 cells or primary myoblasts are stimulated by Dll1 (Delta-like 1) or Dll4, Hesr1 and Hesr3 are upregulated [10, 57]. In addition, we observed premature differentiation and loss of satellite cell pools in Hesr1/3-double knockout mice [10]. Because each single knockout mouse did not show any significant defect in skeletal muscle including satellite cells, these results suggest that Hesr1 and Hesr3 have a redundant effect in maintaining satellite cells downstream of the canonical Notch signal [32].

Like Pax7, Notch signaling might contribute to the realization of cell therapy. Parker et al. compared the in vivo reconstitution potential of transplanted cells stimulated with Notch ligand and control cells and found that the former cells can engraft in vivo more actively than the latter [58]. The mechanism of Pax7 expression induction and the type of ligand/receptor for canonical Notch signaling in adult satellite cells have not been fully determined. Therefore, elucidation of these regulatory mechanisms will lead to the identification of the in vitro maintenance conditions for preparing cells for regenerative medicine.

Except for Pax7 and Notch-related genes knockout mice, decreased numbers of satellite cells are observed in some genetic knockout mice [59–63]. Most gene knockout mice show a loss of satellite cell pools at a relatively young age [31]. However, the phenotypes of Sprouty 1 (an inhibitor of receptor tyrosine kinase signaling) knockout mice are quite different. The loss of Sprouty 1 did not affect the number of satellite cells in uninjured muscle of young mice, but in aged mice (22 months), the satellite cell pool was diminished by half [64]. They also showed that this diminishment of satellite cells resulted from accelerated fibroblast growth factor (FGF) signaling. Therefore, maintenance genes can be divided to two categories: one is a gene for autonomous regulation, and the other is a gene affected by a change of environment. The elucidation of both mechanisms is important for the development of an ideal cell source for muscular disorders.

In addition to coding RNA, noncoding RNA is also essential for maintaining the satellite cell pool in uninjured muscle. Dicer is an enzyme for generating microRNA. When Dicer is conditionally and specifically deleted in adult satellite cells, they start to express proliferative markers and eventually undergo apoptosis [65]. Among quiescent stage-specific microRNA, Cheung et al. demonstrated that mir-489 is critical for a quiescent state of satellite cells through suppressing its target gene, Dek. Notably, mir-489 is located in the intron of the calcitonin receptor expressed specifically in quiescent satellite cells in skeletal muscle [9]. The expressions of both mir-489 and calcitonin receptor are downregulated after activation of satellite cells. During regeneration, re-expression of calcitonin receptors is restricted to the area where regeneration is mostly completed [9]. Although the physiological role of calcitonin receptor is unknown, the common expression mechanism of both mir-489 and calcitonin receptor might be extremely important to unravel the mechanism for establishment of quiescent satellite cells during developmental and regenerative processes.

7.2.1.3 Self-Renewal Mechanism of Satellite Cells

As described above, adult satellite cells are maintained in a dormant and undifferentiated state, but when skeletal muscle is injured, these cells start to enter an activated state. Before proliferating, they begin to express MyoD protein and then enter the cell cycle. Proliferating satellite cells that express both Pax7 and MyoD are called myoblasts. When they become more committed to myogenic differentiation, they start to express myogenin and lose Pax7. Myogenin-expressing cells that can fuse with each other or myotubes and make multinucleated myotubes are called myocytes. After myotubes mature, myofibers are innervated and rebuilt. During the regeneration processes, satellite cells produce self-renewed satellite cells that are indispensable due to their repeated regenerative potentials. The critical mechanism of satellite cell self-renewal is unknown, but two basic models have been proposed. Using cultured single myofibers, Zammit et al. indicated that almost all satellite cells become Pax7^{+}MyoD^{+} cells, and then a part of them return to a Pax7^{+}MyoD^{-} state. On the other hand, Kuang et al. found that satellite cells can be divided into two populations based on YFP expression driven by Myf5-Cre and that the Pax7^{+}Myf5^{-}(YFP^{-}) population has more stem cell-like characteristics than the Pax7^{+}Myf5^{+}(YFP^{+}) population. Intriguingly, when Pax7^{+}Myf5^{-} cells divide on a plane, most cells generated are Pax7^{+}Myf5^{-} cells. On the other hand, when Pax7^{+}Myf5^{-} cells do apical-basal division, both Pax7^{+}Myf5^{-} and Pax7^{+}Myf5^{+} cells (asymmetric division) are generated. However, these cells were observed in regenerating myotubes/myofibers having central nuclei. Furthermore, Wnt7s promote the number of Pax7^{+}Myf5^{-} cells [66], and the effect of Wnt7a was accelerated by fibronectin, which is specifically expressed during myotube/myofiber formation [67]. Therefore, there is a possibility that symmetric and asymmetric division in Pax7^{+}Myf5^{-} might occur after several cell divisions of Pax7^{+}MyoD^{+} cells. The self-renewal mechanism of satellite cells is one of the important issues to be explained.

7.2.2 *Mesenchymal Progenitors*

In 2010, we identified muscle-resident mesenchymal progenitors [3]. Originally, mesenchymal progenitors were identified as cells contributing to pathological changes in skeletal muscle, but, at the same time, we speculated on their support functions in muscle repair because many mesenchymal progenitors proliferate actively even during a successful regeneration process. Intriguingly, recent studies revealed their support functions in muscle regeneration and homeostasis. In this part, we introduce several pathophysiological roles of mesenchymal progenitors on the basis of recent reports.

7.2.2.1 Mesenchymal Progenitors as Villains

Fibrosis is a hallmark of pathological conditions with impaired regeneration in many tissues. In skeletal muscle, accumulation of adipocytes is also observed in progressed muscular dystrophy patients. In order to identify the origin of the cell populations involved in fat accumulation and fibrosis in skeletal muscle, we performed comprehensive FACS-based cell analyses. Although satellite cells were considered the original source of fibrosis and adipogenesis, we found that a non-satellite cell population exclusively contributed to both fat accumulation and fibrosis in skeletal muscle, and this cell population specifically expressed PDGFRα [3, 4]. Besides the potentials to produce adipocytes and fibrogenic cells, they can also differentiate into osteogenic cells [3, 68]. Therefore, we called these cells mesenchymal progenitors.

Our study clearly demonstrated that only PDGFRα$^+$ mesenchymal progenitors differentiate into adipocytes and form ectopic fat tissue in skeletal muscle [3]. This conflicts with the adipogenic potentials of satellite cells proposed by experiments using a myogenic cell line and single isolated myofiber. Myogenic cell lines are extremely useful for investigation of many aspects of myogenic differentiation, but they do not reflect some aspects of characteristics of in vivo satellite cells. Isolated single myofibers are also widely used for studies of satellite cell biology, but we have to pay attention to the risk of contamination by non-satellite cells (including mesenchymal progenitors) attached to the myofiber. Satellite cells were also proposed as a potent cellular source of collagen-producing cells by a study using a myogenic cell line [69]. In fact, fibrosis-related genes are detected even in highly purified primary myogenic cells, but their expression levels in mesenchymal progenitors are much higher than those of myoblasts, and myogenic cells do not contribute to or differentiate into collagen-producing cells in the dystrophic condition [4]. Brack et al. showed that satellite cells in aged mice transdifferentiate into fibroblastic cells in response to canonical Wnt signaling [28]. Therefore, we cannot exclude the potential of satellite cells to become fibroblastic cells. However, given their highly fibrogenic nature, it seems highly plausible that mesenchymal progenitors are the best candidate for fibrosis-initiating cells in skeletal muscle. In addition, we could identify a human counterpart to these progenitors by the expression of PDGFRα [34, 70]. Therefore, their pathological relevance to muscular disorders is further convinced. Taken together, the mesenchymal progenitor is the most potent origin of adipogenesis and fibrosis in skeletal muscle.

7.2.2.2 Mesenchymal Progenitors and Pericytes

Mesenchymal progenitors reside in the muscle interstitium, and thus, their location is also distinct from that of satellite cells. Mesenchymal progenitors are more frequently observed in the perimysium than in the endomysium, particularly in the perivascular space, but they are distinct from pericytes because they locate outside the vessel wall and basement membrane of capillaries [3]. The definition of a pericyte is based exclusively on its anatomic location, where it is bounded by a common basement membrane with endothelial cells [71, 72]; there is no specific pericyte marker. Mesenchymal progenitors account for about 5–10 % of whole mononucleated cells isolated from skeletal muscle [3], but skeletal muscle is known to have an extremely low percentage of pericytes. In skeletal muscle, there is only one pericyte per 100 endothelial cells [71, 73]. This is quite a contrast to pericyte-rich tissues such as the retina or central nervous system, where the pericyte to endothelial cell ratio is 1:1 [71, 73]. Because endothelial cells account for 60–70 %

of total mononuclear cells in skeletal muscle, as described earlier, pericytes should constitute only 0.7 % of all mononuclear cells at most. Although pericytes have been reported to possess myogenic differentiative potential [74], mesenchymal progenitors cannot differentiate into myogenic cells. Where do mesenchymal progenitors arise developmentally? We do not know, but we are sure that they do not originate in bone marrow and that they reside in skeletal muscle before the beginning of inflammation.

7.2.2.3 Mesenchymal Progenitors and Fibroblasts

The morphology of mesenchymal progenitors is similar to that of fibroblasts, and there is no marker that distinguishes fibroblasts and mesenchymal progenitors. Unlike fibroblasts, mesenchymal progenitors have the potential to differentiate into mesenchymal lineage cells including adipocytes, chondrocytes, and osteoblasts. Therefore, the ability to differentiate is the only way to characterize mesenchymal progenitors. Sudo et al. showed that primary fibroblasts derived from various human tissues can differentiate into at least one mesenchymal lineage cell [75], and mesenchymal progenitors and so-called fibroblasts have much more similarity than previously recognized [76]. Therefore, many tissues seem to have their own tissue-resident mesenchymal progenitors which have been considered as fibroblasts.

7.3 Muscular Dystrophy

Duchenne muscular dystrophy (DMD) is a representative inherited muscular disorder that is caused by a mutation in the *DYSTROPHIN* genes [77]. Besides DMD, more than 30 different types and subtypes of muscular dystrophies are known, and most of them lack cell structure-related molecules for sustaining the cell membrane stability of myofibers. DMD patients exhibit progressive muscle weakness, and eventually myofibers are replaced by fibrosis and adipocytes. Although the mechanism of progressive muscle weakness is still unknown, it has been believed that a decline of the ability of muscle regenerative potential results in an increase in the size of pathogenic areas. Therefore, the loss of satellite cell numbers and function is considered to be one reason why many muscular dystrophies exhibit progressive symptoms. In this section, we introduce the relationship between satellite cells and the progression of muscular dystrophies. In addition, we discuss mesenchymal progenitors as therapeutic targets for muscular disorders.

7.3.1 Satellite Cells and Progression of Muscular Dystrophies

In 2010, we found impairment of the repeated regenerative ability in the DBA/2, but not C57BL/6, BALB/c, and C3H/HeN strains, and showed that *mdx* mice having a DBA/2 background exhibit much severe dystrophic phenotypes than C57BL/10-*mdx*, a conventional DMD model mice [78]. The proliferative ability of DBA/2-derived satellite cells is inferior to that of C57BL/6 satellite cells. This phenomenon is not limited to *mdx* mice. Heydemann also observed sever phenotypes in gamma sarcoglycan-deficient mice having a DBA/2 strain background compared to 129SV/J and C57BL/6 J strain mice [79]. The same group employed an unbiased mapping approach and identified a latent TGF-beta-binding protein 4 gene (Ltbp4) as one explanation of the phenotype of DBA/2 J background mice [80]. Ltbp is considered to be a negative factor for TGF-β activity; therefore, accelerated TGF-β signaling likely contributes to the pathological progression in DBA/2-J dystrophic mice. In fact, mutations of LTBP4 are found in humans and result in increased TGF-β activity in cultured human DMD patient-derived fibroblasts [81]. Until now, the phenotype of DAB/2 satellite cells and LTBP4 was unclear because both anti- and pro-proliferative effects of TGF-β signaling have been reported during proliferation of myogenic cells [82]. If we can determine the gene responsible for the low repeated regenerative potential in DBA/2 satellite cells, the progression of muscular dystrophies might be controlled.

Lamin A/C and emerin are known as causal genes of autosomal-Emery-Dreifuss muscular dystrophy (A-EDMD) [83] and X-EDMD [84], respectively. Notably, both molecules are expressed in quiescent satellite cells. In addition, our microarray analyses reveal that satellite cells express *dystroglycan* and *dystrophin* genes [9]. The roles of lamin A/C and emerin in satellite cells are still unknown, but some causative genes of muscular dystrophy may affect the function and survival of satellite cells directly, which might determine the severity of symptoms [85]. The relationship between the causative genes and satellite cell biology is one of the important issues in understanding each muscular dystrophy and development of therapeutic approaches.

7.3.2 Mesenchymal Progenitors as Therapeutic Target

Some studies have indicated or implied that PDGFRα^{+} mesenchymal progenitors are also positive for Sca-1, ADAM12, Tcf4, CD90, and Tie2 [3, 86, 87]. Among them, PDGFRα is not only a specific marker for mesenchymal progenitors but also can be a molecular target for many disorders including muscular dystrophy. Olson and Soriano generated constitutively active PDGFRα mutant mice and observed systemic fibrosis including skeletal muscle in these mice [88]. We showed that PDGF-AA (one ligand of PDGFRα) promotes cell proliferation and expression of fibrosis-related genes in PDGFRα^+ mesenchymal progenitors [4]. Furthermore, we showed that a tryrosine kinase inhibitor, imatinib, inhibits the effect of PDGF-AA on PDGFRα^+ mesenchymal progenitors, and we and others indicated that imatinib ameliorates dystrophic symptoms in the DMD model mice [89–91].

Besides imatinib, many small molecules ameliorate the dystrophic symptoms of *mdx* mice. Intriguingly, mesenchymal progenitors might be a direct target of some of them. Losartan is a blocker of the angiotensin II type I receptor and is widely used for treatment of hypertension. Cohn et al. showed that losartan improves skeletal muscle regeneration in *mdx* and fibrillin-null mice [92]. Fibrillin-1 is a structural component of extracellular matrix microfibrils that is known to be a negative regulator of TGF-β activation and signaling. The effect of losartan is attributed to reduced expression of thrombospondin-1 (TSP-1), which is a downstream target of angiotensin II and has the potential to activate latent TGF-β. In our analyses, mesenchymal progenitors also express TSP-1, and TGF-β induces the expression of fibrosis-related genes (Col1a1, Col3a1, a-SMA, CTNF) in mesenchymal progenitors. Therefore, mesenchymal progenitors might be a direct target of losartan in the dystrophic condition.

Histone deacetylase (HDAC) is a component of the epigenetic regulator. Trichostatin A (TSA) is a chemical compound that selectively inhibits mammalian classes I and II but not class III HDACs. Iezzi et al demonstrated that the expression of follistatin was upregulated in TSA-treated C2C12 cells compared with control C2C12 cells [93]. Follistatin inhibits myostatin, a well-known negative regulator of muscle mass, because myostatin-null mice, cows, and humans exhibit a noticeable increase in skeletal muscle mass. Follistatin was induced by TSA and then promoted C2C12 recruitment and fusion. The same group also showed that TSA induced follistatin in myotubes and ameliorated dystrophic symptoms of *mdx* mice in vivo [94]. Importantly, TSA enhances the ability of mesenchymal progenitors to promote myogenic activity of myoblasts in vitro and in vivo. Mesenchymal progenitors express a much higher level of follistatin than myogenic cells, and the positive effect of mesenchymal progenitors on myogenesis is mediated by follistatin [95]. Therefore, the beneficial effect of an HDAC inhibitor on muscular dystrophy is largely mediated by mesenchymal progenitors. Taken together, PDGFRα^+ mesenchymal progenitors are or will be potent direct targets for the treatment of muscle diseases.

Muscle CD31$^-$CD45$^-$ SP cells [24] are only a small portion of the cells present during regeneration, but they have characteristics similar to those of mesenchymal progenitors; therefore, we consider that muscle CD31$^-$CD45$^-$ SP cells are a type of mesenchymal progenitor. In 2008, we showed that co-transplantation of satellite cells and muscle CD31$^-$CD45$^-$ SP cells results in an increased number of satellite cell-derived myofibers in vivo [96]. Mozzetta et al. reported that co-transplantation of satellite cells with mesenchymal progenitors resulted in an increased number of donor-derived myofibers [95]; therefore, co-transplantation of mesenchymal progenitors might be a promising cell therapy to improve the results of satellite cell transplantation. However, when mesenchymal progenitors are transplanted into a severely dystrophic environment, they differentiate into adipocytes or collagen-producing cells. Therefore, one of the most important issues is the mechanism that controls the behavior of mesenchymal progenitors and affects the myogenic reconstitution of satellite cells. Regulation of the fate of mesenchymal progenitors will be a promising therapeutic strategy to treat muscle dystrophy.

7.4 Homeostasis

As described above, satellite cells are essential for skeletal muscle regeneration. Under conditions of repeated damage like muscular dystrophy, satellite cells undergo repeated proliferation, which is considered to be one reason why some muscular dystrophy patients show progressive symptoms. Thus, there is no doubt that satellite cells are indispensable for sustaining muscle mass and power in conditions in which there is apparent muscle damage. However, the contribution of satellite cells to maintaining muscle mass in a non-injured condition is still controversial. In this section, we discuss the contribution of satellite cells to a steady condition. In addition, the potent roles of mesenchymal progenitors in maintaining muscle mass are described on the basis of recent research.

7.4.1 Contribution of Satellite Cells to Steady Condition

Age-related alterations are observed in many organs and tissues. Skeletal muscle also shows such changes. The age-related loss of skeletal mass is known as sarcopenia, which will become a social problem due to the increasing proportion of aged people. Sarcopenia patients exhibit two characteristic alterations in skeletal muscle. One is the decreased volume of each myofiber, which is referred to atrophy. The other is a decline in the number of myofibers. The physiological capacity for generating new myofibers is limited in satellite cells; therefore, many researchers have considered the relationship between satellite cells and sarcopenia. In fact, many studies have shown a decrease in the number of satellite cells in aged animals and humans. However, many factors seem to be related to the onset of sarcopenia, for example, the nervous system, hormone levels, and availability of nutrients. White et al. estimated that adult satellite cells proliferate once in 51 days [97]. Like cardiomyocytes, myofibers might survive throughout the lifetime if they are not damaged. In this case, satellite cells are not needed to generate new skeletal muscle. Until now, whether the loss of satellite cell results from or causes a decreased number of myofibers is not unclear. The long-term analyses of satellite cell-depleted mice like Pax7-CreER^{T2}::DTA mice will answer this query.

7.4.2 Contribution of Mesenchymal Progenitors to Steady Condition

As a mechanism for sustaining skeletal muscle mass, a new concept has emerged. Roberts et al. demonstrated the essential roles of fibroblast activation protein-α (FAP)-expressing stromal cells in the homeostasis of skeletal muscle by ablating them [36]. Both FAP^+ cells and mesenchymal progenitors express PDGFRα and are localized to the interstitial spaces of muscle. Therefore, FAP^+ stromal cells appear to be almost identical to mesenchymal progenitors. Intriguingly, FAP^+ cell-depleted mice exhibited a loss of skeletal muscle mass, followed by a persistent decrease in follistatin and laminin α2 expression and transitory induction of two muscle-specific ubiquitin ligases, atrogin-1 and MuRF1. Laminin α2 is a component of the basal lamina of myofibers, and mutation in the human *LAMININ α2* gene leads to congenital muscular dystrophy. Although the expression of laminin α2 had been believed to be restricted to myogenic cells, including myofibers, in skeletal muscle, we previously showed that $CD90^+$ interstitial cells (which largely overlap with mesenchymal progenitors) also express laminin α2 protein [86]. Therefore, there are two possible explanations for the decrease in laminin α2 expression in FAP^+ cell-depleted mice. One possibility is that decreased expression of laminin α2 may result directly from a depletion of mesenchymal progenitors. The other is that mesenchymal progenitors may provide factor(s) that sustain the expression of laminin α2 in myofibers and that such factor(s) might be diminished by mesenchymal progenitor ablation. Thus, mesenchymal progenitors may be a vital cellular component in maintaining muscle fibers, even in a steady homeostatic condition [98].

7.5 Cancer Cachexia

Cancer cachexia is a wasting syndrome accompanying the loss of body weight, fatigue, and anorexia. A decrease beyond 5 % of body weight in 12 months or less can be defined as cachexia. Although causative factors for skeletal muscle loss in cancer cachexia patients remain largely unknown, unusual behaviors of both satellite cells and mesenchymal progenitors might be involved in the onset or progress of the loss of muscle weight. Acharyya et al. found fragility of the muscle fiber plasma membrane in cachectic mice and showed that dystrophin-glycoprotein complex dysfunction can cause membrane abnormalities [99]. Myofibers are considered an important cellular component for maintaining the satellite cell pool and therefore might affect the behavior of satellite cells. In fact, Penna et al. found an increased number of satellite cells in a cancer cachexia model mouse [100]. In addition, He et al. found that Pax7 was overexpressed in two types of tumor-bearing mice (mouse models of cancer cachexia) and that non-myogenic cells become $Pax7^+$ cells in the environment of cancer cachexia [101]. The $Pax7^+$ cells also expressed PDGFRα and Sca-1 cells, which were derived from non-Pax7 expressing cells; therefore, the fates of mesenchymal progenitors are altered by cancer cachexia-inducing factors. Intriguingly, Roberts et al. showed that FAP-dependent bioluminescence was decreased in cachectic mice [36]. As described above, diminishment of mesenchymal progenitor numbers may lead to a decrease in muscle mass. Therefore, some cachectic phenomena likely result from the dysfunction of mesenchymal progenitors and satellite cells.

7.6 Prospective

Satellite cells show the highest capacity for myofiber reconstitution. This is not surprising because they function as physiological stem cells during regeneration. However, it is quite difficult to prepare large enough numbers of them for cell therapy. Therefore, we have to expand them in vitro without losing their bona fide potential. In vivo, they are maintained without loss of their capacity during steady and regenerative processes, which is the maintenance mechanism of satellite cells. As described, canonical Notch signaling is one candidate signaling pathway that makes it possible to expand satellite cells while keeping their original potentials, and canonical Notch signaling is essential for maintaining satellite cells. Thus, deep understanding of the physiological mechanisms of satellite cells will lead to successful expansion of an ideal myogenic cell source.

Another cell source for cell therapy is ES/iPS-derived myogenic cells. In this case as well, the molecular mechanisms of satellite cells offer important clues for generation of ES/iPS-derived myogenic cells. Studies of satellite cell biology will continue to provide valuable information to allow the generation of a cell source. On the one hand, mesenchymal progenitors cannot produce myogenic cells. On the other, as described above, they are becoming a bona fide target cell for treatment of muscle dystrophy and other muscle disorders. In addition, they appear to have a promotive effect on regeneration processes. Therefore, their support function may be useful for the expansion of satellite cells or ES/iPS-derived myogenic cells in vitro for effective cell therapy. Furthermore, controlling the properties of mesenchymal progenitors in vivo will be a promising therapeutic strategy to treat muscle dystrophy.

Acknowledgment We thank Katherine Ono for comments on the manuscript. S. F. was supported by JSPS KAKENHI grant, Grants-in-Aid for Young Scientists (A) (25702044), Intramural Research Grant (22-5 and 25-5) for Neurological and Psychiatric Disorders of NCNP. A.U. was supported by JSPS KAKENHI grant (24659687), Kato Memorial Bioscience Foundation, ONO Medical Research Foundation, and The Nakatomi Foundation. The authors indicate no potential conflicts of interest. Both S. F. and A.U. belong to "The Research Center Network for Realization of Regenerative Medicine" of the Japan Science and Technology Agency (JST).

References

1. Segawa M, Fukada S, Yamamoto Y, Yahagi H, Kanematsu M, Sato M, Ito T, Uezumi A, Hayashi S, Miyagoe-Suzuki Y et al (2008) Suppression of macrophage functions impairs skeletal muscle regeneration with severe fibrosis. Exp Cell Res 314:3232–3244
2. Burzyn D, Kuswanto W, Kolodin D, Shadrach JL, Cerletti M, Jang Y, Sefik E, Tan TG, Wagers AJ, Benoist C et al (2013) A special population of regulatory T cells potentiates muscle repair. Cell 155:1282–1295
3. Uezumi A, Fukada S, Yamamoto N, Takeda S, Tsuchida K (2010) Mesenchymal progenitors distinct from satellite cells contribute to ectopic fat cell formation in skeletal muscle. Nat Cell Biol 12:143–152
4. Uezumi A, Ito T, Morikawa D, Shimizu N, Yoneda T, Segawa M, Yamaguchi M, Ogawa R, Matev MM, Miyagoe-Suzuki Y et al (2011) Fibrosis and adipogenesis originate from a common mesenchymal progenitor in skeletal muscle. J Cell Sci 124:3654–3664
5. Collins CA, Olsen I, Zammit PS, Heslop L, Petrie A, Partridge TA, Morgan JE (2005) Stem cell function, self-renewal, and behavioral heterogeneity of cells from the adult muscle satellite cell niche. Cell 122:289–301
6. Sacco A, Doyonnas R, Kraft P, Vitorovic S, Blau HM (2008) Self-renewal and expansion of single transplanted muscle stem cells. Nature 456:502–506
7. Mauro A (1961) Satellite cell of skeletal muscle fibers. J Biophys Biochem Cytol 9:493–495
8. Cornelison DD, Filla MS, Stanley HM, Rapraeger AC, Olwin BB (2001) Syndecan-3 and syndecan-4 specifically mark skeletal muscle satellite cells and are implicated in satellite cell maintenance and muscle regeneration. Dev Biol 239:79–94
9. Fukada S, Uezumi A, Ikemoto M, Masuda S, Segawa M, Tanimura N, Yamamoto H, Miyagoe-Suzuki Y, Takeda S (2007) Molecular signature of quiescent satellite cells in adult skeletal muscle. Stem Cells 25:2448–2459
10. Fukada S, Yamaguchi M, Kokubo H, Ogawa R, Uezumi A, Yoneda T, Matev MM, Motohashi N, Ito T, Zolkiewska A et al (2011) Hesr1 and Hesr3 are essential to generate undifferentiated quiescent satellite cells and to maintain satellite cell numbers. Development 138:4609–4619
11. Irintchev A, Zeschnigk M, Starzinski-Powitz A, Wernig A (1994) Expression pattern of M-cadherin in normal, denervated, and regenerating mouse muscles. Dev Dyn 199:326–337
12. Seale P, Sabourin LA, Girgis-Gabardo A, Mansouri A, Gruss P, Rudnicki MA (2000) Pax7 is required for the specification of myogenic satellite cells. Cell 102:777–786
13. Yamaguchi M, Ogawa R, Watanabe Y, Uezumi A, Miyagoe-Suzuki Y, Tsujikawa K, Yamamoto H, Takeda S, Fukada S (2012) Calcitonin receptor and Odz4 are differently expressed in Pax7-positive cells during skeletal muscle regeneration. J Mol Histol 43: 581–587
14. Yin H, Price F, Rudnicki MA (2013) Satellite cells and the muscle stem cell niche. Physiol Rev 93:23–67
15. Asakura A, Rudnicki MA (2002) Side population cells from diverse adult tissues are capable of in vitro hematopoietic differentiation. Exp Hematol 30:1339–1345
16. Ferrari G, Cusella-De Angelis G, Coletta M, Paolucci E, Stornaiuolo A, Cossu G, Mavilio F (1998) Muscle regeneration by bone marrow-derived myogenic progenitors. Science 279: 1528–1530
17. Fukada S, Miyagoe-Suzuki Y, Tsukihara H, Yuasa K, Higuchi S, Ono S, Tsujikawa K, Takeda S, Yamamoto H (2002) Muscle regeneration by reconstitution with bone marrow or fetal liver cells from green fluorescent protein-gene transgenic mice. J Cell Sci 115: 1285–1293
18. Gussoni E, Soneoka Y, Strickland CD, Buzney EA, Khan MK, Flint AF, Kunkel LM, Mulligan RC (1999) Dystrophin expression in the mdx mouse restored by stem cell transplantation. Nature 401:390–394

19. LaBarge MA, Blau HM (2002) Biological progression from adult bone marrow to mononucleate muscle stem cell to multinucleate muscle fiber in response to injury. Cell 111:589–601
20. Mitchell KJ, Pannerec A, Cadot B, Parlakian A, Besson V, Gomes ER, Marazzi G, Sassoon DA (2010) Identification and characterization of a non-satellite cell muscle resident progenitor during postnatal development. Nat Cell Biol 12:257–266
21. Ojima K, Uezumi A, Miyoshi H, Masuda S, Morita Y, Fukase A, Hattori A, Nakauchi H, Miyagoe-Suzuki Y, Takeda S (2004) Mac-1(low) early myeloid cells in the bone marrow-derived SP fraction migrate into injured skeletal muscle and participate in muscle regeneration. Biochem Biophys Res Commun 321:1050–1061
22. Polesskaya A, Seale P, Rudnicki MA (2003) Wnt signaling induces the myogenic specification of resident CD45+ adult stem cells during muscle regeneration. Cell 113:841–852
23. Tamaki T, Akatsuka A, Ando K, Nakamura Y, Matsuzawa H, Hotta T, Roy RR, Edgerton VR (2002) Identification of myogenic-endothelial progenitor cells in the interstitial spaces of skeletal muscle. J Cell Biol 157:571–577
24. Uezumi A, Ojima K, Fukada S, Ikemoto M, Masuda S, Miyagoe-Suzuki Y, Takeda S (2006) Functional heterogeneity of side population cells in skeletal muscle. Biochem Biophys Res Commun 341:864–873
25. Lepper C, Partridge TA, Fan CM (2011) An absolute requirement for Pax7-positive satellite cells in acute injury-induced skeletal muscle regeneration. Development 138:3639–3646
26. Sambasivan R, Yao R, Kissenpfennig A, Van Wittenberghe L, Paldi A, Gayraud-Morel B, Guenou H, Malissen B, Tajbakhsh S, Galy A (2011) Pax7-expressing satellite cells are indispensable for adult skeletal muscle regeneration. Development 138:3647–3656
27. McCarthy JJ, Mula J, Miyazaki M, Erfani R, Garrison K, Farooqui AB, Srikuea R, Lawson BA, Grimes B, Keller C et al (2011) Effective fiber hypertrophy in satellite cell-depleted skeletal muscle. Development 138:3657–3666
28. Brack AS, Conboy MJ, Roy S, Lee M, Kuo CJ, Keller C, Rando TA (2007) Increased Wnt signaling during aging alters muscle stem cell fate and increases fibrosis. Science 317: 807–810
29. Conboy IM, Conboy MJ, Smythe GM, Rando TA (2003) Notch-mediated restoration of regenerative potential to aged muscle. Science 302:1575–1577
30. Cheung TH, Rando TA (2013) Molecular regulation of stem cell quiescence. Nat Rev Mol Cell Biol 14:329–340
31. Fukada S, Ma Y, Ohtani T, Watanabe Y, Murakami S, Yamaguchi M (2013) Isolation, characterization, and molecular regulation of muscle stem cells. Front Physiol 4:317
32. Yamaguchi M, Fukada S (2013) Regulation of muscle stem cell quiescent and undifferentiated state: roles of Hesr1 and Hesr3 genes. In: Hayat MA (ed) Tumor dormancy, quiescence, and senescence, vol 1. Springer, Dordrecht, pp 107–116
33. Joe AW, Yi L, Natarajan A, Le Grand F, So L, Wang J, Rudnicki MA, Rossi FM (2010) Muscle injury activates resident fibro/adipogenic progenitors that facilitate myogenesis. Nat Cell Biol 12:153–163
34. Uezumi A, Ikemoto-Uezumi M, Tsuchida K (2014) Roles of nonmyogenic mesenchymal progenitors in pathogenesis and regeneration of skeletal muscle. Front Physiol 5:68
35. Mathew SJ, Hansen JM, Merrell AJ, Murphy MM, Lawson JA, Hutcheson DA, Hansen MS, Angus-Hill M, Kardon G (2011) Connective tissue fibroblasts and Tcf4 regulate myogenesis. Development 138:371–384
36. Roberts EW, Deonarine A, Jones JO, Denton AE, Feig C, Lyons SK, Espeli M, Kraman M, McKenna B, Wells RJ et al (2013) Depletion of stromal cells expressing fibroblast activation protein-alpha from skeletal muscle and bone marrow results in cachexia and anemia. J Exp Med 210:1137–1151
37. Fukada S, Higuchi S, Segawa M, Koda K, Yamamoto Y, Tsujikawa K, Kohama Y, Uezumi A, Imamura M, Miyagoe-Suzuki Y et al (2004) Purification and cell-surface marker characterization of quiescent satellite cells from murine skeletal muscle by a novel monoclonal antibody. Exp Cell Res 296:245–255

38. Montarras D, Morgan J, Collins C, Relaix F, Zaffran S, Cumano A, Partridge T, Buckingham M (2005) Direct isolation of satellite cells for skeletal muscle regeneration. Science 309: 2064–2067
39. Rosenblatt JD, Lunt AI, Parry DJ, Partridge TA (1995) Culturing satellite cells from living single muscle fiber explants. In Vitro Cell Dev Biol Anim 31:773–779
40. Shea KL, Xiang W, LaPorta VS, Licht JD, Keller C, Basson MA, Brack AS (2010) Sprouty1 regulates reversible quiescence of a self-renewing adult muscle stem cell pool during regeneration. Cell Stem Cell 6:117–129
41. Schultz E, Gibson MC, Champion T (1978) Satellite cells are mitotically quiescent in mature mouse muscle: an EM and radioautographic study. J Exp Zool 206:451–456
42. Christov C, Chretien F, Abou-Khalil R, Bassez G, Vallet G, Authier FJ, Bassaglia Y, Shinin V, Tajbakhsh S, Chazaud B et al (2007) Muscle satellite cells and endothelial cells: close neighbors and privileged partners. Mol Biol Cell 18:1397–1409
43. Tavazoie M, Van der Veken L, Silva-Vargas V, Louissaint M, Colonna L, Zaidi B, Garcia-Verdugo JM, Doetsch F (2008) A specialized vascular niche for adult neural stem cells. Cell Stem Cell 3:279–288
44. Yoshida S, Sukeno M, Nabeshima Y (2007) A vasculature-associated niche for undifferentiated spermatogonia in the mouse testis. Science 317:1722–1726
45. Lepper C, Conway SJ, Fan CM (2009) Adult satellite cells and embryonic muscle progenitors have distinct genetic requirements. Nature 460:627–631
46. Gunther S, Kim J, Kostin S, Lepper C, Fan CM, Braun T (2013) Myf5-positive satellite cells contribute to Pax7-dependent long-term maintenance of adult muscle stem cells. Cell Stem Cell 13:590–601
47. von Maltzahn J, Jones AE, Parks RJ, Rudnicki MA (2013) Pax7 is critical for the normal function of satellite cells in adult skeletal muscle. Proc Natl Acad Sci U S A 110: 16747–16749
48. Seale P, Ishibashi J, Scime A, Rudnicki MA (2004) Pax7 is necessary and sufficient for the myogenic specification of CD45+:Sca1+ stem cells from injured muscle. PLoS Biol 2, E130
49. Relaix F, Montarras D, Zaffran S, Gayraud-Morel B, Rocancourt D, Tajbakhsh S, Mansouri A, Cumano A, Buckingham M (2006) Pax3 and Pax7 have distinct and overlapping functions in adult muscle progenitor cells. J Cell Biol 172:91–102
50. McKinnell IW, Ishibashi J, Le Grand F, Punch VG, Addicks GC, Greenblatt JF, Dilworth FJ, Rudnicki MA (2008) Pax7 activates myogenic genes by recruitment of a histone methyltransferase complex. Nat Cell Biol 10:77–84
51. Gayraud-Morel B, Chretien F, Flamant P, Gomes D, Zammit PS, Tajbakhsh S (2007) A role for the myogenic determination gene Myf5 in adult regenerative myogenesis. Dev Biol 312:13–28
52. Darabi R, Arpke RW, Irion S, Dimos JT, Grskovic M, Kyba M, Perlingeiro RC (2012) Human ES- and iPS-derived myogenic progenitors restore DYSTROPHIN and improve contractility upon transplantation in dystrophic mice. Cell Stem Cell 10:610–619
53. Lai EC (2004) Notch signaling: control of cell communication and cell fate. Development 131:965–973
54. Iso T, Sartorelli V, Poizat C, Iezzi S, Wu HY, Chung G, Kedes L, Hamamori Y (2001) HERP, a novel heterodimer partner of HES/E(spl) in Notch signaling. Mol Cell Biol 21:6080–6089
55. Bjornson CR, Cheung TH, Liu L, Tripathi PV, Steeper KM, Rando TA (2012) Notch signaling is necessary to maintain quiescence in adult muscle stem cells. Stem Cells 30:232–242
56. Mourikis P, Sambasivan R, Castel D, Rocheteau P, Bizzarro V, Tajbakhsh S (2012) A critical requirement for Notch signaling in maintenance of the quiescent skeletal muscle stem cell state. Stem Cells 30:243–252
57. Buas MF, Kabak S, Kadesch T (2009) Inhibition of myogenesis by Notch: evidence for multiple pathways. J Cell Physiol 218:84–93

58. Parker MH, Loretz C, Tyler AE, Duddy WJ, Hall JK, Olwin BB, Bernstein ID, Storb R, Tapscott SJ (2012) Activation of Notch signaling during ex vivo expansion maintains donor muscle cell engraftment. Stem Cells 30:2212–2220
59. Angione AR, Jiang C, Pan D, Wang YX, Kuang S (2011) PPARdelta regulates satellite cell proliferation and skeletal muscle regeneration. Skelet Muscle 1:33
60. Ge X, McFarlane C, Vajjala A, Lokireddy S, Ng ZH, Tan CK, Tan NS, Wahli W, Sharma M, Kambadur R (2011) Smad3 signaling is required for satellite cell function and myogenic differentiation of myoblasts. Cell Res 21:1591–1604
61. Hosoyama T, Nishijo K, Prajapati SI, Li G, Keller C (2011) Rb1 gene inactivation expands satellite cell and postnatal myoblast pools. J Biol Chem 286:19556–19564
62. Juan AH, Derfoul A, Feng X, Ryall JG, Dell'Orso S, Pasut A, Zare H, Simone JM, Rudnicki MA, Sartorelli V (2011) Polycomb EZH2 controls self-renewal and safeguards the transcriptional identity of skeletal muscle stem cells. Genes Dev 25:789–794
63. Kitamoto T, Hanaoka K (2010) Notch3 null mutation in mice causes muscle hyperplasia by repetitive muscle regeneration. Stem Cells 28:2205–2216
64. Chakkalakal JV, Jones KM, Basson MA, Brack AS (2012) The aged niche disrupts muscle stem cell quiescence. Nature 490:355–360
65. Cheung TH, Quach NL, Charville GW, Liu L, Park L, Edalati A, Yoo B, Hoang P, Rando TA (2012) Maintenance of muscle stem-cell quiescence by microRNA-489. Nature 482:524–528
66. Le Grand F, Jones AE, Seale V, Scime A, Rudnicki MA (2009) Wnt7a activates the planar cell polarity pathway to drive the symmetric expansion of satellite stem cells. Cell Stem Cell 4:535–547
67. Bentzinger CF, Wang YX, von Maltzahn J, Soleimani VD, Yin H, Rudnicki MA (2013) Fibronectin regulates Wnt7a signaling and satellite cell expansion. Cell Stem Cell 12:75–87
68. Oishi T, Uezumi A, Kanaji A, Yamamoto N, Yamaguchi A, Yamada H, Tsuchida K (2013) Osteogenic differentiation capacity of human skeletal muscle-derived progenitor cells. PLoS One 8, e56641
69. Alexakis C, Partridge T, Bou-Gharios G (2007) Implication of the satellite cell in dystrophic muscle fibrosis: a self-perpetuating mechanism of collagen overproduction. Am J Physiol Cell Physiol 293:C661–C669
70. Uezumi A, Fukada S, Yamamoto N, Ikemoto-Uezumi M, Nakatani M, Morita M, Yamaguchi A, Yamada H, Nishino I, Hamada Y et al (2014) Identification and characterization of PDGFRalpha(+) mesenchymal progenitors in human skeletal muscle. Cell Death Dis 5, e1186
71. Armulik A, Abramsson A, Betsholtz C (2005) Endothelial/pericyte interactions. Circ Res 97: 512–523
72. Hudlicka O, Brown MD, Egginton S (2004) Microcirculation in muscle. In: Engel AG, Franzini-Armstrong C (eds) Myology. McGraw-Hill, New York, pp 511–533
73. Shepro D, Morel NM (1993) Pericyte physiology. FASEB J 7:1031–1038
74. Dellavalle A, Sampaolesi M, Tonlorenzi R, Tagliafico E, Sacchetti B, Perani L, Innocenzi A, Galvez BG, Messina G, Morosetti R et al (2007) Pericytes of human skeletal muscle are myogenic precursors distinct from satellite cells. Nat Cell Biol 9:255–267
75. Sudo K, Kanno M, Miharada K, Ogawa S, Hiroyama T, Saijo K, Nakamura Y (2007) Mesenchymal progenitors able to differentiate into osteogenic, chondrogenic, and/or adipogenic cells in vitro are present in most primary fibroblast-like cell populations. Stem Cells 25: 1610–1617
76. Haniffa MA, Collin MP, Buckley CD, Dazzi F (2009) Mesenchymal stem cells: the fibroblasts' new clothes? Haematologica 94:258–263
77. Koenig M, Monaco AP, Kunkel LM (1988) The complete sequence of dystrophin predicts a rod-shaped cytoskeletal protein. Cell 53:219–228
78. Fukada S, Morikawa D, Yamamoto Y, Yoshida T, Sumie N, Yamaguchi M, Ito T, Miyagoe-Suzuki Y, Takeda S, Tsujikawa K et al (2010) Genetic background affects properties of satellite cells and mdx phenotypes. Am J Pathol 176:2414–2424

79. Heydemann A, Huber JM, Demonbreun A, Hadhazy M, McNally EM (2005) Genetic background influences muscular dystrophy. Neuromuscul Disord 15:601–609
80. Heydemann A, Ceco E, Lim JE, Hadhazy M, Ryder P, Moran JL, Beier DR, Palmer AA, McNally EM (2009) Latent TGF-beta-binding protein 4 modifies muscular dystrophy in mice. J Clin Invest 119:3703–3712
81. Urban Z, Hucthagowder V, Schurmann N, Todorovic V, Zilberberg L, Choi J, Sens C, Brown CW, Clark RD, Holland KE et al (2009) Mutations in LTBP4 cause a syndrome of impaired pulmonary, gastrointestinal, genitourinary, musculoskeletal, and dermal development. Am J Hum Genet 85:593–605
82. Charge SB, Rudnicki MA (2004) Cellular and molecular regulation of muscle regeneration. Physiol Rev 84:209–238
83. Bonne G, Di Barletta MR, Varnous S, Becane HM, Hammouda EH, Merlini L, Muntoni F, Greenberg CR, Gary F, Urtizberea JA et al (1999) Mutations in the gene encoding lamin A/C cause autosomal dominant Emery-Dreifuss muscular dystrophy. Nat Genet 21:285–288
84. Bione S, Maestrini E, Rivella S, Mancini M, Regis S, Romeo G, Toniolo D (1994) Identification of a novel X-linked gene responsible for Emery-Dreifuss muscular dystrophy. Nat Genet 8:323–327
85. Gnocchi VF, Ellis JA, Zammit PS (2008) Does satellite cell dysfunction contribute to disease progression in Emery-Dreifuss muscular dystrophy? Biochem Soc Trans 36:1344–1349
86. Fukada S, Yamamoto Y, Segawa M, Sakamoto K, Nakajima M, Sato M, Morikawa D, Uezumi A, Miyagoe-Suzuki Y, Takeda S et al (2008) CD90-positive cells, an additional cell population, produce laminin alpha2 upon transplantation to dy(3k)/dy(3k) mice. Exp Cell Res 314:193–203
87. Wosczyna MN, Biswas AA, Cogswell CA, Goldhamer DJ (2012) Multipotent progenitors resident in the skeletal muscle interstitium exhibit robust BMP-dependent osteogenic activity and mediate heterotopic ossification. J Bone Miner Res 27:1004–1017
88. Olson LE, Soriano P (2009) Increased PDGFRalpha activation disrupts connective tissue development and drives systemic fibrosis. Dev Cell 16:303–313
89. Bizario JC, Cerri DG, Rodrigues LC, Oliveira GL, Nomizo A, de Araujo DD, Fukuhara PS, Ribeiro JC, de Castro FA, Costa MC (2009) Imatinib mesylate ameliorates the dystrophic phenotype in exercised mdx mice. J Neuroimmunol 212:93–101
90. Huang P, Zhao XS, Fields M, Ransohoff RM, Zhou L (2009) Imatinib attenuates skeletal muscle dystrophy in mdx mice. FASEB J 23:2539–2548
91. Ito T, Ogawa R, Uezumi A, Ohtani T, Watanabe Y, Tsujikawa K, Miyagoe-Suzuki Y, Takeda S, Yamamoto H, Fukada S (2013) Imatinib attenuates severe mouse dystrophy and inhibits proliferation and fibrosis-marker expression in muscle mesenchymal progenitors. Neuromuscul Disord 23:349–356
92. Cohn RD, van Erp C, Habashi JP, Soleimani AA, Klein EC, Lisi MT, Gamradt M, ap Rhys CM, Holm TM, Loeys BL et al (2007) Angiotensin II type 1 receptor blockade attenuates TGF-beta-induced failure of muscle regeneration in multiple myopathic states. Nat Med 13:204–210
93. Iezzi S, Di Padova M, Serra C, Caretti G, Simone C, Maklan E, Minetti G, Zhao P, Hoffman EP, Puri PL et al (2004) Deacetylase inhibitors increase muscle cell size by promoting myoblast recruitment and fusion through induction of follistatin. Dev Cell 6:673–684
94. Minetti GC, Colussi C, Adami R, Serra C, Mozzetta C, Parente V, Fortuni S, Straino S, Sampaolesi M, Di Padova M et al (2006) Functional and morphological recovery of dystrophic muscles in mice treated with deacetylase inhibitors. Nat Med 12:1147–1150
95. Mozzetta C, Consalvi S, Saccone V, Tierney M, Diamantini A, Mitchell KJ, Marazzi G, Borsellino G, Battistini L, Sassoon D et al (2013) Fibroadipogenic progenitors mediate the ability of HDAC inhibitors to promote regeneration in dystrophic muscles of young, but not old Mdx mice. EMBO Mol Med 5:626–639

96. Motohashi N, Uezumi A, Yada E, Fukada S, Fukushima K, Imaizumi K, Miyagoe-Suzuki Y, Takeda S (2008) Muscle CD31(-) CD45(-) side population cells promote muscle regeneration by stimulating proliferation and migration of myoblasts. Am J Pathol 173:781–791
97. White RB, Bierinx AS, Gnocchi VF, Zammit PS (2010) Dynamics of muscle fibre growth during postnatal mouse development. BMC Dev Biol 10:21
98. Fukada S, Ma Y, Uezumi A (2014) Adult stem cell and mesenchymal progenitor theories of aging. Front Cell Dev Biol 2:10
99. Acharyya S, Butchbach ME, Sahenk Z, Wang H, Saji M, Carathers M, Ringel MD, Skipworth RJ, Fearon KC, Hollingsworth MA et al (2005) Dystrophin glycoprotein complex dysfunction: a regulatory link between muscular dystrophy and cancer cachexia. Cancer Cell 8:421–432
100. Penna F, Costamagna D, Fanzani A, Bonelli G, Baccino FM, Costelli P (2010) Muscle wasting and impaired myogenesis in tumor bearing mice are prevented by ERK inhibition. PLoS One 5, e13604
101. He WA, Berardi E, Cardillo VM, Acharyya S, Aulino P, Thomas-Ahner J, Wang J, Bloomston M, Muscarella P, Nau P et al (2013) NF-kappaB-mediated Pax7 dysregulation in the muscle microenvironment promotes cancer cachexia. J Clin Invest 123:4821–4835

Chapter 8
Stem Cell-Based Therapy for Duchenne Muscular Dystrophy

Yuko Miyagoe-Suzuki and Shin'ichi Takeda

Abstract In 1978, Partridge et al. first demonstrated that mouse myoblasts intramuscularly transplanted into recipient mice fuse with recipient myofibers. In 1989, the same research group showed that wild-type myoblasts successfully restored dystrophin expression in host *mdx* mice. Based on this report, several clinical trials of myoblast transfer for Duchenne muscular dystrophy (DMD) have been performed, but none has been successful in restoration of muscle function. Meanwhile, information about molecular regulation of satellite cells/myoblasts and cellular and molecular regulation of muscle regeneration has accumulated, and new types of stem cells with multipotency have been identified in skeletal muscle. The mesoangioblast is one such stem cell. Notably, mesoangioblasts have been demonstrated to be deliverable to damaged muscle by intra-arterial injection. In addition to skeletal muscle-resident stem cells, in 2007, Yamanaka and his colleagues reported the induction of embryonic stem (ES) cell-like pluripotent stem cells from human fibroblasts via the ectopic expression of *SOX2, OCT3/4, KLF4*, and *c-MYC* and named them "induced pluripotent stem cells (iPS cells)." The next year, generation of iPS cells from cells of patients with DMD was reported. To utilize iPS cells for regenerative medicine for muscular dystrophies, several protocols for derivation of skeletal muscle from human ES/iPS cells have been developed. Lastly, efficient genome-editing tools have emerged as a technology to obtain genetically corrected autologous cells. To make full use of these new tools in regenerative medicine, we need to understand how skeletal muscle stem cells are born, how they participate in regeneration of muscle fibers, and how the process is impaired in dystrophin-null muscle.

Keywords iPS cells • Skeletal muscle • Duchenne muscular dystrophy • Cell therapy • Dystrophin • MyoD

Y. Miyagoe-Suzuki (✉) • S. Takeda
Department of Molecular Therapy, National Institute of Neuroscience, National Center of Neurology and Psychiatry, 4-1-1 Ogawa-higashi, 187-8502 Kodaira, Tokyo, Japan
e-mail: miyagoe@ncnp.go.jp

S. Takeda et al. (eds.), *Translational Research in Muscular Dystrophy*,
DOI 10.1007/978-4-431-55678-7_8

8.1 Introduction

Stimulated by the discovery of a method to transform ordinary skin fibroblasts into pluripotent stem cells by Nobel laureate Prof. Shinya Yamanaka, research funding in Japan has been drastically weighted toward regenerative medicine. Injured skeletal muscle regenerates well by proliferation and differentiation of skeletal muscle-specific stem cells (muscle satellite cells), and therefore muscular dystrophy is a good target for regenerative medicine. Nonetheless, stem cell transplantation therapy in humans has been unsuccessful until now. In this chapter, the authors would like to briefly review the history, summarize what researchers are currently pursuing, and speculate which way we should go.

8.2 Muscle Satellite Cells/Myoblasts Play Key Roles in Muscle Regeneration

Muscle satellite cells were first identified by electron microscopy in 1961 [1] and have been shown to be skeletal muscle-specific stem cells [2]. In uninjured adult muscle, satellite cells locate between the muscle basal lamina and the sarcolemma of myofibers in a quiescent (G_0) and undifferentiated state. When muscle is injured, satellite cells are activated (and become myoblasts), proliferate, migrate, and fuse with damaged myofibers. A minor subset of satellite cells self-renew and return to their niche (Fig. 8.1). Although endogenous satellite cells are powerful enough to

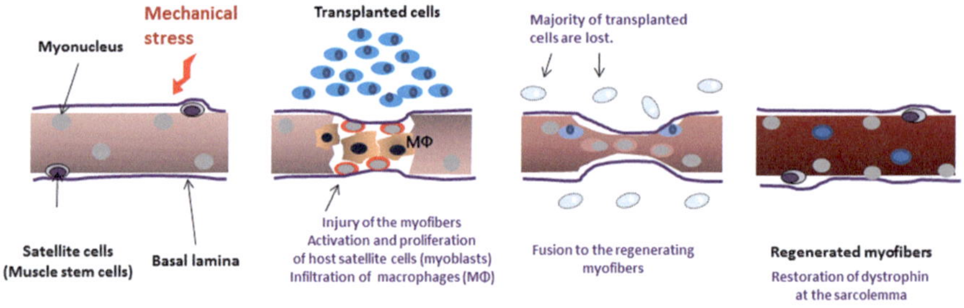

Fig. 8.1 Myoblast transplantation therapy (MMT) for DMD. Endogenous skeletal muscle satellite cells are located between the basal lamina and sarcolemma of myofibers in a dormant state. Upon muscle injury, they are activated, proliferate, migrate, and fuse with injured myofibers to regenerate myofibers. Wild-type myogenic cells injected into degenerating muscle fuse with host dystrophin-deficient myofibers in both animal models and clinical trials. Incorporated nuclei transcribe the normal dystrophin gene, and the hybrid myofibers formed by endogenous and grafted cells become dystrophin-positive and resistant to mechanical stress. When conventional protocols for cell transplantation are used, only a small number of injected satellite cells/myoblasts participate in muscle regeneration, and the engrafted cells are found to fuse only with myofibers near the injection site. The results suggest that the distance injected cells can migrate is limited. Of note, grafted myoblasts fuse with regenerating myofibers but not with undamaged myofibers. This may partly explain the low efficiency of MTT

regenerate injured muscle, satellite cells/myoblasts in DMD muscle are exhausted by repeated muscle degeneration/regeneration cycles [3, 4] and gradually fail to regenerate degenerated muscle, and finally, skeletal muscle tissues are lost and replaced by fibrotic tissue and adipocytes.

8.3 Myoblast Transplantation Therapy (MTT)

8.3.1 Myoblast Transfer in Animal Models

More than 30 years ago, Partridge et al. first demonstrated that mouse myoblasts intramuscularly transplanted into recipient mice fuse with recipient myofibers [5]. In 1989, Partridge et al. reported that normal muscle precursor cells from wild-type mice intramuscularly transplanted into dystrophin-deficient mdx mice fused with preexisting *mdx* myofibers and formed dystrophin-positive myofibers [6]. Based on that report, preclinical and clinical trials of myoblast transplantation began.

8.3.2 MTT (1991–1997)

The studies on MTT for DMD conducted between 1991 and 1997 were disappointing [7–9]. Failure of the trials was ascribed mainly to poor survival and insufficient migration of the transplanted myoblasts. Experiments using animal models suggested that a significant fraction of grafted myoblasts die (or are lost) immediately after transplantation [10]. It was also pointed out that satellite cells had been exhausted by expansion in culture and lost their high regenerative potential [11]. However, some researchers argued that current culture protocols might simply be inappropriate for the expansion of satellite cells/myoblasts, because satellite cells in their niche expand robustly and regenerate injured muscle [12]. In fact, culture conditions mimicking in vivo environments might enhance the survival and proliferation of satellite cells/myoblasts after transplantation [13]. Satellite cells/myoblasts are supposed to migrate quite short distances from the site of injection. Therefore, to produce therapeutic effects, the cells need to be injected at multiple sites at quite small intervals.

8.3.3 High-Density Myoblast Transplantation (2004–2007)

It is widely accepted that satellite cells/myoblasts do not migrate long distances but fuse only with the myofibers in close contact with them. To overcome this limitation, Skuk et al. performed high-density multiple injection of myoblasts into muscles of a Duchenne muscular dystrophy patient at 1–2 mm or smaller intervals under immunosuppression by tacrolimus [14]. Their attempt successfully produced numerous dystrophin-positive fibers in a limited area. Interestingly, the same group has recently reported that transplanted myoblasts can migrate more than several millimeters in nonhuman primate skeletal muscle [15]. The migration of satellite cells might be improved under certain conditions.

8.3.4 Local Injection of Autologous Myoblasts for Oculopharyngeal Muscular Dystrophy (OPMD)

MMT is expected to restore muscle function in myopathies that affect specific muscles, such as oculopharyngeal muscular dystrophy (OPMD). A French group performed a Phase I/IIa clinical study of cell therapy for OPMD (clinicalTrials.gov NCT00773227). Twelve patients received cricopharyngeal myotomy and were injected with autologous myoblasts prepared from unaffected quadriceps or sternocleidomastoid muscles. The study verified the feasibility and safety of the procedures and, importantly, reported cell dose-dependent improvement in swallowing: the patients injected with more than 178 million myoblasts showed improvement in swallowing duration, but the patients transplanted with fewer than 178 million myoblasts did not [16]. The observation suggests that the number of transplanted cells for therapeutic effects has a minimum threshold.

8.3.5 Cell Source Other Than Satellite Cells/Myoblasts

Mesoangioblasts were originally identified as multipotent stem cells associated with the embryonic dorsal aorta [17]. In human skeletal muscle, a subset of pericytes possesses similar properties [18]. In contrast to satellite cells, mesoangioblasts were demonstrated to migrate from the blood into the degenerate muscle and to ameliorate disease phenotypes of two animal models of muscular dystrophy (mouse and dog) after intra-arterial delivery [19, 20]. Clinical trials (Phase I/II) of intra-arterial transplantation of HLA-identical allogeneic mesoangioblasts for DMD are now ongoing (EudraCT no. 2011-000176-33). The regime includes immunosuppression of the host.

8.4 Induced Pluripotent Stem Cells (iPS Cells)

Induced pluripotent stem cells (iPS cells), which show properties almost identical to embryonic stem (ES) cells, can be generated from a wide variety of somatic cells by overexpression of a set of reprogramming factors ([21–23]. Since Park et al. reported generation of iPS cells from DMD patients [24], iPS cells have been

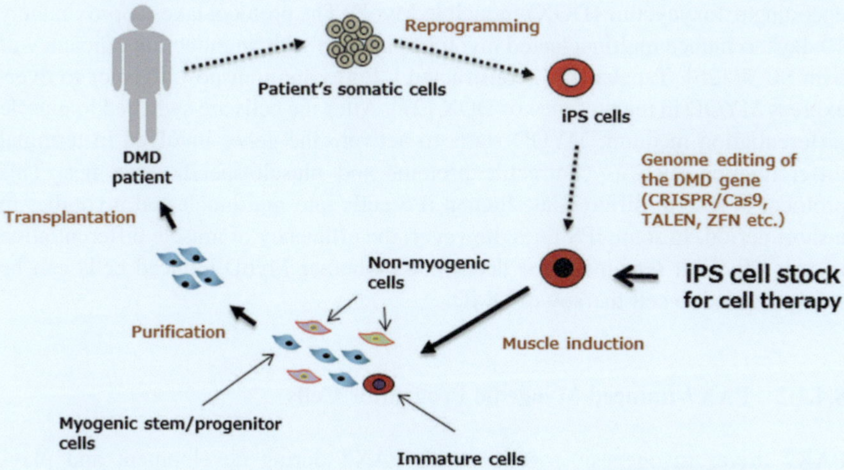

Fig. 8.2 Proposed cell therapy for DMD using patient-specific iPS cells (autologous cell transplantation). Fibroblasts or blood cells from DMD patients are converted into embryonic stem (ES) cell-like pluripotent stem cells by overexpression of reprogramming factors (originally *SOX2, OCT3/4, KLF4,* and *c-MYC*). After correction of gene mutations using genome-editing tools such as CRISPR/Cas9, TALEN, or ZFN, iPS cells are induced to differentiate into myogenic cells. Undifferentiated cells are eliminated to avoid tumor formation, and induced myogenic cells are transplanted back into the patient's muscle, where grafted cells are expected to fuse with dystrophin-deficient myofibers and also migrate into the niche for satellite cells. To circumvent the long process of establishment and evaluation of iPS cells, Yamanaka's team at Kyoto University is constructing a therapeutic iPS bank, a library of iPS cells with major HLA types. "Ready-made iPS cells" require only immunosuppression of the host

expected to be a potential cell source of autologous cell transplantation for DMD (Fig. 8.2).

8.4.1 Advances in Methods of Skeletal Muscle Induction

Although it has long been believed that skeletal muscle cannot be easily induced from ES/iPS cells, several groups have recently reported successful derivation protocols.

8.4.1.1 Direct Reprogramming of Human iPS Cells into Skeletal Muscle by Forced Expression of *MYOD*

More than 25 years ago, *MyoD* was first isolated as a master gene of myogenesis because ectopically expressed MyoD induced differentiation of non-myogenic cells to skeletal muscle [25]. This was the first report of direct reprogramming by transcription factors. Rao et al. transduced human ES cells with a lentiviral vector encoding a doxycycline (DOX)-inducible MyoD. The protocol takes approximately 10 days to induce multinucleated myotubes in vitro with an induction efficiency of over 90 % [26]. Tanaka et al. constructed a PiggyBac transposon vector to overexpress MYOD in the presence of DOX [27]. After the cells are switched to muscle differentiation medium, MYOD starts to activate the genes involved in terminal differentiation such as contractile proteins and muscle-specific enzymes. This protocol is able to differentiate human iPS cells into multinucleated myotubes in a short period. In some iPS lines, however, the efficiency of muscle differentiation is not 100 %. It remains to be determined whether MyoD-induced cells can be safely applied to cell therapy of DMD.

8.4.1.2 PAX7-Induced Myogenic Progenitor Cells

PAX7 drives myogenesis together with PAX3 during development and plays unique roles in postnatal satellite cells (reviewed in [28]). Forced expression of PAX7 during embryoid body (EB) formation successfully induces transplantable myogenic cells from human ES cells [29]. Transplanted PAX7-induced myogenic cells efficiently fuse with host myofibers and restore dystrophin expression and muscle function in immunodeficient *mdx* mice. In contrast to the MRF family (MYOD, MYF5, MRF4, and myogenin), PAX7 alone does not induce fibroblasts to differentiate into skeletal muscle. Therefore, the differentiation stage of the cells and timing of the expression of PAX7 in human ES/iPS cells seem critical.

8.4.1.3 Sphere-Based Culture Method Induces Myogenic Stem/Progenitor Cells from ES/iPS Cells

Recently, Hosoyama et al. reported a new protocol named “EZ-sphere culture” for derivation of myogenic stem/progenitor cells from human ES/iPS cells [30]. iPS cells are cultured in low-attachment poly(2-hydroxyethyl methacrylate)-coated flasks and a medium generally used for formation of neurospheres but supplemented with high concentrations of human fibroblast growth factor 2 (FGF2) and human epidermal growth factor (EGF) (100 ng/ml each). In 1 week, human ES/iPS cells form free-floating spheres and robustly expand (Fig. 8.3). It takes roughly 6 weeks for a sphere to become myogenic. When plated onto Matrigel™-coated dishes, cells forming myospheres start to fuse to form multinucleated myotubes and finally start to twitch. The method is applicable to most human ES and iPS clones including patient-derived iPS cells. We confirmed the myogenic potentials of a variety of disease-specific iPS cells, such as Ullrich congenital muscular dystrophy, Schwartz-Jampel syndrome, congenital myasthenic syndrome, and Duchenne muscular dystrophy (Miyagoe-Suzuki et al. unpublished data). Importantly, some iPS clones fail to form spheres, and some fail to differentiate into the skeletal muscle lineage. This might be correlated to incomplete reprogramming of the iPS cells, but further investigation is needed to determine the cause.

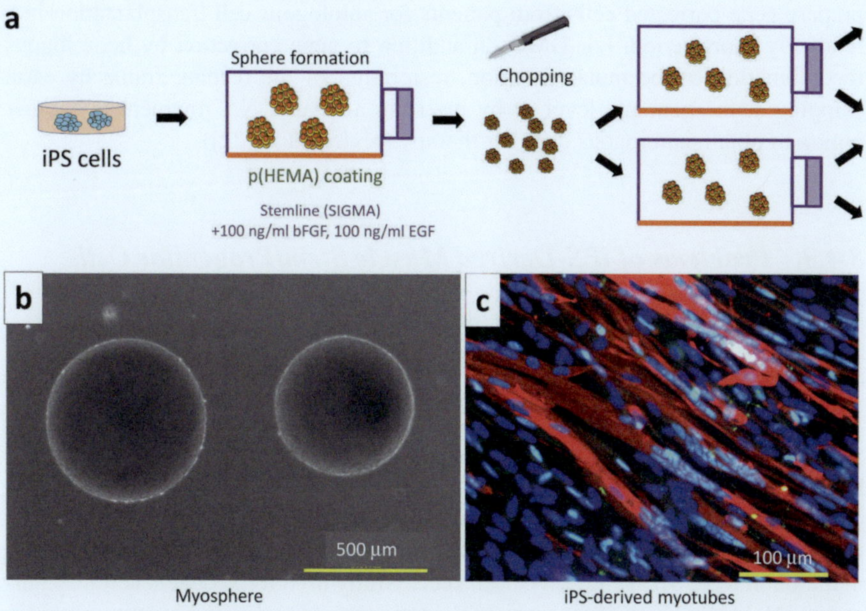

Fig. 8.3 Induction of skeletal muscle from human iPS cells by sphere-based culture (EZ-sphere method). (**a**) EZ-sphere method. iPS cells are cultured in Stemline^{TM} medium (Sigma-Aldrich S-3194) supplemented with 100 ng/ml human FGF-2 and 100 ng/ml human EGF in p(HEMA)-coated flasks, where iPS cells form spherical aggregations and continue to grow. To keep the size of a sphere between 200 and 500 μm, spheres are cut weekly using a McIlwain tissue chopper. (**b**) Spheres are derived from human iPS cells. (**c**) Myosphere cells fuse and form MF20-positive (*red*) multinucleated myotubes on Matrigel^{TM}-coated dishes in differentiation medium (DMEM containing 2 % horse serum and antibiotics). Nuclei (*blue*) are detected with Hoechst 33342

The percentage of myogenic cells produced in cultures using the original protocol described by Hosoyama et al. [30] is not 100 %, and they need purification before transplantation. To increase the efficiency of myogenic differentiation, clarification of the molecular mechanisms by which myogenic cells are induced through sphere formation is required. Myogenic cells induced by the EZ-sphere method fuse with cardiotoxin-injured muscle fibers in host NOD/Scid mice (Miyagoe-Suzuki et al. unpublished data).

8.4.2 Genome-Editing Techniques and Autologous Cell Transplantation

Although whether patient-derived iPS cells and their derivatives are immunogenic or not when transplanted into the same patient remains controversial (discussed in [31]), recent tools for genome editing, such as CRISPR/Cas9, TALE nucleases (TALENs), and zinc finger nuclease (ZFN), are encouraging in that they help us to prepare gene-corrected cells from patients for autologous cell transplantation in a relatively short period. For DMD, in addition to gene correction by homologous recombination of the mutated region, restoration of the reading frame by exon skipping at the genomic level or by inserting a small DNA fragment is another option to obtain autologous cells for therapy (reviewed in [32]).

8.4.3 Problems of iPS-Derived Muscle Stem/Progenitor Cells Remaining to Be Solved

8.4.3.1 Evaluation of Myogenic Potentials of Myogenic Cells Induced from Human iPS Cells in Animal Models

So far a limited number of research groups have reported successful engraftment of human iPS cell-derived myogenic cells in animal models. All studies used immuno-deficient dystrophin-deficient *mdx* mice. Recently *NSG-mdx*^{4Cv} mice, which have triple mutations, i.e., NOD/Scid, IL2 receptor gamma chain deficiency, and a mutation in the DMD gene, have been successfully used for xenogeneic transplantation [33]. However, xenogeneic transplantation might underestimate the myogenic potency of human muscle stem/progenitor cells. On the other hand, in many studies, the leg muscles of recipient mice are X-irradiated to suppress endogenous satellite cells and injected with a high dose of cardiotoxin to damage the whole TA muscle and evoke synchronized muscle regeneration. X-irradiation and cardiotoxin injection are not physiological and cannot be applied in the clinical setting. Thus, currently, the efficiency of cell transplantation is being tested in conditions quite different from clinical settings. The results need to be interpreted with caution.

8.4.3.2 Heterogeneity of iPS Clones in Differentiation Potential

Human iPS cells are heterogeneous in myogenic differentiation potential. Differences are found even among iPS clones from the same donor. One possible reason for the heterogeneity is that some clones are incompletely reprogrammed and retain epigenetic memory of their original cell, which interferes with the differentiation into the intended lineages. Practically, it would be useful to find characteristic gene expression patterns or specific markers of highly myogenic iPS clones instead of empirically testing each iPS clone for myogenic potential.

8.4.3.3 Tumorigenicity of iPS Cell-Derived Myogenic Cells

Human iPS cells vigorously self-renew. Although this property makes them an attractive source for cell transplantation for devastating diseases, the same property seems to be related to tumorigenesis by transplanted undifferentiated cells.

Importantly it is suggested that the risk of tumorigenesis differ greatly among iPS clones. Therefore, primarily, "good" iPS clones should be selected for clinical application. How can we know the quality of iPS cells before transplantation? Koyanagi-Aoi et al. reported the gene expression and methylation patterns of "bad" human iPS clones, which retain a significant number of undifferentiated cells after neural differentiation culture and form teratomas when transplanted into mouse brains [34]. Such a molecular signature would facilitate the selection of therapeutic cells.

For quality control of iPS-derived cells, it is also necessary to develop sensitive methods to detect residual undifferentiated iPS cells in differentiated cells. Kuroda et al. established a qRT-PCR system targeting LIN28 transcripts to detect low levels (as low as 0.002 %) of residual undifferentiated iPS cells in human iPS cell-derived retinal pigment epithelial (RPE) cells [35].

Methods for elimination of contaminated undifferentiated cells are also being developed. The residual undifferentiated iPS cells can be removed by several methods (reviewed in [36]), including sorting out ES-specific marker-expressing cells such as TRA-1-60- or SSEA-3-positive cells. Ben-David and Benvenisty also reported a pharmacological method for ablation of tumor-initiating human ES/iPS cells [36]. Tumors are also formed by iPS-derived progenitor cells at the intermediate stage of differentiation, but are resistant to terminal differentiation. Muscle progenitor-like cells or mesodermal progenitor cells refractory to terminal differentiation might be more troublesome than contaminated pluripotent stem cells because it is not easy to distinguish clearly differentiation-resistant progenitor cells from cells that can differentiate into well-differentiated myofibers.

8.5 Regenerative Activity of Grafted Cells Greatly Depends on Recipient Microenvironments

Survival, proliferation, migration, and differentiation of satellite cells/myoblasts engrafted into host muscle are affected by the microenvironments around the cells. Therefore, it is important to provide supportive microenvironments for engrafted cells.

The extracellular matrix (ECM) is an essential regulator of muscle regeneration. The basal lamina (BL) is especially important. Upon muscle injury, activated satellite cells migrate along and proliferate on BL, where laminin-integrin and laminin-dystroglycan interactions are required for survival and proliferation of satellite cells/myoblasts. Therefore it is natural to speculate that BL or its components promote the survival, proliferation, migration, and differentiation of the grafted cells. Indeed, Goudenege et al. reported that intramuscular injection of myoblasts together with laminin-111 improved the efficiency of myoblast transfer [37].

In response to muscle injury, skeletal muscle-resident mesenchymal progenitor cells or bipotent fibro-adipogenic progenitors (FAPs) in skeletal muscle are activated, proliferate, and facilitate muscle regeneration, but develop into fibrotic tissues and differentiate into adipocytes in pathogenic conditions [38–41]. Interestingly, FAPs never differentiate into adipocytes or fibroblastic cells after successful regeneration of skeletal muscle. Fibrosis and fatty infiltration in DMD muscle are wound-healing mechanisms that compensate for loss of myofibers, but the phenotypes of FAPs in DMD muscle are no longer supportive of transplanted satellite cells/myoblasts. We previously reported that co-transplantation of myoblasts and CD31(−) and CD45(−) side population cells, a subset of FAPs, improves the efficiency of transplantation [42]. These mesenchymal cells are thought to remodel the extracellular matrix via secretion of matrix metalloproteinases and to increase the survival rate and stimulate proliferation and migration by secreting soluble factors. Co-transplantation of myogenic stem/progenitor cells and mesenchymal progenitor cells derived from the same autologous iPS cells are an attractive strategy to improve graft efficiency.

8.6 Systemic Delivery of Myogenic Cells to Musculature Body Wide

Most muscular dystrophies affect skeletal muscle body wide. Therefore, the final goal of regenerative medicine for muscular dystrophy is to deliver myogenic stem/progenitor cells to the whole musculature. So far, mesoangioblasts are the most promising stem cells because they have already shown therapeutic effects in murine and canine models of muscular dystrophy by systemic delivery [19, 20]. Human mesoangioblasts are now in clinical trials for the treatment of patients with Duchenne muscular dystrophy (https://www.clinicaltrialsregister.eu/ctr-search/trial/2011-000176-33/IT). However, like satellite cells/myoblasts, mesoangioblasts have a limited ability to proliferate; therefore, it would be difficult to prepare mesoangioblasts in good condition on a scale sufficient for clinical trials. To overcome this limitation, Tedesco et al. tried to induce mesoangioblast-like myogenic cells from iPS cells. The authors overexpressed MyoD-ER in iPS cell-derived mesoangioblasts and induced myogenic differentiation in vivo by tamoxifen administration after intramuscular transplantation [43].

8.7 Conclusion

Satellite cells/myoblasts play central roles in muscle regeneration, and the contribution of cells other than satellite cells/myoblasts to regeneration of myofibers is negligible. However, transplantation of satellite cells/myoblasts has two major limitations: (1) it is difficult to prepare satellite cells/myoblasts with high myogenic potential on a large scale and (2) the migration distance of satellite cells/myoblasts is limited, and thus they cannot be delivered body wide. In contrast, mesoangioblasts can be delivered systemically. However, mesoangioblasts also reach senescence in culture, inhibiting the preparation of therapeutic cells on a large scale. Human iPS cells are an attractive cell source for cell therapy of muscular dystrophy in that they self-renew almost infinitely. Recent progress in methods of induction of myogenic cells from iPS cells and a lineup of efficient gene-editing tools ensure the clinical application of iPS cells in the near future. To avoid tumor formation, establishment of a protocol for quality control of iPS cells and their derivatives is required.

Muscle regeneration is a dynamic temporally and spatially regulated process, involving many types of cells and numerous soluble and insoluble factors. For successful stem cell-based therapy, complete understanding of the roles of the microenvironments around satellite cells/myoblasts in muscle regeneration is required. Especially, investigation of the mechanisms of fibrosis and fat deposition seen in DMD muscle are required for realization of cell therapy for muscular dystrophies.

Acknowledgments YS and ST are supported by grants from the Research Center Network for Realization of Regenerative Medicine (Japan Science and Technology Agency), Intramural Research Grants for Neurological and Psychiatric Disorders of NCNP(24–9), and Grants-in-Aid for Scientific Research (C) (24590497) (Japan Society for the Promotion of Science).

References

1. Mauro A (1961) Satellite cell of skeletal muscle fibers. J Biophys Biochem Cytol 9:493–495
2. Schultz E, Gibson MC, Champion T (1978) Satellite cells are mitotically quiescent in mature mouse muscle: an EM and radioautographic study. J Exp Zool 206:451–456
3. Blau HM, Webster C, Pavlath GK (1983) Defective myoblasts identified in Duchenne muscular dystrophy. Proc Natl Acad Sci U S A 80:4856–4860
4. Blau HM, Webster C, Pavlath GK, Chiu CP (1985) Evidence for defective myoblasts in Duchenne muscular dystrophy. Adv Exp Med Biol 182:85–110
5. Partridge TA, Grounds M, Sloper JC (1978) Evidence of fusion between host and donor myoblasts in skeletal muscle grafts. Nature 273:306–308
6. Partridge TA, Morgan JE, Coulton GR, Hoffman EP, Kunkel LM (1989) Conversion of mdx myofibers from dystrophin negative to dystrophin positive by injection of normal myoblasts. Nature 337:176–179
7. Law PK, Goodwin TG, Fang Q et al (1992) Feasibility, safety, and efficacy of myoblast transfer therapy on Duchenne muscular dystrophy boys. Cell Transplant 1:235–244
8. Mendell JR, Kissel JT, Amato AA et al (1995) Myoblast transfer in the treatment of Duchenne muscular dystrophy. N Engl J Med 333:832–838
9. Tremblay JP, Malouin F, Roy R et al (1993) Results of a triple blind clinical study of myoblast transplantations without immunosuppressive treatment in young boys with Duchenne muscular dystrophy. Cell Transplant 2:99–112
10. Mouly V, Aamiri A, Périé S et al (2005) Myoblast transfer therapy: is there any light at the end of the tunnel? Acta Myol 24:128–133

11. Ikemoto M, Fukada S, Uezumi A et al (2007) Autologous transplantation of SM/C-2.6(+) satellite cells transduced with micro-dystrophin CS1 cDNA by lentiviral vector into mdx mice. Mol Ther 15:2178–2185
12. Collins CA, Olsen I, Zammit PS et al (2005) Stem cell function, self-renewal, and behavioral heterogeneity of cells from the adult muscle satellite cell niche. Cell 122:289–301
13. Gilbert PM, Havenstrite KL, Magnusson KE et al (2010) Substrate elasticity regulates skeletal muscle stem cell self-renewal in culture. Science 329:1078–1081
14. Skuk D, Goulet M, Roy B et al (2007) First test of a "high-density injection" protocol for myogenic cell transplantation throughout large volumes of muscles in a Duchenne muscular dystrophy patient: eighteen months follow-up. Neuromuscul Disord 17:38–46
15. Skuk D, Goulet M, Trembley JP (2011) Transplanted myoblasts can migrate several millimeters to fuse with damaged myofibers in nonhuman primate skeletal muscle. J Neuropathol Exp Neurol 70:770–778
16. Périé S, Trollet C, Mouly V et al (2014) Autologous myoblast transplantation for oculopharyngeal muscular dystrophy: a phase I/IIa clinical study. Mol Ther 22:219–225
17. De Angelis L, Berghella L, Coletta M et al (1999) Skeletal myogenic progenitors originating from embryonic dorsal aorta coexpress endothelial and myogenic markers and contribute to postnatal muscle growth and regeneration. J Cell Biol 147:869–878
18. Dellavalle A, Sampaolesi M, Tonlorenzi R et al (2007) Pericytes of human skeletal muscle are myogenic precursors distinct from satellite cells. Nat Cell Biol 9:255–267
19. Sampaolesi M, Torrente Y, Innocenzi A et al (2003) Cell therapy of alpha-sarcoglycan null dystrophic mice through intra-arterial delivery of mesoangioblasts. Science 301:487–492
20. Sampaolesi M, Blot S, D'Antona G et al (2006) Mesoangioblast stem cells ameliorate muscle function in dystrophic dogs. Nature 444:574–579
21. Takahashi K, Yamanaka S (2006) Induction of pluripotent stem cells from mouse embryonic and adult fibroblast cultures by defined factors. Cell 126:663–676
22. Takahashi K, Tanabe K, Ohnuki M, Narita M, Ichisaka T et al (2007) Induction of pluripotent stem cells from adult human fibroblasts by defined factors. Cell 131:861–872
23. Yu J, Vodyanik MA, Smuga-Otto K et al (2007) Induced pluripotent stem cell lines derived from human somatic cells. Science 318:1917–1920
24. Park IH, Arora N, Huo H et al (2008) Disease-specific induced pluripotent stem cells. Cell 134:877–886
25. Weintraub H, Tapscott SJ, Davis RL et al (1989) Activation of muscle-specific genes in pigment, nerve, fat, liver, and fibroblast cell lines by forced expression of MyoD. Proc Natl Acad Sci U S A 86:5434–5438
26. Rao L, Tang W, Wei Y et al (2012) Highly efficient derivation of skeletal myotubes from human embryonic stem cells. Stem Cell Rev 8:1109–1119
27. Tanaka A, Woltjen K, Miyake K et al (2013) Efficient and reproducible myogenic differentiation from human iPS cells: prospects for modeling Miyoshi Myopathy in vitro. PLoS One 8, e61540
28. Buckingham M, Rigby PW (2014) Gene regulatory networks and transcriptional mechanisms that control myogenesis. Dev Cell 28:225–238
29. Darabi R, Arpke RW, Irion S et al (2012) Human ES- and iPS-derived myogenic progenitors restore dystrophin and improve contractility upon transplantation in dystrophic mice. Cell Stem Cell 10:610–619
30. Hosoyama T, McGivern JV, Van Dyke JM et al (2014) Derivation of myogenic progenitors directly from human pluripotent stem cells using a sphere-based culture. Stem Cells Transl Med 3:564–574
31. Cao J, Li X, Lu X, Zhang C, Yu H, Zhao T (2014) Cells derived from iPSC can be immunogenic – yes or no? Protein Cell 5:1–3
32. Lisa Li H, Nakano T, Hotta A (2014) Genetic correction using engineered nucleases for gene therapy applications. Dev Growth Differ 56:63–77

33. Arpke RW, Darabi R, Mader TL et al (2013) A new immuno-, dystrophin-deficient model, the NSG-mdx(4Cv) mouse, provides evidence for functional improvement following allogeneic satellite cell transplantation. Stem Cells 31:1611–1620
34. Koyanagi-Aoi M, Ohnuki M, Takahashi K et al (2013) Differentiation-defective phenotypes revealed by large-scale analyses of human pluripotent stem cells. Proc Natl Acad Sci U S A 110:20569–20574
35. Kuroda T, Yasuda S, Kusakawa S et al (2012) Highly sensitive in vitro methods for detection of residual undifferentiated cells in retinal pigment epithelial cells derived from human iPS cells. PLoS One 7, e37342
36. Ben-David U, Benvenisty N (2014) Chemical ablation of tumor-initiating human pluripotent stem cells. Nat Protoc 9:729–740
37. Goudebege S, Lamarre Y, Dumont N et al (2010) Laminin-111: a potential therapeutic agent for Duchenne muscular dystrophy. Mol Ther 18:2155–2163
38. Joe AW, Yi L, Natarajan A, Le Grand F, So L et al (2010) Muscle injury activates resident fibro/adipogenic progenitors that facilitate myogenesis. Nat Cell Biol 12:153–163
39. Judson RN, Zhang RH, Rossi FM (2013) Tissue-resident mesenchymal stem/progenitor cells in skeletal muscle: collaborators or saboteurs? FEBS J 280:4100–4108
40. Uezumi A, Fukada S, Yamamoto N et al (2010) Mesenchymal progenitors distinct from satellite cells contribute to ectopic fat cell formation in skeletal muscle. Nat Cell Biol 12: 143–152
41. Uezumi A, Ito T, Morikawa D et al (2011) Fibrosis and adipogenesis originate from a common mesenchymal progenitor in skeletal muscle. J Cell Sci 124:3654–3664
42. Motohashi N, Uezumi A, Yada E et al (2008) Muscle CD31(−) CD45(−) side population cells promote muscle regeneration by stimulating proliferation and migration of myoblasts. Am J Pathol 173:781–791
43. Tedesco FS, Gerli MF, Perani L et al (2012) Transplantation of genetically corrected human iPSC-derived progenitors in mice with limb-girdle muscular dystrophy. Sci Transl Med 4: 140ra89

Chapter 9
Therapeutic Approach of iPS Cell Technology for Treating Muscular Dystrophy

Hidetoshi Sakurai

Abstract Most genetic disorders of skeletal muscle do not have curative treatment and are limited to palliative care that fails to curb progression. Additionally, for many myopathies, the pathology remains unclear, although the causative genes have been identified. Thus, research attempts are underway to develop new treatments for these intractable myopathies, including those based on induced pluripotent stem (iPS) cells. In general, iPS cell strategies can be divided into two groups: those focused on cell transplant therapies in the hope of finding a curative treatment and those seeking to elucidate the underlying pathology to develop effective drugs.

The transplantation of muscle progenitor cells derived from mouse iPS cells promotes muscle regeneration in a muscular dystrophy mouse model and restores muscle strength. Similarly, research using human iPS cells has led to several methods for inducing muscle engraftable progenitors. Though reports on pathology studies using patient-derived iPS cells are few, they have shown successful recapitulation of the disease. Here I explain how the induction of differentiation of human iPS cells into muscle cells with exceptional efficiency and high reproducibility will boost drug development and therapeutic efforts along with providing detailed understanding of myopathies.

Keywords iPS cell • Cell therapy • Disease modeling • Drug screening

9.1 Introduction

Pluripotent stem cells are capable of considerable proliferation and are theoretically able to differentiate into any kind of somatic cell, which gives them promise as a source of cells for various transplant therapies. Induced pluripotent stem cells (iPS cells) are pluripotent stem cells that were derived by introducing and expressing specific genes into somatic cells [1, 2]. They share many properties with another

H. Sakurai (✉)
Department of Clinical Application, Center for iPS Cell Research and Application (CiRA), Kyoto University, 53 Shogoin-Kawahara-cho, Sakyo-ku, Kyoto 606-8507, Japan
e-mail: hsakurai@cira.kyoto-u.ac.jp

S. Takeda et al. (eds.), *Translational Research in Muscular Dystrophy*,
DOI 10.1007/978-4-431-55678-7_9

pluripotent stem cell, embryonic stem cells (ES cells), but have two significant advantages: (1) in transplantation therapy, the rejection reactions can be much lower since iPS cells are derived from patient's cells whereas ES cells come from another source, and (2) iPS cells have fewer ethical concerns since fertilized eggs are not destroyed in the process. Already, research on iPS cells in cell transplant therapies is being carried out for many intractable diseases such as age-related macular degeneration [3] and spinal cord injuries [4].

There is now a concerted effort to expand the use of iPS cells in cell transplant therapies to skeletal muscle diseases, including intractable myopathies such as muscular dystrophy. Currently, satellite cells, which are in vivo skeletal muscle stem cells, are considered the best source of cells for transplant therapy [5, 6]; however, current culturing methods cause satellite cells to differentiate into myoblasts, which have limited regenerative ability and therefore compromises their use for cell transplant therapy [5]. Alternatively, there has been an effort to transplant the embryonic origin of satellite cells, namely, muscle progenitor cells, into host skeletal muscle and then induce their differentiation into normal satellite cells in vivo. ES [7] and iPS cells are recognized as potential sources for generating muscle progenitor cells. If ES/iPS cell-derived muscle progenitor cells could form satellite cells and repeatedly regenerate and proliferate when transplanted into the skeletal muscle, effective muscle regeneration would be possible even with only few transplants.

Another therapeutic approach using iPS cells is drug screening and drug development. Because iPS cells are derived from patients with intractable diseases, inducing them to differentiate into a specific cell type, i.e., the diseased cell type, offers a new human model that reproduces the pathology in vitro for drug testing [8]. To date, knockout mice have been used as primary disease models; however, knocking out human orthologous genes in these models often fails to reproduce the disease pathology. Further, drugs developed using mouse models are too frequently ineffective in humans. Consequently, pathology models constructed from human cells are quintessential for future drug development. Presently, myoblasts from Duchenne muscular dystrophy (DMD) patients are the most common cell source for modeling the pathological condition [9]. Yet DMD patient myoblasts show certain phenotypes that make them unreliable for disease modeling. For example, patient skeletal muscles vary in nature from individual to individual depending on various factors such as genetic background, age, and medical history. Furthermore, muscle cell differentiation from DMD patient myoblasts is delayed and has poor proliferation capacity compared to those of healthy individuals [10–12]. Finally, the repetitive regeneration of DMD muscle could reduce the proliferation potential of the muscle satellite cells, again making the model design difficult [13, 14]. These DMD myoblast phenotypes are considered secondary effects of chronic inflammation and therefore may not well represent the actual primary pathogenesis. On the other hand, since the establishment of human iPS cells in 2007 [2], iPS cell-based disease models have become invaluable resources for the study of disease mechanisms and drug screening [15, 16]. Because of their unlimited proliferation potential, patient-derived human iPS cells have tremendous advantages in drug screening over patient-derived somatic cells such as myoblasts or fibroblasts.

Myoblasts induced from patient-derived iPS cells allow us to investigate primary pathogenesis which is generated by the loss of dystrophin itself without the conflation of secondary effects due to chronic inflammation. Additionally, myogenic differentiation from iPS cells allows us to repeatedly produce a large number of intact and homogeneous myotubes from healthy subjects and DMD patients in vitro.

Just as it was possible to identify a drug target through the accurate understanding of pathology in a genetic disease such as a sialic acid for GNE myopathy [17], a detailed analysis of pathogenesis in other intractable myopathies is also warranted. The majority of intractable myopathies are genetic disorders, and there is a high expectation that their pathology can be reproduced using in vitro models drawing on genetic information contained in patient-derived iPS cells.

This chapter will discuss how iPS cells are being used in cell transplant therapy and drug discovery for myopathies as well as studying the pathology of the disease.

9.2 Approaches for Cell Therapy

9.2.1 Basic Studies of Cell Therapy Using Mouse ES/iPS Cells

Using mouse models, muscle regeneration therapies based on the induction of mouse pluripotent stem cells to differentiate into skeletal muscle progenitor cells are being developed for transplantation experiments. Various methods have been reported to induce mouse ES cell differentiation to skeletal muscle. Darabi et al. were the first to successfully treat muscular dystrophy in a mouse model [18]. They produced skeletal muscle progenitor cells with high efficiency by forcing the expression of an indispensable transcription factor in the formation of skeletal muscle, Pax3, in ES cells using a tetracycline induction system. However, when whole differentiated cells were transplanted into mice, teratomas, a major adverse effect of ES cell transplants, occurred due to mixing with undifferentiated cells. Using a DMD mouse model (*mdx* mice), they transplanted a purified cell fraction that included PDGFRa positive and Flk1 negative, which are markers for somite and paraxial mesoderm [19], which is the embryonic origin of skeletal muscle [20]. The transplanted cells fused to host myofibers and the muscle fibers expressed dystrophin which is encoded by *Dmd*, a causative gene of DMD. Furthermore, the contractile force of isolated skeletal muscle and motor function of treated mouse improved. Additionally, engraftment and regeneration were found not only with direct administration to the skeletal muscle but also via vascular administration. However, it was still unclear at that time whether the transplanted cells were engrafted as satellite cells or were just fused to host myofiber like myoblasts.

In the same year, I and colleagues induced the differentiation of mouse ES cells into mesoderm cells in 2D culture without forcing gene expression and found that the PDGFRa-positive fraction contained skeletal muscle progenitor cells [21].

In vivo differentiation into satellite cells was reported when these PDGFRa-positive cells were transplanted into mice with muscle damage. A portion of the transplanted, ES cell-derived cells expressed Pax7, which is a known molecular marker for satellite cells, and differentiated into multinucleated, mature muscle fibers when isolated from live mice and cultured, although the efficiency of the differentiation was low. Chang et al. induced the differentiation of mouse ES cells into mesoderm cells by embryoid body formation and succeeded in isolating cells with a high capacity for muscle regeneration [22] by using markers specific to resting-state satellite cells called SM/C-2.6 [23]. Dystrophin expression was restored by locally transplanting these cells into the skeletal muscle of *mdx* mice, and their differentiation into satellite cells was confirmed. Additionally, when the ES cell-derived satellite cells were isolated from skeletal muscle and transplanted again, they fused to skeletal muscle as expected, confirming their differentiation into satellite cells in vivo. This work is the first published report to show mouse ES cell-derived cells differentiated into functional satellite cells and to demonstrate repeated muscle regeneration in vivo. In 2011, Darabi et al. showed that mouse ES cells could be induced to become skeletal muscle progenitor cells through forced expression of not only Pax3 but also Pax7 [24]. In this report, the transplanted ES cell-derived cells differentiated into Pax7-positive cells in vivo and exhibited regenerative capacity, indicating that the Pax7-mediated ES cell-derived muscle progenitors were engrafted as functional satellite cells.

Following the development of mouse iPS cells [1], SM/C-2.6-positive cells were isolated from mouse iPS cells and found to engraft as satellite cells in vivo the same way as mouse ES cells [25]. Later, it was discovered that mouse iPS cells could also be induced to differentiate into skeletal muscle progenitor cells by the forced expression of Pax7 [26]. Moreover, mouse iPS cells were induced to differentiate into PDGFRa-positive/Flk1-negative cells without genetic recombination and found to engraft as satellite cells in vivo following transplantation [27]. Thus, the myogenic progenitor production found in mouse ES cells was reproduced in mouse iPS cells, demonstrating that mouse iPS cells are equivalent to mouse ES cells in their ability to differentiate into muscle cell lineages based on the induction of satellite cells.

9.2.2 Basic Studies of Cell Therapy Using Human ES/iPS Cells

Parallel to the mouse studies above, research on the induction of human pluripotent stem cells for differentiation into satellite cells is being conducted for clinical application in cell transplant therapies. These studies are expected to be especially effective, because human iPS cells can be obtained from the patients themselves, which reduces the immune rejection response. However, since muscular dystrophy is a genetic disease, patient cells cannot be used as a treatment strategy without gene repair. Although the dystrophin gene, the causative factor of DMD, is a very large gene, which makes complete repair difficult, Kazuki et al. succeeded in patient-derived iPS cells using artificial human chromosome techniques [28]. Due to this advancement, expectations for research in the development of muscle stem cell transplant therapies using iPS cells have grown.

The first induction of human ES cells to differentiate into myoblast cells was reported in 2007 [29]. In that paper, surface marker molecules such as CD73 and NCAM were used to isolate myoblast cells, which were obtained approximately 50 days after induction. Although these cells did not turn into satellite cells upon transplantation, they did show similar local regenerative capability. However, the differentiation potential varied tremendously between human pluripotent stem cell clones, including those established from the same donor [30]. Although a very interesting finding, because this method is difficult to reproduce, alternative induction protocols have been sought. Two include using either a TGF-beta signal inhibitor, SB-431542 [31], or retinoic acid [32]. However, while both promote the differentiation of skeletal muscle, neither could be used to induce differentiation into satellite cells nor to achieve successful engraftment. Subsequently, similar to mouse ES/iPS cells, it was reported that progenitor cells, including those derived from human iPS cells, with the ability to differentiate into muscle are present in the PDGFRa-positive/Flk1-negative population, although again, differentiation into satellite cells and engraftment in vivo was not observed [27]. Awaya et al. succeeded to induce differentiation into skeletal muscle progenitor cells using an improved culturing method and marker-based separation without performing forced gene expression [33]. They found that human iPS cell-derived muscle progenitors differentiated into Pax7-positive satellite cells in vivo when transplanted into cardiotoxin treated regeneration model muscle of immunocompromised mice.

Since then, many important reports on cell transplant therapy using muscular dystrophy mouse models have been published. Darabi et al. applied a method originally used to induce skeletal muscle progenitor cells from mouse ES/iPS cells on human ES/iPS cells and succeeded in obtaining skeletal muscle progenitor cells with high efficiency by forced Pax7 expression [34]. There, human ES/iPS cells were first differentiated into mesoderm cells using the embryoid body (EB) method, and then time-specific expression of Pax7 was forced using a tetracycline-inducible system. After purifying Pax7 positive cells, the cells were induced to become muscle progenitor cells at a purity of 99 % when cultured with continuous forced expression of Pax7. When these skeletal muscle progenitor cells were transplanted into immunocompromised *mdx* mice, human nucleus-positive/human dystrophin-positive muscle fibers were formed, and it was found that the transplanted cells participated in the muscle regeneration. Additionally, some of the transplanted cells engrafted into muscle fibers as Pax7-positive satellite cells, and as much as a year after transplantation, human/dystrophin-positive muscle fibers were confirmed, suggesting that the transplanted cells participated in the repair as satellite cells for long term in vivo. Unfortunately, despite these promising results, this method involved a lentivirus vector for recombination into the genome, which is considered unsafe for clinical purposes.

Similarly, Tedesco et al. reported successful muscle regeneration by inducing human iPS cells to differentiate into cells that had characteristics similar to fetal-stage vascular progenitor cells called mesoangioblasts and subsequently transplanting these cells into diseased muscles of limb-girdle muscular dystrophy 2D model mice [35]. They reported that human iPS cells could differentiate into mesoangioblast-like cells that were previously established from human periarterial cells [36] by changing the culture conditions at four different stages over a 1-month period. Though these iPS cell-derived mesoangioblast-like cells rarely produced skeletal muscle spontaneously in vitro, if the master gene for skeletal muscle differentiation, myogenic differentiation 1 (MyoD1), was forcibly expressed during transplantation into a mouse model, the cells could adhere to the mouse muscle fibers and participate in the muscle regeneration. Furthermore, engraftment in the skeletal muscle was verified not only by intramuscular injection but also by administration into the arteries, suggesting that the iPS cell-derived mesoangioblast-like cells are excellent progenitor cells capable of systemic administration into model animals. The same team also succeeded in inducing mesoangioblast-like cells in iPS cells derived from muscular dystrophy patients. However, differentiation into satellite cells in vivo was not obtained. Following that work, Goudenege et al. reported that by inducing differentiation of human ES/iPS cells into mesenchymal cells over approximately a week and then forcing the expression of MyoD1 using an adenovirus vector, skeletal muscle progenitor cells could be generated with an efficiency of approximately 40–60 % [37]. They showed that, through intramuscular injection, iPS cell-derived skeletal muscle progenitor cells could provide a similar level of muscle regeneration to myoblast cells. They also succeeded in inducing differentiation in iPS cells derived from muscular dystrophy patients. However, differentiation into satellite cells in vivo was again not obtained. Additionally, while adenovirus vectors offer the advantage of avoiding recombination with the genome, they are considerably immunogenic such that a different vector is desirable for clinical use. The above studies show that successful muscular regeneration following transplantation can be achieved by inducing muscle progenitor cells through the forced expression of Pax7 or MyoD1. More recently, however, Xu et al. induced the differentiation of engraftable muscle progenitor cells to skeletal muscle following transplantation without any gene modification by using a differentiation culture with additives including the respective bFGF and Wnt signal agonists Bio and forskolin [38].

These findings demonstrate the use of human iPS cell-derived cells for muscle regeneration in mouse dystrophy models. The discovery of markers such as Pax7 will be instrumental in verifying whether satellite cells can be induced from hiPSCs and whether posttransplant engrafted cell populations really function as satellite cells. Future work is also required to evaluate the efficacy and safety of these transplant therapies by analyzing the motor function of individual mice and expanding the long-term observations of these transplantations in animal models with long life-spans such as dog.

9.3 Approaches for Drug Screening Followed by Disease Modeling Using Patient-Derived iPS Cells

9.3.1 Establishment of Efficient and Reproducible Differentiation Methods from Human iPS Cells to Muscle Cells

Drug development research using patient-derived iPS cells requires a highly efficient and reproducible method for inducing the differentiation to the target tissue. However, even as research into skeletal muscle progresses, most reports to date about the induction of human ES/iPS cells for differentiation into skeletal muscle cells are poor in these metrics. In order to initiate skeletal muscle differentiation, we forcibly expressed the master transcription gene, MyoD1, in undifferentiated human iPS cells to achieve an efficiency approaching 90 % [39]. MyoD1 expression was controlled by using a tetracycline-responsive vector in an extremely simple method that involved only the addition of doxycycline to the culture medium. The reproducibility and efficiency of this method is extremely high even when carried out on various iPS cell lines including patient-derived iPS cells [39]. Moreover, the cells induced by this protocol showed promising phenotypes, including fusion with each other and contraction upon electrical stimuli, indicating mature muscle cells [39]. Through comprehensive gene expression analysis and structural analysis using electron microscopy, we showed that these iPS cell-derived muscle cells exhibited similarities to primary myoblasts obtained through human biopsies [39]. Utilizing the above results, we carried out studies to reproduce pathologies in muscle cells differentiated from patient-derived iPS cells, as described below.

9.3.2 Modeling Muscular Dystrophy Using Patient-Derived iPS Cells

9.3.2.1 Modeling Miyoshi Muscular Dystrophy

Miyoshi myopathy is an autosomal recessive, hereditary distal myopathy that was first reported by Miyoshi et al. in 1986 [40]. The disease may present itself from the age of 10 years and causes difficulty in walking or standing on the toes. It is a progressive disease with gradual muscle loss, and the causative gene was identified as the dysferlin gene [41]. It was confirmed that dysferlin functions to repair muscle cell membranes [42], and it is believed that the muscle cells become damaged due to delayed membrane repair, which leads to the onset of the myopathy [43]. However, the mechanism by which the delayed membrane repair causes the degeneration and death of muscle cells is not well understood. We aimed to reproduce this abnormal muscle cell membrane repair pathology using iPS cells derived from Miyoshi myopathy patients. Adopting the forced expression of

MyoD1 described above, we induced mature muscle cells from Miyoshi myopathy patient-derived iPS cells with high efficiency [39]. Compared to healthy control cells, there was no difference in the induction efficiency, rate of differentiation, or marker molecule expression in the cells obtained. Next, to reproduce the muscle repair pathology, a membrane damage experiment was performed using two-photon laser confocal microscopy, whereby the differentiated muscle cells were perforated by laser irradiation. The time required for membrane repair was calculated by measuring the time taken for a fluorescent dye added to the culture medium to be taken into the cells. Because repair of the muscle cell membrane occurs on a timescale of a few seconds for healthy control iPS cell-derived muscle cells, we found that these cells did not increase their uptake of fluorescent compounds after 1 min. However, for muscle cells from Miyoshi myopathy patient-derived iPS cells, the intake of fluorescent compounds continued even after 5 min [39]. As mentioned earlier, clones of human iPS cells show a large variation in differentiation potential [30]. To verify that the differences between healthy control cells and patient-derived cells were not due to the variation between clones, gene-repaired, new patient-derived iPS cells were produced whereby dysferlin was restored by the forced expression of dysferlin cDNA. These cells were made to differentiate into skeletal muscle cells, and, on carrying out similar membrane damage experiments, it was found that the prolonged fluorescent compound uptake was shortened compared to that before the restoration [39]. In other words, we successfully reproduced the pathology of the lengthened membrane repair time and found that it was clearly due to dysferlin deficiency.

Based on these results, we are developing new methods of a membrane damage-inducing system which can be adopted for multi-well plate-based drug screening. It is expected that in the near future, drug screening using muscle cells from patient-derived iPS cells to augment muscle cell membrane repair will be possible.

9.3.2.2 Modeling Duchenne Muscular Dystrophy

DMD is a severely debilitating and intractable disease that occurs in 1 of every 3,500 male children born [44]. It is caused by damage or mutation of the dystrophin gene on the X chromosome [45], which leads to muscle degeneration caused by progressive inflammation and necrosis of the skeletal muscle. The disease has an exceptionally poor prognosis, with management using artificial respirators by the time the patient is in his 20s and death in his 30s. At present, there is no curative treatment, with steroids being the only drug used to slow progression [46]. Collaborative international clinical trials using antisense oligonucleotides for exon skipping in DMD are underway [47]; however, only limited number of DMD patients who have specific exon deletions can be applied by this treatment. Thus, a drug treatment that shows positive effects in all DMD patients is preferred. However, more than a quarter century since the identification of dystrophin [45], the question of why dystrophin deficiency causes serious, chronic inflammation in skeletal muscle remains unanswered.

Continued research using the DMD mouse model, *mdx*, has suggested an excess flow of Ca^{2+} within muscle cells as a likely cause [48]. This hypothesis argues that if a state of high intracellular Ca^{2+} concentration continues unabated, not only do the mitochondria become damaged [49], which increases oxidative stress, but abnormal activation of the NF-kB pathway leads to chronic inflammation [50]. Indeed, when genetic modifications were made to restrain the activity of a stretch-activated ion channel, transient receptor potential vanilloid 2 (TRPV2), in *mdx* mice, a reduction in muscle tissue inflammation was reported [51]. In contrast, in healthy mice expressing dystrophin, overexpression of another stretch-activated ion channel, transient receptor potential canonical 6 (TRPC6), reproduced the pathology of muscular dystrophy [52].

On the suspicion that this excess in intracellular Ca^{2+} flow triggers the DMD pathology, we undertook recapitulating the pathology in DMD patient-derived iPS cells (DMD-iPSCs). Using electrical stimuli, we contracted these differentiated skeletal muscle cells, and, using Ca^{2+} imaging and a fluorescent probe, we measured the Ca^{2+} concentrations during the contraction [53]. DMD-iPSC derived myocytes demonstrated higher Ca^{2+} influx than control iPS-derived myocytes [53]. Furthermore, when dystrophin expression was restored by exon-skipping in DMD-iPSCs, excess Ca^{2+} influx was attenuated [53]. Based on these results, we successfully demonstrated that excessive Ca^{2+} influx is one of the earliest events to occur in dystrophin-deficient muscle during contraction [53]. We have been investigating to apply our DMD modeling system as a screening method for drugs that target the excess Ca^{2+} flow.

9.3.2.3 Modeling Facial Scapular Humeral Muscular Dystrophy (FSHD)

Facioscapulohumeral muscular dystrophy (FSHD) is an autosomal dominant muscular dystrophy that inflicts 1 in 20,000 people and, as its name suggests, is characterized by progressive and often asymmetric weakness and atrophy of facial, shoulder girdle, and upper arm muscles [54]. The most common form of FSHD, FSHD1, is caused by the deletion of a subset of D4Z4 macrosatellite repeat units in the subtelomeric region of chromosome 4q35 [55]. The general healthy population normally has 11–100 D4Z4 repeat units, whereas the FSHD1 patient population has 1–10 repeat units [54]. The only 4q35-localized protein-coding gene found to be dysregulated in FSHD is DUX4, a retrogene located within each D4Z4 repeat unit [56]. Because the contracted D4Z4 repeat units induce mRNA stabilization by a polyadenylation signal, the FSHD-specific full-length mRNA of the *DUX4* gene (*DUX4-fl*) is transcribed [56]. No animal models for investigating the FSHD pathogenesis caused by DUX4 have been designed, because DUX4 is not coded in rodents, dogs, or pigs. Snider et al., however, showed that *DUX4-fl* is expressed in undifferentiated human iPS cells and the testis of healthy individuals [57]. They further demonstrated that *DUX4-fl* expression in human iPS cells derived from healthy individuals using the embryoid body method disappears upon differentiation into the three embryonic germ layers, but that the expression continues in FSHD patient-derived iPS cells even after the induction of differentiation [57]. This disease model may elucidate the mechanism of the dysregulated splicing of the

DUX4 gene that causes aberrant expression of full-length DUX4 in skeletal muscle. Additionally, human iPS cells have an advantage that they provide a large amount of human early embryonic cells in which *DUX4-fl* is normally expressed.

9.3.2.4 Modeling Myotonic Dystrophy Type 1 (DM1)

Myotonic dystrophy is an autosomal dominant muscular dystrophy and the most common form of adult onset-muscular dystrophy. While skeletal muscle deterioration and delayed relaxation after contraction (myotonia) are the most obvious characteristics of the disease, other multisystemic dysfunctions include cardiac conduction defects, insulin resistance, cataracts, smooth muscle dysfunction, and neuropsychiatric disturbances [58]. The most common form of myotonic dystrophy is type 1 (DM1), which is caused by expanded CTG triplet repeats in the 3′ UTR of the *DMPK1* gene [59, 60]. DM1 patients may have between 50 and 5,000 CTG repeats in their pathogenic allele, while normal alleles have between 6 and 34 repeats [61]. Toxic gain-of-function CUG RNA produced by the expanded CTG repeats interferes with the function of RNA-binding proteins to cause impaired RNA splicing and abnormal expression of a large number of genes [62, 63]. It was found that the number of CTG repeats expands in myotonic dystrophy type 1 (DM1) in progeny [64], with children of patients having more serious complications than their parents. Using DM1 patient-derived iPS cells, Du et al. reported that CTG repeats in the causative gene, DMPK1, expanded with each subculture, suggesting that, for this model, it is possible to use patient-derived undifferentiated human iPS cells to analyze the mechanism of the CTG repeat expansion [65].

9.4 Prospective

9.4.1 Prospective for Cell Therapy

Human iPS cells show tremendous promise as curative cell transplant therapies for muscular dystrophy. Already, they have been differentiated into satellite cells that successfully engrafted and regenerated muscle in animal experiments. However, since in vitro cultivation and proliferation methods that maintain the stem cell properties of the satellite cells are not yet established, it is difficult to analyze at present whether human iPS cell-derived satellite cells in vivo indeed have the same capacity as intrinsic satellite cells. Therefore, further research must be done not only on satellite cells differentiated from human iPS cells, but also on the characteristics of adult human satellite cells.

Even if the iPS cell-generated satellite cells adequately recapitulate endogenous satellite cell properties, iPS cells have other concerns. One is their carcinogenic effect. To minimize this risk, scientists are selecting appropriate iPS cell clones that show no resistance to differentiation. Financially, it is not feasible to perform gene modifications in patient-derived iPS cells and then select safe iPS cells that also have high capacity for differentiation based on animal experiments. Therefore, the transplantation of iPS cells from donors after HLA-type matching is being investigated. At the Center for iPS Cell Research and Application at Kyoto University, research into the construction of high common HLA homozygous donor-derived iPS cell stocks for clinical use has already begun. By producing iPS cells from homozygous donors with HLA types that are common in the Japanese population and evaluating their quality before use, it is expected that iPS cell clones will be available for clinical use.

9.4.2 Prospective for Drug Screening with Patient-Derived iPS Cells

Human iPS cells are expected to become beneficial tools for new curative treatments. We have established a reliable, highly efficient method for inducing their differentiation into skeletal muscle, including iPS cells derived from patients with muscular dystrophy [39]. Using this same method, we recapitulated the pathology by inducing the patient-derived iPS cells to differentiate into skeletal muscle cells and applied suitable stress that initiated the disease pathogenesis. As a pathology model for muscular dystrophy, these cells can be used for detailed pathologic analysis and are expected to play a fundamental role in drug development by providing an abundant source of cells for drug screening. In fact, even if the detailed mechanism of the pathology is not understood, iPS cell-based models can screen for compounds by visualizing the disease phenotype. For example, if a pathologic model is achieved whereby the cells of a healthy individual are nonfluorescent, but the cells of a patient are, then screening for compounds that result in a loss of fluorescence could suggest positive drug candidates, and subsequent analysis of the functions of the individual compounds could further elucidate the mechanism of the pathology.

References

1. Takahashi K, Yamanaka S (2006) Induction of pluripotent stem cells from mouse embryonic and adult fibroblast cultures by defined factors. Cell 126(4):663–676
2. Takahashi K, Tanabe K, Ohnuki M, Narita M, Ichisaka T, Tomoda K, Yamanaka S (2007) Induction of pluripotent stem cells from adult human fibroblasts by defined factors. Cell 131(5):861–872
3. Osakada F, Hirami Y, Takahashi M (2010) Stem cell biology and cell transplantation therapy in the retina. Biotechnol Genet Eng Rev 26:297–334
4. Tsuji O, Miura K, Okada Y, Fujiyoshi K, Mukaino M, Nagoshi N, Kitamura K, Kumagai G, Nishino M, Tomisato S, Higashi H, Nagai T, Katoh H, Kohda K, Matsuzaki Y, Yuzaki M, Ikeda E, Toyama Y, Nakamura M, Yamanaka S, Okano H (2010) Therapeutic potential of

appropriately evaluated safe-induced pluripotent stem cells for spinal cord injury. Proc Natl Acad Sci U S A 107(28):12704–12709. doi:10.1073/pnas.09101061070910106107

5. Montarras D, Morgan J, Collins C, Relaix F, Zaffran S, Cumano A, Partridge T, Buckingham M (2005) Direct isolation of satellite cells for skeletal muscle regeneration. Science 309(5743): 2064–2067
6. Cerletti M, Jurga S, Witczak CA, Hirshman MF, Shadrach JL, Goodyear LJ, Wagers AJ (2008) Highly efficient, functional engraftment of skeletal muscle stem cells in dystrophic muscles. Cell 134(1):37–47. doi:10.1016/j.cell.2008.05.049S0092-8674(08)00755-1
7. Thomson JA, Itskovitz-Eldor J, Shapiro SS, Waknitz MA, Swiergiel JJ, Marshall VS, Jones JM (1998) Embryonic stem cell lines derived from human blastocysts. Science 282(5391): 1145–1147
8. Grskovic M, Javaherian A, Strulovici B, Daley GQ (2011) Induced pluripotent stem cells—opportunities for disease modelling and drug discovery. Nat Rev Drug Discov 10(12): 915–929. doi:10.1038/nrd3577nrd3577
9. van Deutekom JC, Bremmer-Bout M, Janson AA, Ginjaar IB, Baas F, den Dunnen JT, van Ommen GJ (2001) Antisense-induced exon skipping restores dystrophin expression in DMD patient derived muscle cells. Hum Mol Genet 10(15):1547–1554
10. Blau HM, Webster C, Pavlath GK (1983) Defective myoblasts identified in Duchenne muscular dystrophy. Proc Natl Acad Sci U S A 80(15):4856–4860
11. Delaporte C, Dautreaux B, Rouche A, Fardeau M (1990) Changes in surface morphology and basal lamina of cultured muscle cells from Duchenne muscular dystrophy patients. J Neurol Sci 95(1):77–88
12. Delaporte C, Dehaupas M, Fardeau M (1984) Comparison between the growth pattern of cell cultures from normal and Duchenne dystrophy muscle. J Neurol Sci 64(2):149–160
13. Decary S, Hamida CB, Mouly V, Barbet JP, Hentati F, Butler-Browne GS (2000) Shorter telomeres in dystrophic muscle consistent with extensive regeneration in young children. Neuromuscul Disord 10(2):113–120, doi:S0960896699000930
14. Webster C, Blau HM (1990) Accelerated age–related decline in replicative life-span of Duchenne muscular dystrophy myoblasts: implications for cell and gene therapy. Somat Cell Mol Genet 16(6):557–565
15. Hirata S, Takayama N, Jono-Ohnishi R, Endo H, Nakamura S, Dohda T, Nishi M, Hamazaki Y, Ishii E, Kaneko S, Otsu M, Nakauchi H, Kunishima S, Eto K (2013) Congenital amegakaryocytic thrombocytopenia iPS cells exhibit defective MPL-mediated signaling. J Clin Invest 123(9):3802–3814. doi:10.1172/JCI6472164721
16. Kondo T, Asai M, Tsukita K, Kutoku Y, Ohsawa Y, Sunada Y, Imamura K, Egawa N, Yahata N, Okita K, Takahashi K, Asaka I, Aoi T, Watanabe A, Watanabe K, Kadoya C, Nakano R, Watanabe D, Maruyama K, Hori O, Hibino S, Choshi T, Nakahata T, Hioki H, Kaneko T, Naitoh M, Yoshikawa K, Yamawaki S, Suzuki S, Hata R, Ueno S, Seki T, Kobayashi K, Toda T, Murakami K, Irie K, Klein WL, Mori H, Asada T, Takahashi R, Iwata N, Yamanaka S, Inoue H (2013) Modeling Alzheimer's disease with iPSCs reveals stress phenotypes associated with intracellular Abeta and differential drug responsiveness. Cell Stem Cell 12(4):487–496. doi:10.1016/j.stem.2013.01.009S1934-5909(13)00012-X
17. Malicdan MC, Noguchi S, Hayashi YK, Nonaka I, Nishino I (2009) Prophylactic treatment with sialic acid metabolites precludes the development of the myopathic phenotype in the DMRV-hIBM mouse model. Nat Med 15(6):690–695. doi:10.1038/nm.1956nm.1956
18. Darabi R, Gehlbach K, Bachoo RM, Kamath S, Osawa M, Kamm KE, Kyba M, Perlingeiro RC (2008) Functional skeletal muscle regeneration from differentiating embryonic stem cells. Nat Med 14(2):134–143. doi:10.1038/nm1705nm1705
19. Sakurai H, Era T, Jakt LM, Okada M, Nakai S, Nishikawa S (2006) In vitro modeling of paraxial and lateral mesoderm differentiation reveals early reversibility. Stem Cells 24(3): 575–586, doi:2005–0256
20. Relaix F, Rocancourt D, Mansouri A, Buckingham M (2005) A Pax3/Pax7-dependent population of skeletal muscle progenitor cells. Nature 435(7044):948–995. doi:10.1038/nature03594

21. Sakurai H, Okawa Y, Inami Y, Nishio N, Isobe K (2008) Paraxial mesodermal progenitors derived from mouse embryonic stem cells contribute to muscle regeneration via differentiation into muscle satellite cells. Stem Cells 26(7):1865–1873. doi:10.1634/stemcells.2008-01732008-0173
22. Chang H, Yoshimoto M, Umeda K, Iwasa T, Mizuno Y, Fukada S, Yamamoto H, Motohashi N, Miyagoe-Suzuki Y, Takeda S, Heike T, Nakahata T (2009) Generation of transplantable, functional satellite-like cells from mouse embryonic stem cells. Faseb J 23(6):1907–1919. doi:10.1096/fj.08-123661fj.08-123661
23. Fukada S, Higuchi S, Segawa M, Koda K, Yamamoto Y, Tsujikawa K, Kohama Y, Uezumi A, Imamura M, Miyagoe-Suzuki Y, Takeda S, Yamamoto H (2004) Purification and cell-surface marker characterization of quiescent satellite cells from murine skeletal muscle by a novel monoclonal antibody. Exp Cell Res 296(2):245–255. doi:10.1016/j.yexcr.2004.02.018S0014482704000886
24. Darabi R, Santos FN, Filareto A, Pan W, Koene R, Rudnicki MA, Kyba M, Perlingeiro RC (2011) Assessment of the myogenic stem cell compartment following transplantation of Pax3/Pax7-induced embryonic stem cell-derived progenitors. Stem Cells 29(5):777–790. doi:10.1002/stem.625
25. Mizuno Y, Chang H, Umeda K, Niwa A, Iwasa T, Awaya T, Fukada S, Yamamoto H, Yamanaka S, Nakahata T, Heike T (2010) Generation of skeletal muscle stem/progenitor cells from murine induced pluripotent stem cells. Faseb J 24(7):2245–2253. doi:10.1096/fj.09-137174fj.09-137174
26. Darabi R, Pan W, Bosnakovski D, Baik J, Kyba M, Perlingeiro RC (2011) Functional myogenic engraftment from mouse iPS cells. Stem Cell Rev 7(4):948–957. doi:10.1007/s12015-011-9258-2
27. Sakurai H, Sakaguchi Y, Shoji E, Nishino T, Maki I, Sakai H, Hanaoka K, Kakizuka A, Sehara-Fujisawa A (2012) In vitro modeling of paraxial mesodermal progenitors derived from induced pluripotent stem cells. PLoS One 7(10), e47078. doi:10.1371/journal.pone.0047078 PONE-D-12-02501
28. Kazuki Y, Hiratsuka M, Takiguchi M, Osaki M, Kajitani N, Hoshiya H, Hiramatsu K, Yoshino T, Kazuki K, Ishihara C, Takehara S, Higaki K, Nakagawa M, Takahashi K, Yamanaka S, Oshimura M (2010) Complete genetic correction of ips cells from Duchenne muscular dystrophy. Mol Ther 18(2)):386–393. doi:10.1038/mt.2009.274
29. Barberi T, Bradbury M, Dincer Z, Panagiotakos G, Socci ND, Studer L (2007) Derivation of engraftable skeletal myoblasts from human embryonic stem cells. Nat Med 13(5):642–648
30. Osafune K, Caron L, Borowiak M, Martinez RJ, Fitz-Gerald CS, Sato Y, Cowan CA, Chien KR, Melton DA (2008) Marked differences in differentiation propensity among human embryonic stem cell lines. Nat Biotechnol 26(3):313–315
31. Mahmood A, Harkness L, Schroder HD, Abdallah BM, Kassem M (2010) Enhanced differentiation of human embryonic stem cells to mesenchymal progenitors by inhibition of TGF–beta/activin/nodal signaling using SB-431542. J Bone Miner Res 25(6):1216–1233. doi:10.1002/jbmr.34
32. Ryan T, Liu J, Chu A, Wang L, Blais A, Skerjanc IS (2012) Retinoic acid enhances skeletal myogenesis in human embryonic stem cells by expanding the premyogenic progenitor population. Stem Cell Rev 8(2):482–493. doi:10.1007/s12015-011-9284-0
33. Awaya T, Kato T, Mizuno Y, Chang H, Niwa A, Umeda K, Nakahata T, Heike T (2012) Selective development of myogenic mesenchymal cells from human embryonic and induced pluripotent stem cells. PLoS One 7(12), e51638. doi:10.1371/journal.pone.0051638PONE-D-12-18790
34. Darabi R, Arpke RW, Irion S, Dimos JT, Grskovic M, Kyba M, Perlingeiro RC (2012) Human ES– and iPS-derived myogenic progenitors restore DYSTROPHIN and improve contractility upon transplantation in dystrophic mice. Cell Stem Cell 10(5):610–619. doi:10.1016/j.stem.2012.02.015
35. Tedesco FS, Gerli MF, Perani L, Benedetti S, Ungaro F, Cassano M, Antonini S, Tagliafico E, Artusi V, Longa E, Tonlorenzi R, Ragazzi M, Calderazzi G, Hoshiya H, Cappellari O, Mora M,

Schoser B, Schneiderat P, Oshimura M, Bottinelli R, Sampaolesi M, Torrente Y, Broccoli V, Cossu G (2012) Transplantation of genetically corrected human iPSC-derived progenitors in mice with limb-girdle muscular dystrophy. Sci Transl Med 4(140):140ra189. doi:10.1126/scitranslmed.30035414/140/140ra89
36. Dellavalle A, Sampaolesi M, Tonlorenzi R, Tagliafico E, Sacchetti B, Perani L, Innocenzi A, Galvez BG, Messina G, Morosetti R, Li S, Belicchi M, Peretti G, Chamberlain JS, Wright WE, Torrente Y, Ferrari S, Bianco P, Cossu G (2007) Pericytes of human skeletal muscle are myogenic precursors distinct from satellite cells. Nat Cell Biol 9(3):255–267
37. Goudenege S, Lebel C, Huot NB, Dufour C, Fujii I, Gekas J, Rousseau J, Tremblay JP (2012) Myoblasts derived from normal hESCs and dystrophic hiPSCs efficiently fuse with existing muscle fibers following transplantation. Mol Ther 20(11):2153–2167. doi:10.1038/mt.2012.188mt2012188
38. Xu C, Tabebordbar M, Iovino S, Ciarlo C, Liu J, Castiglioni A, Price E, Liu M, Barton ER, Kahn CR, Wagers AJ, Zon LI (2013) A zebrafish embryo culture system defines factors that promote vertebrate myogenesis across species. Cell 155(4):909–921. doi:10.1016/j.cell.2013.10.023S0092-8674(13)01299-3
39. Tanaka A, Woltjen K, Miyake K, Hotta A, Ikeya M, Yamamoto T, Nishino T, Shoji E, Sehara-Fujisawa A, Manabe Y, Fujii N, Hanaoka K, Era T, Yamashita S, Isobe K, Kimura E, Sakurai H (2013) Efficient and reproducible myogenic differentiation from human iPS cells: prospects for modeling Miyoshi myopathy in vitro. PLoS One 8(4), e61540. doi:10.1371/journal.pone.0061540PONE-D-12-35707
40. Miyoshi K, Kawai H, Iwasa M, Kusaka K, Nishino H (1986) Autosomal recessive distal muscular dystrophy as a new type of progressive muscular dystrophy. Seventeen cases in eight families including an autopsied case. Brain 109(Pt 1):31–54
41. Liu J, Aoki M, Illa I, Wu C, Fardeau M, Angelini C, Serrano C, Urtizberea JA, Hentati F, Hamida MB, Bohlega S, Culper EJ, Amato AA, Bossie K, Oeltjen J, Bejaoui K, McKenna-Yasek D, Hosler BA, Schurr E, Arahata K, de Jong PJ, Brown RH Jr (1998) Dysferlin, a novel skeletal muscle gene, is mutated in Miyoshi myopathy and limb girdle muscular dystrophy. Nat Genet 20(1):31–36. doi:10.1038/1682
42. Bansal D, Miyake K, Vogel SS, Groh S, Chen CC, Williamson R, McNeil PL, Campbell KP (2003) Defective membrane repair in dysferlin-deficient muscular dystrophy. Nature 423 (6936):168–172. doi:10.1038/nature01573nature01573
43. Han R (2011) Muscle membrane repair and inflammatory attack in dysferlinopathy. Skelet Muscle 1(1):10. doi:10.1186/2044-5040-1-102044-5040-1-10
44. Hoffman EP, Knudson CM, Campbell KP, Kunkel LM (1987) Subcellular fractionation of dystrophin to the triads of skeletal muscle. Nature 330(6150):754–758. doi:10.1038/330754a0
45. Hoffman EP, Brown RH Jr, Kunkel LM (1987) Dystrophin: the protein product of the Duchenne muscular dystrophy locus. Cell 51(6):919–928. doi:10.1016/0092-8674(87)90579-4
46. Nowak KJ, Davies KE (2004) Duchenne muscular dystrophy and dystrophin: pathogenesis and opportunities for treatment. EMBO Rep 5(9):872–876. doi:10.1038/sj.embor.7400221
47. Cirak S, Arechavala-Gomeza V, Guglieri M, Feng L, Torelli S, Anthony K, Abbs S, Garralda ME, Bourke J, Wells DJ, Dickson G, Wood MJ, Wilton SD, Straub V, Kole R, Shrewsbury SB, Sewry C, Morgan JE, Bushby K, Muntoni F (2011) Exon skipping and dystrophin restoration in patients with Duchenne muscular dystrophy after systemic phosphorodiamidate morpholino oligomer treatment: an open-label, phase 2, dose-escalation study. Lancet 378(9791):595–605. doi:10.1016/S0140-6736(11)60756-3
48. Constantin B, Sebille S, Cognard C (2006) New insights in the regulation of calcium transfers by muscle dystrophin-based cytoskeleton: implications in DMD. J Muscle Res Cell Motil 27(5–7):375–386. doi:10.1007/s10974-006-9085-2
49. Robert V, Massimino ML, Tosello V, Marsault R, Cantini M, Sorrentino V, Pozzan T (2001) Alteration in calcium handling at the subcellular level in mdx myotubes. J Biol Chem 276(7): 4647–4651. doi:10.1074/jbc.M006337200M006337200

50. Acharyya S, Villalta SA, Bakkar N, Bupha-Intr T, Janssen PM, Carathers M, Li ZW, Beg AA, Ghosh S, Sahenk Z, Weinstein M, Gardner KL, Rafael-Fortney JA, Karin M, Tidball JG, Baldwin AS, Guttridge DC (2007) Interplay of IKK/NF-kappaB signaling in macrophages and myofibers promotes muscle degeneration in Duchenne muscular dystrophy. J Clin Invest 117(4):889–901. doi:10.1172/JCI30556
51. Iwata Y, Katanosaka Y, Arai Y, Shigekawa M, Wakabayashi S (2009) Dominant-negative inhibition of Ca^{2+} influx via TRPV2 ameliorates muscular dystrophy in animal models. Hum Mol Genet 18(5):824–834. doi:10.1093/hmg/ddn408
52. Millay DP, Goonasekera SA, Sargent MA, Maillet M, Aronow BJ, Molkentin JD (2009) Calcium influx is sufficient to induce muscular dystrophy through a TRPC-dependent mechanism. Proc Natl Acad Sci U S A 106(45):19023–19028. doi:10.1073/pnas.0906591106
53. Shoji E, Sakurai H, Nishino T, Nakahata T, Heike T, Awaya T, Fujii N, Manabe Y, Matsuo M, Sehara-Fujisawa A (2015) Early pathogenesis of Duchenne muscular dystrophy modelled in patient-derived human induced pluripotent stem cells. Sci Rep 5:Article 12831. doi: 10.1038/srep12831
54. Tawil R, Van Der Maarel SM (2006) Facioscapulohumeral muscular dystrophy. Muscle Nerve 34(1):1–15. doi:10.1002/mus.20522
55. Wijmenga C, Hewitt JE, Sandkuijl LA, Clark LN, Wright TJ, Dauwerse HG, Gruter AM, Hofker MH, Moerer P, Williamson R et al (1992) Chromosome 4q DNA rearrangements associated with facioscapulohumeral muscular dystrophy. Nat Genet 2(1):26–30. doi:10.1038/ng0992-26
56. Lemmers RJ, van der Vliet PJ, Klooster R, Sacconi S, Camano P, Dauwerse JG, Snider L, Straasheijm KR, van Ommen GJ, Padberg GW, Miller DG, Tapscott SJ, Tawil R, Frants RR, van der Maarel SM (2010) A unifying genetic model for facioscapulohumeral muscular dystrophy. Science 329(5999):1650–1653. doi:10.1126/science.1189044science.1189044
57. Snider L, Geng LN, Lemmers RJ, Kyba M, Ware CB, Nelson AM, Tawil R, Filippova GN, van der Maarel SM, Tapscott SJ, Miller DG (2010) Facioscapulohumeral dystrophy: incomplete suppression of a retrotransposed gene. PLoS Genet 6(10), e1001181. doi:10.1371/journal.pgen.1001181
58. Turner C, Hilton-Jones D (2014) Myotonic dystrophy: diagnosis, management and new therapies. Curr Opin Neurol 27(5):599–606. doi:10.1097/WCO.0000000000000128
59. Brook JD, McCurrach ME, Harley HG, Buckler AJ, Church D, Aburatani H, Hunter K, Stanton VP, Thirion JP, Hudson T et al (1992) Molecular basis of myotonic dystrophy: expansion of a trinucleotide (CTG) repeat at the 3′ end of a transcript encoding a protein kinase family member. Cell 69(2):385
60. Mahadevan M, Tsilfidis C, Sabourin L, Shutler G, Amemiya C, Jansen G, Neville C, Narang M, Barcelo J, O'Hoy K et al (1992) Myotonic dystrophy mutation: an unstable CTG repeat in the 3′ untranslated region of the gene. Science 255(5049):1253–1255
61. Lopez Castel A, Nakamori M, Tome S, Chitayat D, Gourdon G, Thornton CA, Pearson CE (2011) Expanded CTG repeat demarcates a boundary for abnormal CpG methylation in myotonic dystrophy patient tissues. Hum Mol Genet 20(1):1–15. doi:10.1093/hmg/ddq427ddq427
62. Osborne RJ, Lin X, Welle S, Sobczak K, O'Rourke JR, Swanson MS, Thornton CA (2009) Transcriptional and post-transcriptional impact of toxic RNA in myotonic dystrophy. Hum Mol Genet 18(8):1471–1481. doi:10.1093/hmg/ddp058ddp058
63. Ranum LP, Cooper TA (2006) RNA-mediated neuromuscular disorders. Annu Rev Neurosci 29:259–277. doi:10.1146/annurev.neuro.29.051605.113014
64. Ashizawa T, Anvret M, Baiget M, Barcelo JM, Brunner H, Cobo AM, Dallapiccola B, Fenwick RG Jr, Grandell U, Harley H et al (1994) Characteristics of intergenerational contractions of the CTG repeat in myotonic dystrophy. Am J Hum Genet 54(3):414–423
65. Du J, Campau E, Soragni E, Jespersen C, Gottesfeld JM (2013) Length-dependent CTG.CAG triplet-repeat expansion in myotonic dystrophy patient-derived induced pluripotent stem cells. Hum Mol Genet 22(25):5276–5287. doi:10.1093/hmg/ddt386ddt386

Chapter 10
Clinical Aspects of GNE Myopathy and Translational Medicine

Madoka Mori-Yoshimura

Abstract Prior to recent advances in therapeutics, various aspects of rare diseases, such as their etiology, natural history, and evaluation items, were not well understood. Yet, in reality, only a few studies have been conducted on rare diseases, given the difficulty of obtaining a sufficient patient sample size for data collection. In this study, we performed questionnaire and retrospective medical record surveys, as well as a prospective natural history study of patients with UDP-N-acetylglucosamine-2-epimerase/N-acetylmannosamine kinase gene (GNE) myopathy, which is also referred to as distal myopathy with rimmed vacuoles (DMRV). This study aimed to identify evaluation tools for use in upcoming clinical trials and to clarify the natural history of GNE myopathy and life-threatening risk factors related to disease progression in a historical control. Moreover, in order to inform patients with GNE myopathy, physicians, researchers, and companies of progress in clinical research, we established a patient registry system. Our efforts are aimed not only at preparing for upcoming clinical trials, but also to provide information regarding the nature of the disease and advice on preferable patient care. International cooperation will improve the understanding of GNE myopathy and promote clinical progress by providing access to a larger cohort.

Keywords GNE myopathy • Natural history • Translational medicine • Patient registry

10.1 Introduction

Clinical progress can present challenges to physicians, who need to adapt and accurately diagnose and evaluate diseases in view of new developments. To date, many clinical trials have been conducted to evaluate the natural history of muscle disorders.

M. Mori-Yoshimura (✉)
Department of Neurology, National Center Hospital, National Center of Neurology and Psychiatry, 4-1-1 Ogawahigashi, 187-8551 Kodaira, Tokyo, Japan
e-mail: yoshimur@ncnp.go.jp

S. Takeda et al. (eds.), *Translational Research in Muscular Dystrophy*,
DOI 10.1007/978-4-431-55678-7_10

GNE myopathy, also known as distal myopathy with rimmed vacuoles (DMRV), is an early adult-onset myopathy with slow progression that preferentially affects the tibialis anterior muscle and commonly spares the quadriceps femoris muscles [1, 2]. The disease is caused by a mutation in the *GNE* gene, which encodes a bifunctional enzyme [uridine diphosphate-*N*-acetylglucosamine (UDP-GlcNAc) 2-epimerase (GNE) and N-acetylmannosamine kinase (NMK)] that catalyzes two rate-limiting reactions in cytosolic sialic acid synthesis [3–7]. Oral sialic acid metabolite treatment prevents muscle atrophy and weakness in a mouse GNE myopathy model [8]. A recent phase I clinical trial with oral sialic acid was conducted in Japan (ClinicalTrials.gov; identifier, NCT01236898), and a phase II study is currently underway in the United States and Israel (ClinicalTrials.gov; identifier, NCT01517880).

To prepare for global phase III clinical trials, we believe it is necessary to gain a better understanding of the natural history of GNE, as well as its progression. To this end, we first conducted questionnaire and medical record surveys among patients with GNE to obtain a rough understanding of the natural history of the disease. Second, we performed a prospective study on the natural history of patients with confirmed GNE myopathy in order to identify evaluation items that can be used to monitor disease progression. Finally, we generated a patient registry of Japanese patients with GNE myopathy with the aim of recruiting patients to clinical trials and as an information tool on healthcare and research progress for patients, physicians, researchers, and companies. Through these efforts, we provide a view of the clinical progress in GNE myopathy and discuss the significance of rare-disease translational research for physicians.

10.1.1 Retrospective Questionnaire and Medical Record Surveys

10.1.1.1 Aims

To date, no natural history study has been conducted on the genetics of the GNE gene. Indeed, some studies to date have denied significant genotype–phenotype correlations in GNE myopathy [7]. However, we suspected that disease severity might be related to the genotype of the GNE gene, given the existence of severely affected, early onset patients, as well as mildly affected, late onset patients. Some patients also exhibit respiratory dysfunction, although there have been no reports on the involvement of respiratory dysfunction in GNE myopathy. Against this backdrop, we assessed (1) disease onset, ambulatory status, and respiratory dysfunction and (2) genotype–phenotype correlations. This study was approved by the Medical Ethics Committee of the National Center of Neurology and Psychiatry (NCNP).

10.1.1.2 Study Design

We first performed a questionnaire survey of patients with confirmed GNE myopathy. The questionnaire was provided to patients by physicians at eight hospitals specializing in neuromuscular diseases, including the NCNP. This study was a retrospective and cross-sectional analysis and involved 71 patients with genetically confirmed GNE myopathy. Clinical information was collected from patients using the questionnaire, and genetic information was acquired from available medical records. We then conducted a medical record survey of NCNP patients in order to obtain their clinical characteristics. The presence or absence of respiratory failure was of particular interest in this aspect of the study.

10.1.1.3 Results

Mean age at symptom onset was 25.2 ± 9.2 years (range, 12–58 years; median, 24.5 years), 52.0 % (n = 37/71) were ambulant (41.3 ± 12.8 years), 15.5 % (n = 11/71, 40.0 ± 13.6 years) could walk without assistance, and 35.2 % required assistance (n = 25/71, 41.8 ± 12.7 years). The median age at which assistance was required for walking was 30.0 ± 1.4 years, the median age of wheelchair users was 36.0 ± 2.7 years, and the median age at loss of ambulation was 45.0 ± 4.2 years. Durations from disease onset to walking with assistance, wheelchair use, and loss of ambulation were 7.0 ± 0.4 years, 11.5 ± 1.2 years, and 17.0 ± 2.1 years, respectively. We also identified potential genotype–phenotype correlations. V572L homozygotes (i.e., mutation in the NMK domain), the most frequent mutation in Japan, had more severe phenotypes than V572L/D176V (i.e., mutations in both GNK/MNK domains) compound heterozygotes, the most frequent type of compound heterozygote in Japan. It was unclear whether each individual mutation contributed to these differences or whether the combination of mutations was important; GNK/MNK mutations tended to be more severely affected. The medical record survey revealed that some patients had respiratory dysfunction which correlated with disease severity. Some reports have suggested that patients with advanced disease may require respiratory support [8, 9]. Differences in disease severity between V572L homozygotes and D176V/V572L compound heterozygotes were also found in a study using the NCNP muscle bank [10].

Unresolved questions include genotype–phenotype correlations in patients with mutations other than V572L and D176V/V572L, as well as genotype–phenotype relationships with respect to cardiac impairment observed in the mouse GNE model [11].

10.1.2 Prospective Natural History Study

10.1.2.1 Aims

This study aimed to identify evaluation tools for use in upcoming clinical trials. As mentioned above, a phase II study is currently underway in the United States and Israel. We believe that further insight into the natural history of the disease will be beneficial for preparing for phase III clinical trials. Thus, we aimed to identify evaluation items that can be used to detect disease progression within a year, with respect to observation duration of clinical trials.

10.1.2.2 Patients and Methods

A total of 24 Japanese patients (9 men and 15 women) participated in this study. Two women were siblings and the rest were unrelated. Mean age at the time of data collection was 43.0 ± 12.9 years (mean ± SD), and mean age at disease onset was 25.9 ± 10.3 years (range, 15–58 years; median, 24 years). Of the 24 patients, 9 (36.0 %) were ambulant, 8 completed the 6-min walk test (6MWT) without assistance, 1 required assistance (e.g., cane and/or ankle brace) and could not complete the 6MWT, and 15 (64.0 %) had lost ambulation.

All patients rested for more than 2 h before each muscle strength test. Measurements using a handheld dynamometer for knee extension in the sitting position, grip power, and pinch power were repeated three times on both the right and left sides, and all six measurements were averaged for data analysis. Muscle strength tests, including manual muscle testing (MMT) and gross motor function measure (GMFM, Japanese version; range, 0–100 [%]), were performed to examine 17 muscle groups (neck flexion, truncal flexion, shoulder abduction, shoulder adduction, shoulder flexion, shoulder extension, elbow flexion, elbow extension, wrist flexion, wrist extension, hip flexion, thigh adduction, thigh abduction, knee extension, knee flexion, ankle dorsiflexion, and plantar flexion). Results of right and left MMTs were averaged, except for those corresponding to neck and truncal flexion. The summed MMT value (range, 0–85) was obtained from the sum of the 17 muscle groups. The 6MWT was performed among patients who were able to walk without assistance.

10.1.2.3 Results

At baseline, eight, eight, and six patients were too weak to complete measurements for HHD, grip power, and pinch power, respectively. In two patients, noninvasive positive pressure ventilation (NPPV) for respiratory failure was started at night due to newly diagnosed respiratory dysfunction and hypoxemia during hospitalization for baseline evaluation. None of the patients presented with disease-specific cardiac dysfunction.

A significant reduction in summed MMT ($p < 0.01$), grip power ($p = 0.034$), and the percentage of forced vital capacity (%FVC) ($p = 0.030$) and a nonsignificant reduction in 6MWT ($p = 0.061$) scores, GMFM ($p = 0.089$), and CK ($p = 0.087$) were observed (Fig. 10.1). Among all muscles examined, shoulder extension ($p = 0.017$) and abduction ($p = 0.029$) and knee flexion ($p = 0.010$) showed significant annual decreases. Seven of eight ambulant patients showed deteriorations in 6 MW distance within 1 year (Fig. 10.1a). Changes in %FVC ($p = 0.034$) were greater in nonambulant patients than in ambulant patients [12].

10.1.2.4 Limitations and Conclusions

Summed MMT, grip power, and %FVC significantly changed over the course of a year. Although results of the 6MWT were not significant, which likely reflects the small number of ambulant patients, a larger cohort may clearly detect the deterioration. The 6MWT and summed MMT are important end-point item candidates for clinical trials because they can be used to determine annual changes in disease progression. Our study showed reductions in respiratory function, especially among nonambulant patients, suggesting that %FVC is a useful outcome measure for nonambulant patients. Our data suggest that GNE myopathy does not involve cardiomyopathy, although cardiac involvement was previously implicated in a mouse model [11].

Limitations include the small number of patients and short study period. In rare diseases such as GNE myopathy, large-scale studies tend to be difficult.

In conclusion, 6MWT, summed MMT, GMFM, grip power tests, and %FVC may be good clinical evaluation tools for clinical trials and to correlate with disease progression, although %FVC and grip power should be used according to ambulation status.

10.1.3 Patient Registry Development

10.1.3.1 Aims

Our previous studies made clear the limitations of natural history studies, which involved small sample populations. In order to gain further insight into GNE myopathy for the purpose of improving therapy and care, more patient data are required. To this end, we aimed to develop a nationwide patient registry for GNE myopathy in order to facilitate the planning of clinical trials and recruitment of candidates and to disseminate standard care and current information to patients, physicians, and researchers.

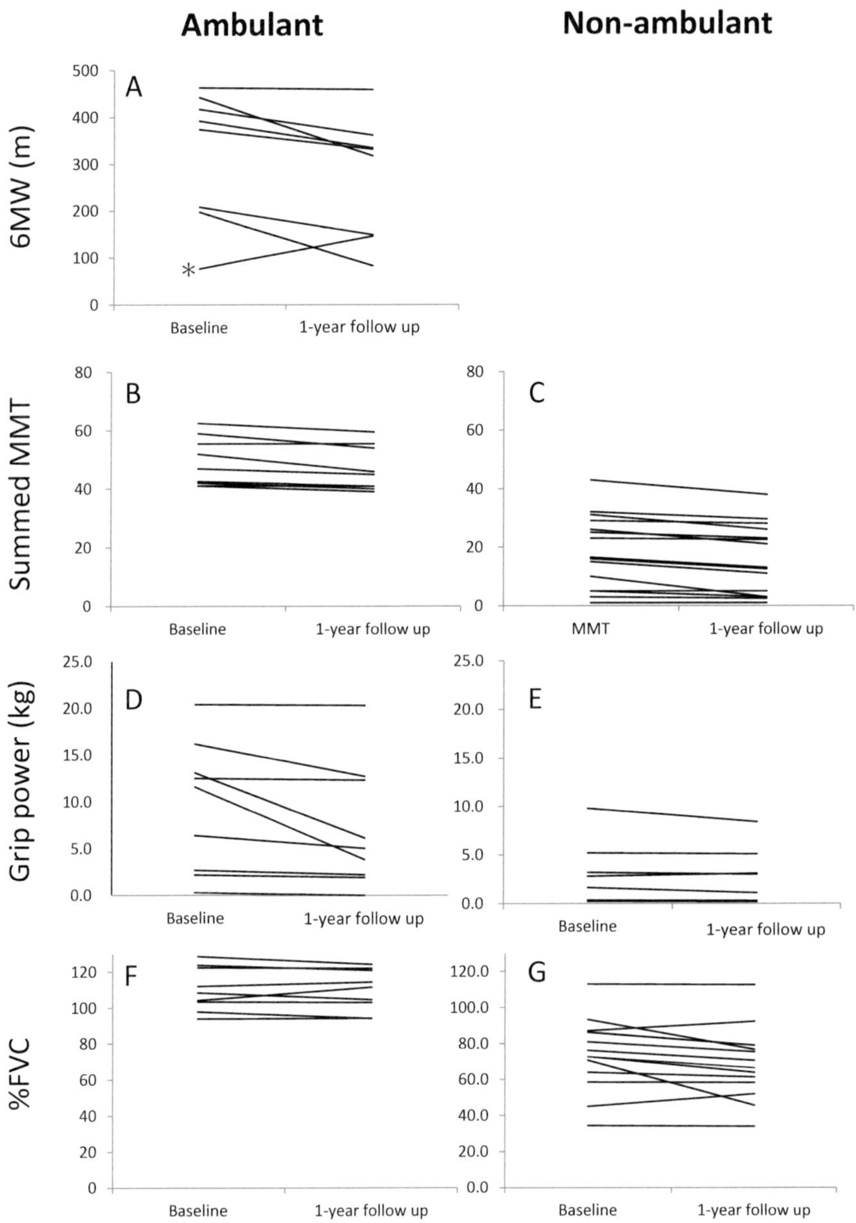

Fig. 10.1 Annual changes in motor function. *Right column*, ambulant patients; *left column*, nonambulant patients. **a** 6MWT; **b**, **c** summed MMT; **d**, **e** grip power; and **f**, **g** %FVC. All patients, with the exception of one (*), showed deterioration in 6MWT. (**a**) Only one patient with improved 6MWT succeeded in weight control and had more opportunities to walk relative to baseline. Both ambulant (**b**) and nonambulant (**c**) patients showed deterioration in summed MMT. The decrease in grip power was greater in ambulant patients (**d**, **e**), whereas the decrease in %FVC was greater in nonambulant patients

10.1.3.2 Study Design

Medical records of genetically confirmed patients with GNE myopathy at the NCNP were retrospectively reviewed in order to obtain data reflecting the severity and progression of the disease. Items selected for the registration sheet included age, sex, age at onset, past history and complications, family history, body weight and height, pathological findings from muscle biopsy, grip power, walking ability, respiratory function, cardiac function, willingness to join upcoming clinical trials, and participation in patient associations. A copy of the original genetic analysis report was required of each patient.

10.1.3.3 Institution, Organization, Registration Method, Data Collection, and Ethical Approval

In 2009, we developed a national registry for neuromuscular diseases (Registry of Muscular Dystrophy, Remudy; http://www.Remudy.jp/, see also Chap. 11) in Japan in collaboration with the TREAT-NMD Alliance in order to aid in the recruitment of eligible patients for clinical trials, provide information regarding the natural history and epidemiology of diseases, and serve as a source of information on current clinical care [13]. Remudy is supported by Intramural Research Grants (23-4/26-7) for Neurological and Psychiatric Disorders from the NCNP. Registry information was provided to interested individuals and their informed consent was obtained. Individuals whose data were included were informed that inclusion in the database confers no obligation to the patient and that they will be removed from the registry immediately upon request. They were also told that refusal to participate would not affect subsequent medical care. Study objectives, design, risks, and benefits of participation were explained to all patients, and their written informed consent was obtained prior to enrollment.

10.1.3.4 Results

As of the end of October 2013, a total of 121 Japanese patients with GNE myopathy (55 men and 66 women) had registered. Mean ages at data collection and disease onset were 44.9 ± 13.2 years (median, 43 years; range, 21–85 years) and 27.9 ± 9.6 years (median, 26 years; range, 12–61 years), respectively. The registry included patients from throughout Japan (38/47 prefectures) who were recruited through a collaboration with 92 attending physicians from 73 institutes (Fig. 10.2). Three patients had a past history of idiopathic thrombocytopenia (ITP).

Thirty-nine of 121 patients (32.3 %) harbored a homozygous mutation in *GNE*, and 78 of 121 (64.5 %) had a compound heterozygous mutation. Only one heterozygous mutation was found in four (3.3 %) patients. Among those with a homozygous mutation, 82 % (32/39), 8 % (3/39), and 5 % (2/39) harbored p. V572L,

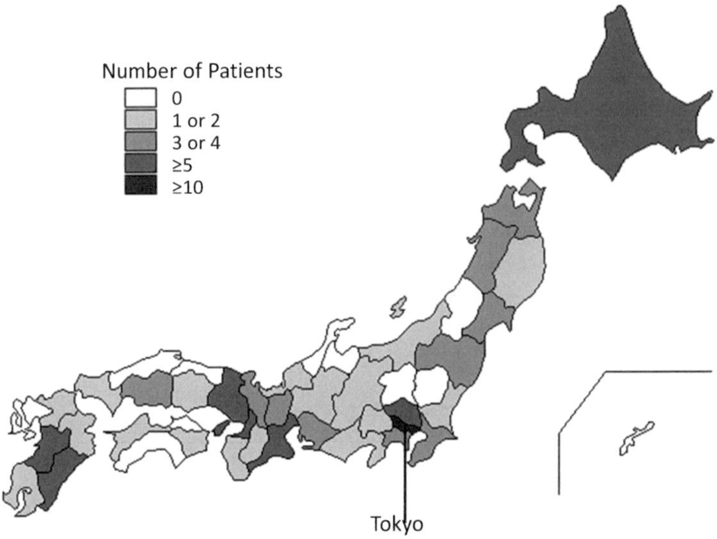

Fig. 10.2 Patient distribution. Patients were distributed throughout Japan (38/47 prefectures), and 92 physicians at 73 institutes agreed to contribute to the registry

p. C13S, and p. M172T mutations, respectively. A homozygous mutation of p. D176V was identified in only one patient. Of those carrying two heterozygous mutations, 31 % (24/78) had p. D176V/p. V572L mutations, while the remaining patients had other combinations of mutations.

Mean age at disease onset was 27.7 ± 9.6 years (median, 27.5 years; interquartile range, 15–61), 20 % (24/121) were ambulant without assistance, 37 % (45/121) required assistance (e.g., canes and/or braces), and 43 % (52/121) had lost ambulation. Mean age at loss of ambulation was 35.4 ± 11.3 years. Kaplan–Meier analysis revealed median durations from disease onset to walking with assistance, wheelchair use, and loss of ambulation of 8.9 years (95 % CI, 6.3–9.7), 14.0 years (95 % CI, 11.8–16.2), and 21.0 years (95 % CI, 15.4–26.6), respectively.

Information on pulmonary and cardiac function was available for 65 % (79/121) and 34 % (41/121) of patients, respectively. Of those examined, 33 % (26/79) had respiratory dysfunction (%FVC < 80), and two were using nocturnal NPPV. %FVC was significantly correlated with disease duration ($\rho = 0.479$, $p < 0.01$) and serum CK levels ($\rho = 0.573$, $p < 0.01$). None of those who underwent ultrasound cardiographic examination had cardiac dysfunction (ejection fraction, 50–82 %; fraction shortening (FS), 25–50 %). Mean serum CK level was 459.1 ± 355.0 IU/L (median, 202; range, 11–3133).

The patient registry is useful in that it allows for recruiting patients and resolving data deviation in comparison with analyses by isolated institutions. For example, the age at disease onset in the Remudy cohort was later than that determined from an analysis of medical records at the NCNP Hospital (26.8 ± 9.0 years). In a previous questionnaire-based study of core muscle disease center patients, we reported median durations from disease onset to walking with assistance, wheelchair use, and loss of ambulation of 7.0 ± 0.4 years, 11.5 ± 1.2 years, and 17.0 ± 2.1 years, respectively [8], which were all shorter than the durations determined in the present study. We speculate that this discrepancy reflects the more advanced disease status of patients at neuromuscular disease-specialized center hospitals. Patients with GNE myopathy were widely distributed throughout Japan, with 1.7 patients per hospital and 1.3 patients per physician. There were fewer patients per physician or per hospital than for dystrophinopathy (5.8 patients per hospital and 3.6 per physician). Thus, while patients with GNE myopathy appeared to be dispersed throughout Japan, those with dystrophinopathy were concentrated in specialized hospitals, given the need for cardiopulmonary care.

We have been publishing bulletins every 3 months and sending them to patients and physicians who join Remudy. The bulletin includes useful information regarding clinical care, translational medicine, and clinical trials, as well as articles introducing specialists and specialized hospitals for muscle diseases. These contents are available on the Remudy home page. Patient recruitment has also started for additional phase I clinical trials via the Remudy GNE myopathy registry home page [14].

10.2 Discussion

Through the three studies presented herein, we revealed various new aspects of GNE myopathy. First, unlike previous reports, we found that GNE myopathy is associated with respiratory dysfunction. Indeed, some patients required a respirator, indicating that respiratory dysfunction can be life threatening in this population. Physicians should take careful note of any abnormalities in respiratory function, which may serve as an evaluation tool for disease progression and therapeutic effects in the late stages of the disease. Notably, respiratory failure was not considered to be associated with GNE myopathy, despite GNE myopathy being one of the most common muscle diseases in Japan. One reason for this is that physicians may be of the mindset that respiratory failure does not derive from myopathy itself, given the small number of affected patients they see. Second, given that GNE myopathy is progressive, walk tests such as the 6MWT and other quantitative methods, and respiratory function for nonambulant patients, may be useful evaluation items for annual disease progression and clinical trials. Finally, patient registries are useful for rare diseases such as GNE myopathy, as it allows for the building of a larger cohort, which can be used to assess more accurately etiologic aspects of the disease compared to medical record surveys from specialized hospitals. Such registries are also useful in that they allow for recruiting patients and resolving data deviation in comparison with analyses by isolated institutions.

The direct motivation to conduct these studies stemmed from the need to prepare for upcoming clinical trials and follow the development of new therapies and improved care methods. Comparisons with animal disease models will also provide insight into new symptoms, which in turn may provide insight into patient care. We note that our patients were very cooperative, as they were aware of the importance of these studies in driving the development of new therapies.

We recognize that a large cohort study is essential to gain a better understanding of rare diseases, including progression and potential risk factors. Yet our data were not sufficient to make conclusive genotype–phenotype correlations, so this will be an important aspect for further elucidation of the disease pathogenesis. Thus, studies similar to those described herein with a larger cohort are warranted.

Similar to our collaborations with the dystrophinopathy registry, we are currently in discussions to join the international registry of GNE myopathy of the TREAT-NMD Alliance [ClinicalTrials.gov; identifier, NCT01784679, http://www.treat-nmd.eu/gne/patient-registries/patient-registries/]. Our Japanese registry and the TREAT-NMD Alliance registry work in close collaboration and will serve as irreplaceable infrastructures that accelerate research, therapy development, and trial readiness, in addition to increasing opportunities for collaboration and improving global patient care.

Acknowledgments We thank members of the Patients Association for Distal Myopathies (PADM) in Japan. This work was partly supported by Health and Labor Sciences Research Grants for research on rare and intractable diseases from the Ministry of Health, Labor, and Welfare and Intramural Research Grants (26-7) for Neurological and Psychiatric Disorders from the NCNP.

References

1. Nonaka I, Sunohara N, Satoyoshi E et al (1985) Autosomal recessive distal muscular dystrophy: a comparative study with distal myopathy with rimmed vacuole formation. Ann Neurol 17:51–59
2. Argov Z, Yarom R (1984) "Rimmed vacuole myopathy" sparing the quadriceps. a unique disorder in Iranian Jews. J Neurol Sci 64:33–43
3. Nishino I, Noguchi S, Murayama K et al (2002) Distal myopathy with rimmed vacuoles is allelic to hereditary inclusion body myopathy. Neurology 59:1689–1693
4. Eisenberg I, Avidan N, Potikha T et al (2001) The UDP-N-acetylglucosamine 2-epimerase/N-acetylmannosamine kinase gene is mutated in recessive hereditary inclusion body myopathy. Nat Genet 29:83–87
5. Kayashima T, Matsuo H, Satoh A et al (2002) Nonaka myopathy is caused by mutations in the UDP-N-acetylglucosamine-2-epimerase/N-acetylmannosamine kinase gene (GNE). J Hum Genet 47:77–79
6. Keppler OT, Hinderlich S, Langner J et al (1999) UDP–GlcNAc 2-epimerase: a regulator of cell surface sialylation. Science 284:1372–1376
7. Malicdan MC, Noguchi S, Hayashi YK et al (2009) Prophylactic treatment with sialic acid metabolites precludes the development of the myopathic phenotype in the DMRV-hIBM mouse model. Nat Med 15:690–695
8. Mori-Yoshimura M, Monma K, Suzuki N et al (2012) GNE myopathy (distal myopathy with rimmed vacuoles) patients with mutations in the UDP-GlcNAc 2-epimerase and in the *N*-acetylmannosamine kinase domains of the GNE gene exhibit less severe phenotypes than patients with mutations only in MNK domain. J Neurol Sci 318(1–2):100–105

9. Mori-Yoshimura M, Oya Y, Hayashi YK, Noguchi S, Nishino I, Murata M (2013) Respiratory dysfunction in patients severely affected by GNE myopathy (distal myopathy with rimmed vacuoles). Neuromuscul Disord 23:84–88
10. Cho A, Hayashi YK, Monma K et al (2014) Mutation profile of the GNE gene in Japanese patients with distal myopathy with rimmed vacuoles (GNE myopathy). J Neurol Neurosurg Psychiatry 85:914–917
11. Malicdan MC, Noguchi S, Nonaka I et al (2007) A Gene knockout mouse expressing human GNE D176V mutation develops features similar to distal myopathy with rimmed vacuoles or hereditary inclusion body myopathy. Hum Mol Genet 16:2669–2682
12. Mori-Yoshimura M, Oya Y, Yajima H et al (2014) GNE myopathy: a prospective natural history study of disease progression. Neuromuscul Disord 24:380–386
13. Nakamura H, Kimura E, Mori-Yoshimura M, Komaki H, Matsuda Y, Goto K, Hayashi YK, Nishino I, Takeda SI, Kawai M (2013) Characteristics of Japanese Duchenne and Becker muscular dystrophy patients in a novel Japanese national registry of muscular dystrophy (Remudy). Orphanet J Rare Dis 19:60
14. UMIN CTR website. https://upload.umin.ac.jp/cgi-open-bin/ctr/ctr.cgi?function=brows&action=brows&type=summary&recptno=R000013489&language=J

Chapter 11
Patient Registries for International Harmonized Clinical Development

En Kimura and Harumasa Nakamura

Abstract In this chapter, the role of patient registry and importance of the international harmonization to make a step toward progress in clinical development in orphan diseases are discussed. Remudy, Registry of Muscular Dystrophy, operated by the NCNP, National Center of Neurology and Psychiatry, Japan, runs two national registries for dystrophinopathy and GNE myopathy under the collaboration with the TREAT-NMD alliance. The aim of Remudy is to construct clinical research infrastructure and accelerate clinical development research for these rare diseases in Japan. We successfully disclose data sets for the feasibility studies in response to enquiries, send out appropriate information of clinical trials for the candidates to gear up for recruitment, as well as present the natural history and epidemiological data of the rare diseases with a new "registry-based" research style. Remudy provides a prototype of the clinical research infrastructure to overcome rare and incurable diseases.

Keywords Remudy • Patient registry • Rare disease • International harmonization • TREAT-NMD

11.1 Introduction

"Ichi-nichi mo hayaku" means "longing for the day" by Dr. Hisanobu Kaiya, administrative director of the Japanese Muscular Dystrophy Association, Corp., JMDA (http://www.jmda.or.jp), which is a slogan of the JMDA and also an official journal title of this 51-year-old patient's advocacy organization. To deliver curative treatment for patients and family of the rare, orphan, and incurable diseases is a wish of all concerned in this field. Based on the remarkable progress of basic research in molecular biology field, researchers have successfully clarified pathomechanism and achieved the "proof-of-concept" of treatment using animal models of the diseases. Following these successes, clinical applications of these results have been expected, related especially to molecular target strategies such as

E. Kimura (✉) • H. Nakamura
Translational Medical Center, National Center of Neurology and Psychiatry, 4-1-1 Ogawa-Higashi, 187-8551 Kodaira, Tokyo, Japan
e-mail: enkimura@ncnp.go.jp

S. Takeda et al. (eds.), *Translational Research in Muscular Dystrophy*,
DOI 10.1007/978-4-431-55678-7_11

development of read-through agents [1] and exon-skipping therapies [2, 3] as curative treatments, which people really desire to be approved as the medication of the rare and incurable diseases, especially for Duchenne and Becker muscular dystrophies (DMD/BMD, dystrophinopathy). Actually, some clinical trials for new therapeutic strategies for dystrophinopathy are currently in operation or being planned. During the process, many challenges still exist in the planning and conducting of a clinical trial for rare diseases, in which dystrophinopathy is classified. The epidemiological data, the total number of patients, natural history, and clinical outcome measures are unclear or less well understood, although an adequate number of patients are needed to achieve significant results in clinical trials.

11.2 Rising of Global Tides of the Clinical Research Infrastructure Development with International Harmonization

To solve these problems, a patient registry is considered as an important infrastructure worldwide. In 2007, TREAT-NMD (*T*ranslational *R*esearch in *E*urope: *A*ssessment and *T*reatment of *N*euro*m*uscular *D*iseases), as a network of excellence for neuromuscular diseases, was established with the aim of "reshaping the research environment" in the neuromuscular field and to support translational research [4], by the original Sixth Framework Programme (FP6) grant from the European Union (EU) between 2007 and 2011. The National Institutes of Health (NIH) in the United States of America and the national institutes in Asian and Oceanian countries participated in TREAT-NMD. From 2012, it evolved into the international TREAT-NMD alliance with worldwide activity. TREAT-NMD developed a global database for DMD/BMD (dystrophinopathy) [5] and spinal muscular atrophy (SMA) patients [6] both in and out of Europe, to obtain epidemiological data, examine the total number of patients, determine the natural history of the disease, determine appropriate clinical outcome measures, collect adequate numbers of patients needed to achieve significant results in clinical trials, and inform patients of new drug development. This was achieved in part by the formation of a harmonized set of national DMD patient registries with a common data-sharing philosophy, comprising both new registries set up to follow the TREAT-NMD guidelines and existing national registries who agreed to follow them. Information collected follows a mandatory or highly encouraged set of questions agreed on by the TREAT-NMD global database oversight committee. As a result, information can be shared and compared between the different national registries, with the ultimate goal of all national registries eventually linking into a centralized global DMD registry. Actually, at the international level, the registries had been used for feasibility and recruitment in at least ten studies, following enquiries from researchers and industries.

As of 2014, in addition to DMD/BMD (dystrophinopathy) and SMA, the list of ten different disease patient registries was found on the TREAT-NMD website (http://www.treat-nmd.eu). Internationally, myotonic dystrophy (DM), congenital muscular dystrophies (CMD), congenital myasthenic syndrome (CMS), Charcot-Marie-Tooth disease (CMT), facioscapulohumeral muscular dystrophy (FSHD), hereditary inclusion body myopathy (GNE/HIBM), limb-girdle muscular dystrophy (LGMD) including fukutin-related protein (FKRP), myotubular and centronuclear myopathy (MTM/CNM), and dysferlinopathy are in operation.

11.3 Establishment and Operation of Japanese National Registry for Dystrophinopaty

In Japan, muscular dystrophy research groups have a history of close to 50 years, which were funded by the Nervous and Mental Disorders from the Ministry of Health, Labour, and Welfare (by March 2011) and are now by Intramural Research Grant for Neurological and Psychiatric Disorders of the National Center of Neurology and Psychiatry, Japan (NCNP, from April 2011), and achieved distinguished and world-leading researches in this field. To date, several Japanese dystrophinopathy databases have been developed; however, these have not been on a broad national scale. For instance, some were on a single-center basis, and others encompassed only a small local area or several hospital sites [7–9]. Some others were restricted to inpatients only [10]. Despite these early efforts, no national registry has been developed with the purpose of focusing on clinical trials.

In 2009, Dr. Mitsuru Kawai with his national research group and the NCNP developed a national registry of Japanese dystrophinopathy patients, Remudy (*Re*gistry of *Mu*scular *Dy*strophy) (http://www.remudy.jp/), in collaboration with the Japanese national muscular dystrophy research groups, 27 traditional muscular dystrophy wards, and hospitals belonging to the National Hospital Organization (NHO) and the NCNP, the Japanese Muscular Dystrophy Association, and finally the TREAT-NMD [11]. This project has been funded by the Nervous and Mental Disorders from the Ministry of Health, Labour, and Welfare (20B-12; between 2008 and 2011), and by Intramural Research Grant for Neurological and Psychiatric Disorders of the NCNP (23-4; 2011–2014, 26-7; 2014-) and supported by helpful cooperation with the JMDA. The development and management of the registry is led by the principal investigator of the Japanese muscular dystrophy research group. Steering committee members include scientists, clinicians, and representatives of patient organizations. The registry office was set up in the NCNP. The purpose of this registry was to effectively recruit eligible patients to new clinical trials and provide timely information to patients about upcoming trials. The data included clinical and molecular genetic information as well as all items required for the TREAT-NMD global patient registry. Registry data also provides more detailed knowledge about the natural history and epidemiology of the disease, as well as information about clinical care.

The database includes dystrophinopathy patients whose genetic status was confirmed by genetic analysis throughout Japan. As the cost of sequencing analysis of the DMD gene is not covered by the public health insurance in Japan, for patients who intend to register but are not genetically confirmed by the multiplex ligation-dependent probe amplification (MLPA) for *dystrophin* gene, Remudy provides free service of sequencing analysis of the *dystrophin* gene. Information about the registry was provided to interested individuals, who could easily access to the "case report form" and the "informed consent form" in the Remudy website or at the registry office. Provision of all data by patients is voluntary and is not shared with any third party without the permission of the committee responsible for disclosing the information. Inclusion in the database confers no obligation on the patient, and they may be removed from the registry immediately on request. It was stated that refusal to participate would not affect the subsequent medical care of the patient. The National Center of Neurology and Psychiatry Ethics Committee approved this registration system. Data obtained via the registry form included clinical symptoms, results of biochemistry, muscle biopsy, other laboratory analysis, and description of the genetic mutation. Epidemiological information provided includes walking capability, cardiac and respiratory functions, serum creatine kinase, history of scoliosis surgery, and steroid therapy status. All items were confirmed by their attending physicians and, finally, by molecular and clinical curators in Remudy (three active molecular and clinical curators each). Information was annually updated by registrant's self-report with their physician's confirmation following reminder from registration office. To decide whether a patient was classified as DMD or BMD, first, the attending physician made a diagnosis whether a patient was DMD or BMD by the clinical and molecular information. Then, our clinical and genetic curators double-checked their classification by reviewing clinical information and also data from pathological (including dystrophin immunohistchemical staining, if applicable) and genetic analysis.

As of May 2014, 1,293 patients were registered in the Remudy dystrophinopathy registry from all over Japan (Figs. 11.1 and 11.2). To analyze the data from July 2009 to May 2014, information of 1,173 patients were confirmed by the curators. Data from 1,171 patients, who agreed to participate in this study, were analyzed. It comprises of 940 DMD, 201 BMD, and 30 IMD patients, respectively (Fig. 11.3). All the registrants in Remudy database got genetic diagnosis as dystrophinopathy by MLPA for *dystrophin* gene and/or direct sequencing analysis of the *dystrophin* gene which was provided by Remudy. At the end of December 2013, we have well analyzed the *dystrophin* gene in 340 out of 342 cases. In case of single exon deletion/duplication reported by the MLPA methods, the corresponding exon and the neighbor exons were sequenced (41 %). In case of no deletion/duplication reported by the MLPA methods, whole 79 exons were sequenced (59 %). Based on the precise curation system, distribution of mutation in the registrants with dystrophinopathy was shown in Table 11.1. Most frequent mutation was deletion (60.6 % of DMD, 76.9 % of BMD, and 47.1 % of IMD). Second frequent was other

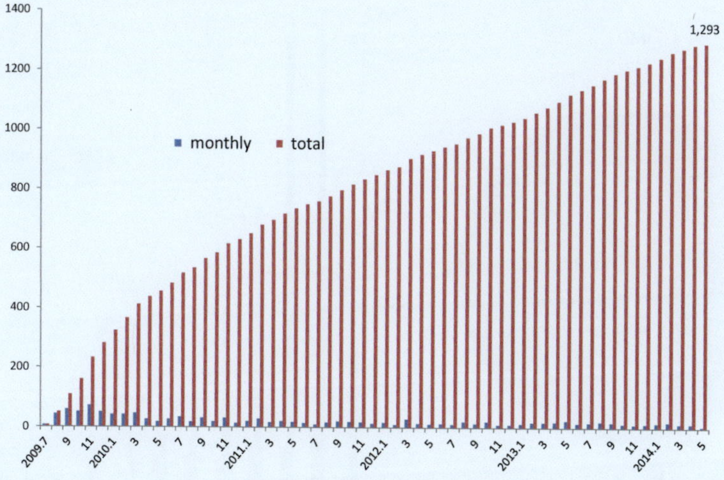

Fig. 11.1 Number of registrants in Remudy national dystrophinopathy registry. As of May 2014, 1,293 patients were registered in this national registry from all over Japan. *Blue bars* show monthly registered number; *red bars* show total number accumulated since the start of the registry. Total number of registrants is still increasing

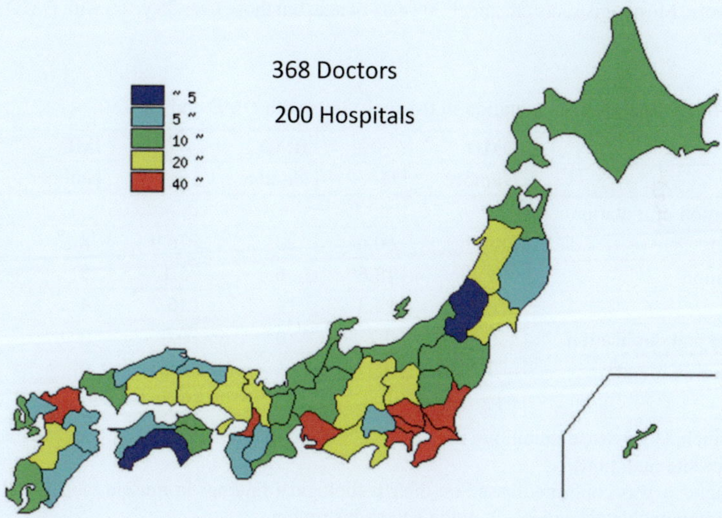

Fig. 11.2 Prefectural distribution of registrants in Remudy national dystrophinopathy registry. Dystrophinopathy patients from every prefecture in Japan are registered in this registry by cooperation of 368 doctors in 200 hospitals. Most registrants were concentrated in populated area: Fukuoka, Osaka, Aichi, and Kanto region

mutations (24.3 % of DMD, 16.2 % of BMD, and 23.5 % of IMD) which included nonsense mutations, small insertion/deletion mutations, deep intronic mutations, and splice site mutations. Then third frequent was duplication (13.6 % of DMD,

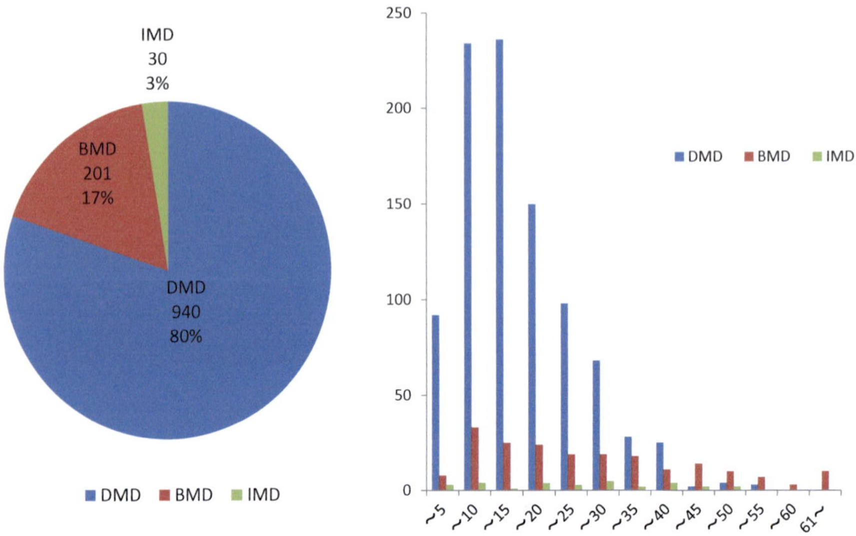

Fig. 11.3 Diagnosis and age distribution of registered individuals. Data from 1,171 patients who have agreed to participate in this study and confirmed by molecular and clinical curators were analyzed. It comprises of 940 (80 %) DMD, 201 (17 %) BMD, and 30 (3 %) IMD patients, respectively. Most registrants are under 20 years of age, but those over 35 years with DMD are also registered

Table 11.1 Distribution of mutation in the registrants with DMD and BMD

	DMD		BMD		IMD	
	Number	%	Number	%	Number	%
Distribution of mutation						
Deletion	388	60.6	90	76.9	8	47.1
Duplication	87	13.6	6	5.1	5	29.4
Others[a]	163	24.3	19	16.2	4	23.5
Deletion and duplication	1	0.2	0	0.0	0	0.0
No mutation found[b]	1	0.2	2	1.7	0	0.0
	640	100	117	100	17	100

[a]Others include nonsense mutations, small insertion/deletion mutations, deep intronic mutations, and splice site mutations

[b]The diagnosis was confirmed based on their pathological findings in muscle biopsy including a negative immunohistochemical staining against dystrophin

5.1 % of BMD, and 29.4 % of IMD, Fig. 11.3). Clinical features of Japanese dystrophinopathy patients are shown in Table 11.2, which are available on the Remudy website to all concerned, including patients, family, and doctors who care for the dystrophinopathy patients, for download. Frequency of individual exon deletions was shown in Fig. 11.4.

Remudy already supplied the epidemiological data for 11 feasibility studies, and provided timely information about two independent clinical trials to registrants who

Table 11.2 Clinical manifestations of Japanese dystrophinopathy patients in Remudy database

	DMD		BMD		IMD	
	Number	%	Number	%	Number	%
Walking capacity						
Normal walking	328	40.2	125	74.4	7	26.9
Not able to walk and sit without support	252	30.9	38	22.6	10	38.5
Not able to sit without support	229	28.1	5	3.0	9	34.6
Before development	6	0.7	0	0.0	0	0.0
Cardiac function						
Normal	516	63.3	120	71.4	13	50.0
Dysfunction	277	34.0	47	28.0	13	50.0
Not performed	22	2.7	1	0.6	0	0.0
Respiratory function						
Normal	619	76.0	163	97.0	17	65.0
Dysfunction	162	20.0	3	2.0	6	23.0
Not performed	34	4.0	2	1.0	3	11.0
Steroid use						
Current	264	32.4	8	4.8	6	23.1
Used to	103	12.6	6	3.6	3	11.5
Never	447	54.8	154	91.7	17	65.4
Total	815	100	168	100	26	100

Detailed information is available on the Remudy website (http://www.remudy.jp)

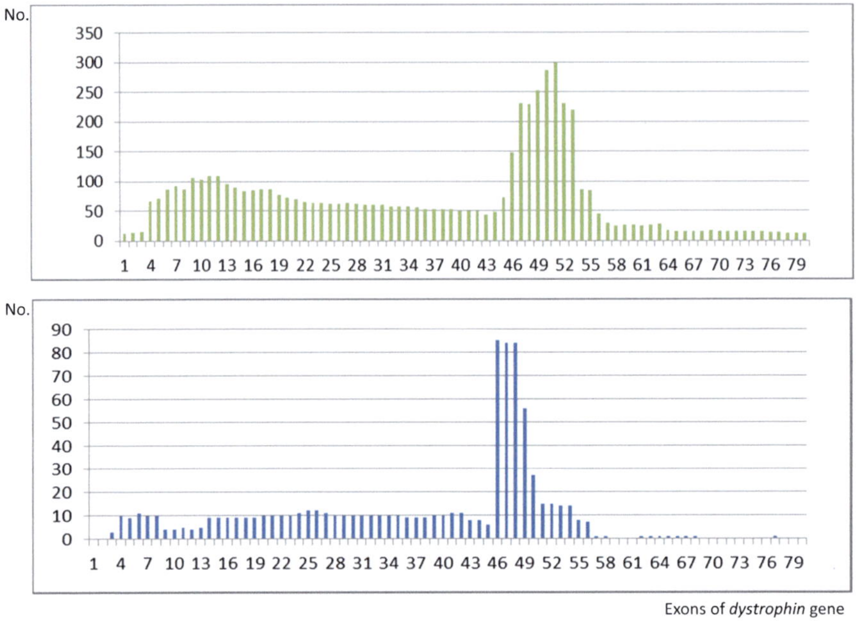

Fig. 11.4 Frequency of individual exon deletions. The distribution of exon deletion shows common hot spot regions in exon 45–54 in DMD and BMD

might be eligible for upcoming clinical trials, and accelerated the effective recruitment of eligible patients as expected. To inform the public of the activity of Remudy, we sent a paper version of "Remudy news," "Remudy news letter" by e-mail, and frequently renewed news page on Remudy website. Remudy news volume 11 was published with 1,781 copies in June 2014, Remudy news letter volume 50 was sent out to 648 subscribers, and the Remudy website traffic count was 1,845 during June 2014. We also hosted local lecture meetings for medical experts and patients all over Japan. In 2013, we sent out the questionnaires for medical providers throughout Japan in 2013 to clarify how Remudy was well known. We found nearly 75 % of medical providers knew about the Remudy activity.

11.4 Importance of Clinical Research Arisen from Registry Data Analysis

This registry data also provides more detailed knowledge about natural history, epidemiology, and clinical care. Especially, a natural history data regarding ambulation of DMD patients in 2013 was reported to solve a research question which arose from the Japanese DMD guideline committee [12]. In this study, we evaluated

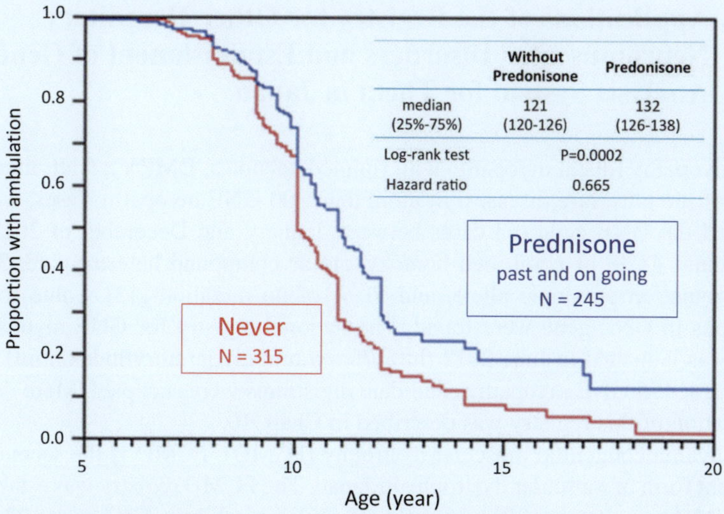

Fig. 11.5 Long-term efficacy of prednisolone (PSL) for prolonging ambulation among genetically confirmed DMD patients in Japanese dystrophinopathy national registry (Remudy). Of the 560 patients included, 245 (43.8 %) were in PSL treatment group, and 315 (56.2 %) were without PSL treatment. Both groups consist of ambulant patients aged 5, 10, and 15 years, and the number breakdown by age was 242, 136, and 8 for the PSL treatment group and 311, 145, and 10 for without-PSL group, respectively. The median age at loss of ambulation was 10.1 years for the patients in without-PSL treatments group and 11.0 years in the PSL treatment group. Patients treated with PSL were able to ambulate significantly 11 months longer than those without PSL

the long-term efficacy of prednisolone (PSL) for prolonging ambulation among 560 Japanese DMD patients who were genetically confirmed. The time of loss of ambulation in patients with prednisolone (PSL) treatment (n = 245) was 11 months longer than that of those without PSL treatment (n = 315) (Fig. 11.5). This is the largest cross-sectional objective study in the world. This research spun off into another survey research to ask the effective resume of steroid treatment for DMD, such as dosage, intervals, starting age, and adverse side effect if any, since there was no registry item regarding these.

In our research group, Dr. Kawai estimated the number of DMD patients in Japan would be about 3,500 at the end of March 2013, according to the annual numbers of boy's birth data in Japan and the life chart data of DMD from the NHO hospital database, which closed to the number expected from Akita prefecture's data on Remudy. This information is frequently asked and needed by pharmaceutical companies when considering new products for DMD and also demanded by persons in charge of neuromuscular field in the regulatory agency, Pharmaceuticals and Medical Devices Agency, Japan.

11.5 Applications of the Registry for Other Hereditary Neuromuscular Disorders and Establishment of Gene Analysis System for Them in Japan

GNE myopathy (distal myopathy with rimmed vacuoles, DMRV): GNE myopathy is one of the ultra-rare diseases. In more than 300 GNE myopathy cases, we have analyzed the GNE gene (63 cases between January and December of 2013) and have found 41 % of confirmed homozygote or compound heterozygote, 3 % of single mutation on single allele, and 51 % of no mutation [13]. Some frequent mutations in GNE gene were found. The national registry for GNE myopathy in Japan was launched in June 2012 (http://www.remudy.jp/dmrv/index.html). As of June 2014, 155 GNE myopathy candidate registrants were accepted. More detailed information of this registry was described in Chap. 10.

Fukuyama congenital muscular dystrophy (FCMD): FCMD is the second most prevalent form of muscular dystrophy in Japan. The FCMD registry was established by the JMDA on October 2011 (http://www.jmda.or.jp/kiko/). By January 23, 2014, 165 candidate registrants were accepted. Every year, the questionnaires for registrants were sent out, and those results were reported at the research group meeting and JMDA website and then were reflected to the activity of the branch meeting for FCMD patients in the JMDA.

Myotonic dystrophy and other myotonia syndromes: The arrangement meeting for the myotonic dystrophy registry started at February 2012. We have planned the curators training, set up the registry items, and collected and regulated experts' opinions. We prepared the DM registry office at the Department of Neurology, Osaka University. The application of DM registry has been reviewed by the ethical committee in Osaka University and is currently under review at the NCNP. DM registry will be launched in October 1, 2014. This DM registry may cover other myotonia syndromes. The advanced gene analysis methods for Myotonic dystrophy type 1 and 2 were also examined in the NCNP.

Spinal muscular atrophy (SMA): SMA registry was launched in August 2012 and run by the Institute of Medical Genetics, Tokyo Women's Medical University (Prof. Kayoko Saito, http://www.sma-rt.org). As of July 2013, more than 100 candidate registrants were accepted.

Oculopharyngeal muscular dystrophy (OPMD): The *PABPN1* gene mutations were detected in 99 patients (84 families), according to Dr. Narihiro Minami in the NCNP [14]. The opposite correlation was found between GCN repeat numbers and the age of onset. Japanese OPMD national registry is now in preparation with nationwide collaboration.

Dysferlinopathy (Miyoshi myopathy, limb-girdle muscular dystrophy type 2B, LGMD2B, anterior tibial myopathy): Dr. Toshiaki Takahashi in the NHO Sendai Nishitaga National Hospital reported that 42 independent mutations among affected 91 families were determined by PCR-SSCP method and then 31 independent mutations among affected 45 families by whole 55 exon sequencing method [15]. Also, the next-generation sequencing for dysferlinopathy, considered as a useful tool as well as for other LGMD, will be ready to use in several institutes in Japan. Dysferlinopathy national registry is also planned with Remudy research group.

In addition, registries for congenital muscular dystrophies (CMD) [16], congenital myasthenic syndrome (CMS) [17], facioscapulohumeral muscular dystrophy (FSHD) [18], and limb-girdle muscular dystrophy (LGMD) have been planned as well.

Preparation of the new advanced web registration system: We studied safe and efficient way of patient self-registry and developed a new web-based registration system under collaborations with Hitachi Solutions, Ltd. Because of high-standard security within ethical guidelines, in addition, stability, and applicability, this excellent system will be useful for other rare diseases as well as many common disorders.

11.6 International and Nationwide Research Harmonization for Rare Diseases

From 1999, the Cooperative International Neuromuscular Research Group (CINRG) was developed as a consortium of medical and scientific investigators from over 20 international academic and research centers. The CINRG coordinating center is located in the Children's Research Institute of Children's National Medical Center in Washington, DC, USA. The goal of CINRG is to contribute to the research and the treatment of neuromuscular diseases by studying the causes, pathogenesis, and clinical outcomes of the diseases and also by conducting well-controlled clinical studies that examine promising therapeutic interventions that may improve or extend quality of life for patients. To date, CINRG has completed six [19, 20] and is currently running four clinical studies. Both in and out of Europe, TREAT-NMD alliance has developed a global database for dystrophinopathy patients to promote clinical trials for new therapeutic strategies, as tools to study the epidemiology [5], burden of the DMD [21], as well as other neuromuscular disorders, as described above. CARE-NMD (http://en.care-nmd.eu), a European project improving care for DMD, led by Dr. Janbernd Kirschner, Freiburg University, part-funded by the EU between May 2010 and April 2013, brought together leading care centers to disseminate information about best-practice DMD care and to implement international consensus care standards. The CARE-NMD patient survey of care and quality of life to the national dystrophinopathy registries across seven partner countries in EU, already collecting almost 1,100 responses, expanded to other national registries belongs to TREAT-NMD, internationally. In 2013, the CARE-NMD family survey in Japan was carried out under collaboration with CARE-NMD project and the Muscular Disease Center at the NCNP directed by Dr. Hirofumi Komaki. This survey presented the current conditions and problems of DMD patients and families, clarified some similarities and differences among the countries including western and eastern European countries and Japan, and was also useful for providing the patients information about the care and cure for DMD.

We have also discussed the role of the Remudy as a prototype among the rare disease infrastructure for the clinical research. We participated in every related meetings, such as the meeting for rare and intractable diseases held every other month with the concerned persons in some pharmaceutical companies and the preparation meetings for patient registries in January and February 2013, led by Dr. Tomonori Tateishi (former NCNP, present PMDA). In the first international workshop in Japan for rare disease registries in July 2013, the international key speakers from Europe, the United States, and China were invited, and domestic speakers working for each patient registry discussed the collaboration among the rare disease registries, followed by a second domestic workshop for rare disease registries in July 2014, both managed by Dr. Hiroshi Mizushima and our group (http://www.remudy.jp). At the symposium in the 34th Annual Meeting of The Japanese Society of Clinical Pharmacology and Therapeutics, we discussed the roles and the recent status of patient registries in clinical research in Japan. Among these activities, we confirmed importance of the harmonization of patients and families, medical providers, and other stakeholders, such as pharmaceutical industries, researchers, patient advocacies, and the regulatory agency.

11.7 Discussion and Plan for Next Step

Today in the drug development field, operation of international clinical trials have been discussed across the world. In Japan, various international trials have already been done or are in operation. Information regarding adequate dosage, administration, efficacy, and safety of the candidate agents in Japanese people are important for review and approval in Japan, even though clinical trials do not have to be done as international trials. It was impossible to recruit participants who met inclusion criteria of each study in a single country. For example, 174 nonsense mutation DMD patients participated in an international late phase II trial for ataluren (PTC124, Translarna™), and more than 300 DMD patients who had particular mutation altered by exon 51 skipping therapy from 25 countries participated in 5 clinical trials to develop drisapersen. Now, it is an important strategy to plan and operate international harmonization at the early phase of development and to investigate racial variation of drug efficacy and safety concurrently in many hereditary neuromuscular diseases, which are classified into rare diseases. At the present day, some other international clinical trials for DMD patients are running, such as phase II/III study of coenzyme Q10 and lisinopril and phase III study of tadalafil. Domestic clinical trials for unique drug development in Japan are also running such as phase II study of arbekacin sulfate (NPC-14) as a read-through agent and exploratory study of NS-065/NCNP-01 as an exon 53 skip agent. In addition, clinical development of medical devices draws an awful lot of attention at the moment. One major example is the currently ongoing multicenter clinical trial of a robot suit HAL being designed as a tool for neuromuscular rehabilitation.

Recently, in June 2014, Prosensa, a leading company developing exon-skipping agents for DMD, announced regulatory path forward for drisapersen as a potential treatment for DMD, with a plan to submit a new drug application to the FDA in 2014. Dialogue with EMA continues with the intent to seek approval. In August 2014, PTC Therapeutics received conditional approval in the EU for Translarna™ (ataluren) for the treatment of nonsense mutation DMD.

To conclude, Remudy, the patient registry for the neuromuscular disorders, is the first national registry for rare diseases including both clinical and molecular information in Japan to lead to the clinical developmental studies and to enable revealing nationwide epidemiological data. We run the Remudy successfully so far, because of the accurate gene analysis system, cooperation of patients, families, advocacy groups, medical providers, and carefully planned operation system including the steering committee as well as international collaboration. We continue to run this system, to expand the target diseases, and to step forward to develop a new system covering the whole rare and intractable diseases with other research groups. The patient registries are now recognized as a useful tool to accelerate clinical research of various rare diseases. Further, we will promote this infrastructure for clinical research to complement the pitfall of the national intractable disease registries now being planned as one of the effective measures to overcome the diseases by the Ministry of Health, Labour, and Welfare, Japan, especially prepared for deduction of patient's medical expenses. Our proposed new registry system will make the healthcare administration of the government more satisfactory.

Acknowledgments We thank all the registered patients and their families, their cooperative doctors, the Japanese Muscular Dystrophy Association and other patient advocacy groups, members of the Remudy office and gene analysis department, and supportive administrative persons, especially Dr. Mitsuru Kawai, chair of NHO Higashi-Saitama Hospital, and Prof. Shin'ichi Takeda, chair of Translational Medical Center, the National Center of Neurology and Psychiatry, Japan. The Remudy and its research projects have been supported by the Nervous and Mental Disorders from the Ministry of Health, Labour, and Welfare (20B-12, 2008–2011), Intramural Research Grant for Neurological and Psychiatric Disorders of the NCNP (23-4, 2011–2014, 26-7, 2014-), and the Policy Research for Intractable Diseases, Health and Labour Sciences Research Grant, Ministry of Health, Labour, and Welfare.

References

1. Welch EM, Barton ER, Zhuo J et al (2007) PTC124 targets genetic disorders caused by nonsense mutations. Nature 447:87–91
2. Mann CJ, Honeyman K, Cheng AJ et al (2001) Antisense-induced exon skipping and synthesis of dystrophin in the mdx mouse. Proc Natl Acad Sci U S A 98:42–47
3. Yokota T, Lu QL, Partridge T et al (2009) Efficacy of systemic morpholino exon-skipping in Duchenne dystrophy dogs. Ann Neurol 65:667–676

4. Mercuri E, Mayhew A, Muntoni F et al (2008) Towards harmonisation of outcome measures for DMD and SMA within TREAT-NMD; report of three expert workshops: TREAT-NMD/ENMC workshop on outcome measures, 12th–13th May 2007, Naarden; TREAT-NMD workshop on outcome measures in experimental trials for DMD, 30th June–1st July 2007, Naarden; conjoint Institute of Myology TREAT-NMD meeting on physical activity monitoring in neuromuscular disorders, 11th July 2007, Paris, Neuromuscul Disord 18:894–903
5. Bladen CL, Rafferty K, Straub V et al (2013) The TREAT-NMD Duchenne muscular dystrophy registries: conception, design, and utilization by industry and academia. Hum Mutat 34:1449–1457
6. Bladen CL, Thompson R, Jackson JM et al (2014) Mapping the differences in care for 5,000 spinal muscular atrophy patients, a survey of 24 national registries in North America, Australasia and Europe. J Neurol 261:152–163
7. Takeshima Y, Yagi M, Okizuka Y et al (2010) Mutation spectrum of the dystrophin gene in 442 Duchenne/Becker muscular dystrophy cases from one Japanese referral center. J Hum Genet 55:379–388
8. Matsumura T, Saito T, Fujimura H, Shinno S, Sakoda S (2012) Lung inflation training using a positive end-expiratory pressure valve in neuromuscular disorders. Intern Med 51:711–716
9. Ishikawa Y, Miura T, Ishikawa Y et al (2011) Duchenne muscular dystrophy: survival by cardio-respiratory interventions. Neuromuscul Disord 21:47–51
10. Saito T, Tatara K (2012) Database of wards for patients with muscular dystrophy in Japan. In: Hegde M, Ankala A (eds) Muscular dystrophy. Intech, Rijeka, pp 247–260
11. Nakamura H, Kimura E, Mori-Yoshimura M et al (2013) Characteristics of Japanese Duchenne and Becker muscular dystrophy patients in a novel Japanese national registry of muscular dystrophy (Remudy). Orphanet J Rare Dis 8:60
12. Takeuchi F, Yonemoto N, Nakamura H et al (2013) Prednisolone improves walking in Japanese Duchenne muscular dystrophy patients. J Neurol 260:3023–3029
13. Mori-Yoshimura M, Okuma A, Oya Y et al (2012) Clinicopathological features of centronuclear myopathy in Japanese populations harboring mutations in dynamin 2. Clin Neurol Neurosurg 114:678–683
14. Nagashima T, Kato H, Kase M et al (2000) Oculopharyngeal muscular dystrophy in a Japanese family with a short GCG expansion (GCG)(11) in PABP2 gene. Neuromuscul Disord 10:173–177
15. Takahashi T, Aoki M, Suzuki N et al (2013) Clinical features and a mutation with late onset of limb girdle muscular dystrophy 2B. J Neurol Neurosurg Psychiatry 84:433–440
16. Yonekawa T, Komaki H, Okada M et al (2013) Rapidly progressive scoliosis and respiratory deterioration in Ullrich congenital muscular dystrophy. J Neurol Neurosurg Psychiatry 84:982–988
17. Ohkawara B, Cabrera-Serrano M, Nakata T et al (2014) LRP4 third beta-propeller domain mutations cause novel congenital myasthenia by compromising agrin-mediated MuSK signaling in a position-specific manner. Hum Mol Genet 23:1856–1868
18. Goto K, Nishino I, Hayashi YK (2006) Rapid and accurate diagnosis of facioscapulohumeral muscular dystrophy. Neuromuscul Disord 16:256–261
19. Henricson EK, Abresch RT, Cnaan A et al (2013) The cooperative international neuromuscular research group Duchenne natural history study: glucocorticoid treatment preserves clinically meaningful functional milestones and reduces rate of disease progression as measured by manual muscle testing and other commonly used clinical trial outcome measures. Muscle Nerve 48:55–67
20. Escolar DM, Buyse G, Henricson E et al (2005) CINRG randomized controlled trial of creatine and glutamine in Duchenne muscular dystrophy. Ann Neurol 58:151–155
21. Landfeldt E, Lindgren P, Bell CF et al (2014) The burden of Duchenne muscular dystrophy: an international, cross-sectional study. Neurology 83:529–536

Chapter 12
Muscular Dystrophy Clinical Trial Network in Japan

Katsuhisa Ogata

Abstract Muscular dystrophy is a rare disease, affecting less than 0.01 % of the population. The establishment of clinical trial networks between medical institutes reportedly helps to improve readiness for trials on rare diseases such as muscular dystrophy. Some networks for clinical research on neuromuscular diseases have already been established in other parts of the world. The Muscular Dystrophy Clinical Trial Network (MDCTN) was established in 2012 to promote and activate clinical research on neuromuscular diseases in Japan. This network was organized based on an existing study group for clinical myology funded by a Japanese national research grant and is a network of national hospitals with wards specifically for patients with progressive neuromuscular disorders. As of April 2015, 33 medical institutions had joined this network. Site registry queries have revealed that approximately 6000 patients with neuromuscular diseases visit the member hospitals annually. The work of the MDCTN includes sharing updates in healthcare information, developing standardized means of evaluation through workshops, supporting clinical trials with feasibility surveys and patient recruitment, and conducting collaborative research. Working closely with patient registries is one of the keys to the functioning of this network. The MDCTN has collaborated with one patient registry, Remudy, to support remarkably rapid recruitment of subjects with Duchenne muscular dystrophy who meet criteria of specific genetic mutations and conditions for some clinical trials. The goal of MDCTN is to be a model for developing pharmaceuticals and medical devices for rare diseases in Japan.

Keywords Muscular Dystrophy Clinical Trial Network • Rare disease • Neuromuscular disease • Clinical trial network • Patient registry • Remudy

---

K. Ogata (✉)
Institute of Clinical Research, National Hospital Organization Higashisaitama Hospital, 4147 Kurohama, Hasuda, Saitama 349-0196, Japan
e-mail: ogataneu@nhs.hosp.go.jp

S. Takeda et al. (eds.), *Translational Research in Muscular Dystrophy*,
DOI 10.1007/978-4-431-55678-7_12

12.1 The Importance of Organizing a Network of Clinical Sites for Studies on Muscular Dystrophy

Muscular dystrophy is a rare disease, affecting less than 0.01 % of the population [1]. The elucidation of molecular pathophysiology in many subtypes of muscular dystrophies has enabled the introduction of various therapeutic approaches, such as antisense oligonucleotide drugs and stop codon readthrough therapy [2]. Clinical trials of epochal drugs for muscular dystrophy have been planned and are running [3–5].

Rare diseases pose many challenges that are specific to their scarcity. Improvement in readiness for clinical trials for muscular dystrophy is desirable to facilitate progress in research and new drug development.

The establishment of clinical trial networks between medical institutes reportedly helps to improve readiness for trials on rare diseases such as muscular dystrophy for the following reasons: it facilitates recruitment of patients and standardization of clinical backgrounds and trial procedures, improves efficiency and effectiveness of clinical trial management, and is a step toward establishing a global network [6].

Because it is difficult to conduct meaningful clinical studies with few subjects, the accumulation of disease information is important in that it can inform the design of clinical trial protocols. For this reason, collaboration between the clinical trial network and patient registry is indispensable.

Standardization of clinical background is necessary for reliable evaluation of safety and efficacy of new drugs. Guidelines for care and therapeutic procedures are useful in this respect [7]. Naturally, standardized outcome measures are also needed for effective clinical trials. Planning of good outcome measures and mastering them are essential for good trial design and operation.

Because there are few clinics with experience in caring for patients with rare diseases and conducting research in the field, establishing a specialized professional network improves clinical trial readiness and facilitates cooperation with a global network. A well-organized network enables efficient operation and management of clinical trials.

12.2 Existing Clinical Trial Networks for Neuromuscular Diseases

12.2.1 TREAT-NMD

Initially established in 2007, TREAT-NMD is an EU-funded network for reshaping the research environment in the neuromuscular field [8]. Many projects have been established within this network, including patient registries, support for molecular diagnosis, care and trial site registries, outcome measures research and validation, standards of care guidelines, advisory committee for therapeutics, animal models, a biobank, engagement with regulatory authorities, a regulatory affairs database, and advisory support for industry.

The TREAT-NMD Care and Trial Site Registry (CTSR), an online self-registration database of information on clinical sites, was established in 2007 [6]. As of October 2014, 320 centers for neuromuscular diseases in 48 countries had joined this registry.

This network has developed from its European roots to become a global organization that brings together leading specialists, patient groups, and industry representatives to ensure preparedness for trials and therapies of the future while promoting best practice today.

12.2.2 Cooperative International Neuromuscular Research Group (CINRG)

The CINRG was established in 1999 as a consortium of medical and academic investigators from academic and research centers in the USA for the purpose of contributing to improvement in therapies for neuromuscular diseases by conducting further observational studies and well-controlled clinical trials [9]. Today, CINRG is a global, state-of-the-art clinical research network, with 28 sites from 12 countries worldwide.

12.2.3 Australasian Neuromuscular Network (ANN)

Established in 2010, ANN is an alliance between Australia and New Zealand for diagnosis, research, therapy, and advocacy of patients with neuromuscular diseases; it collaborates with TREAT-NMD and CINRG [10]. The goal of ANN is to improve health outcomes of patients with neuromuscular diseases by providing best practice in diagnosis, care, and treatment, ready access to standards of care, a unified approach to ethical approvals and consent, improved communication, integrated training programs for clinicians and researchers, assistance for setting up multidisciplinary services, providing a single voice to advocate for patients, and notification of opportunities to participate in registries, research studies, and clinical trials.

12.3 The History of Clinical Research on Muscular Dystrophy in Japan

From 1964, wards specifically for patients with progressive neuromuscular disorders have been established in 27 national hospitals in Japan, including the National Center of Neurology and Psychiatry (NCNP) [11]. National research grants for muscular dystrophy from the Ministry of Health and Welfare of Japan were also initiated in 1964. Four study groups were established with these grants: basic myology, pathology and molecular pathophysiology, clinical myology, and multidisciplinary care for patients. These study groups have formed an alliance that functions as an integrated network for research on muscle and muscular diseases.

Clinical research on muscular dystrophy in Japan has developed in collaboration with universities and national hospitals contributing to myology, with financial support by the government.

With the transformation of the national hospitals and NCNP into independent administrative institutions in 2004 and reorganization of national research grants for muscular dystrophy in 2010, establishing a clinical research network for neuromuscular diseases was necessary.

12.4 Muscular Dystrophy Clinical Trial Network (MDCTN): A Clinical Trial Network for Neuromuscular Diseases in Japan

The MDCTN was established in 2012 based on the preexisting experiences and network of wards specifically for persons with muscular dystrophy and a clinical myology research group [12]. It is the first clinical research network for neuromuscular diseases in Asia.

The four main purposes of the MDCTN are to improve patient recruitment, develop an infrastructure for clinical trials, cooperate with and support clinical studies, and improve communication about research among member institutes (Fig. 12.1).

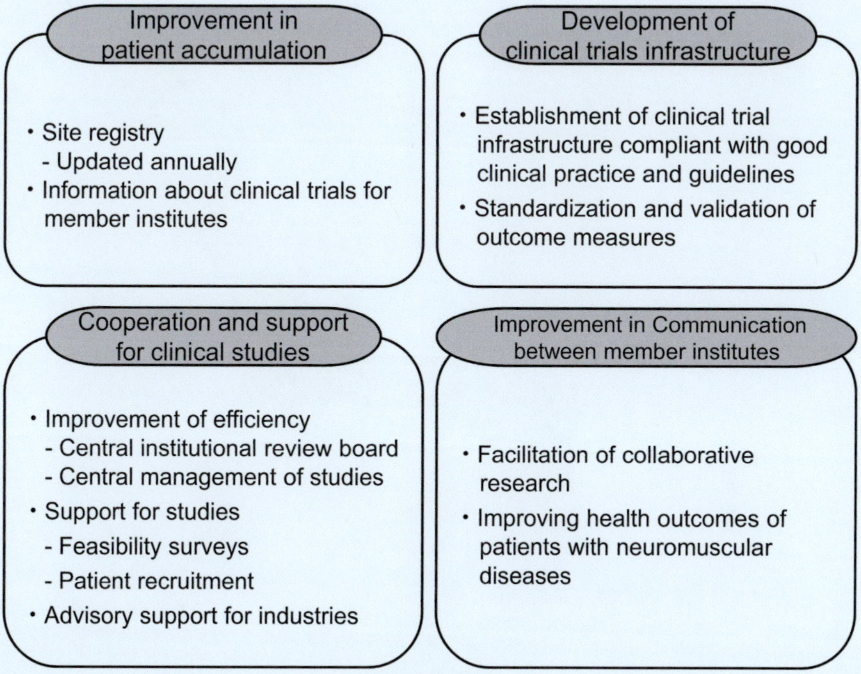

Fig. 12.1 Main purposes and resources of the MDCTN

As of April 2015, 33 clinical institutes distributed over all four main islands of Japan have joined the MDCTN (Fig. 12.2); these comprise 17 hospitals of the National Hospital Organization, one national center (NCNP), 12 university hospitals and institutes, one prefectural hospital, one hospital of a local welfare organization, and one private hospital.

According to the data from the annual site registry as of December 2014, approximately 6000 patients with neuromuscular diseases visit MDCTN member hospitals annually. In decreasing order, their neuromuscular diseases are Duchenne muscular dystrophy 29 %, myotonic dystrophy type 1 21 %, limb-girdle muscular dystrophy 11 %, Becker muscular dystrophy 10 %, facioscapulohumeral muscular dystrophy 6 %, Fukuyama congenital muscular dystrophy 6 %, spinal muscular atrophy 6 %, congenital myopathy 4 %, mitochondrial disorder 4 %, congenital

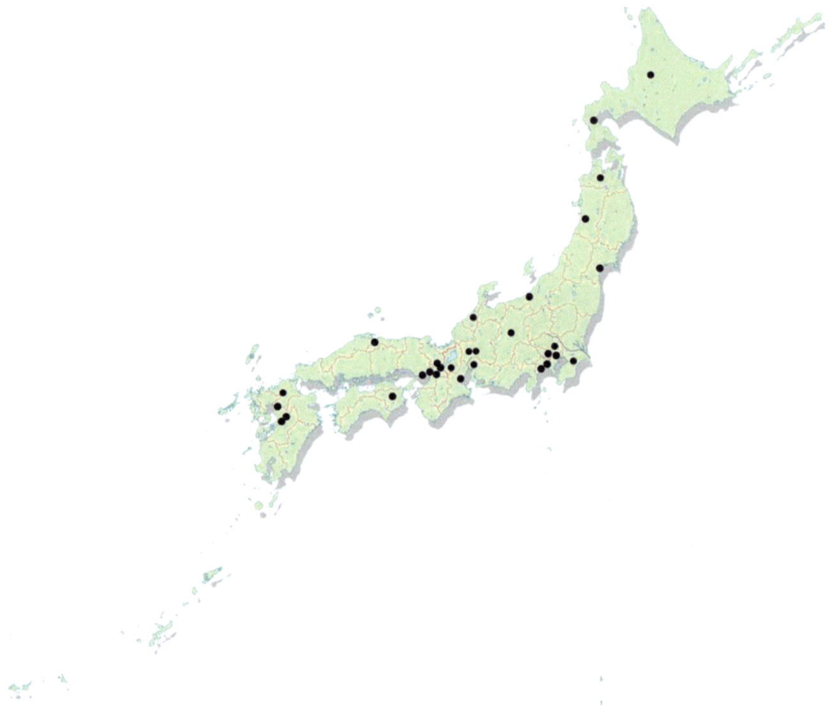

Fig. 12.2 Locations of the member institutes of the MDCTN. As of April 2015, 33 institutes located on all four main islands of Japan had joined the MDCTN

muscular dystrophy excluding Fukuyama type 3 %, and GNE myopathy 2 % (Fig. 12.3).

Pulmonary function testing, continuous pulse oximetry, standard 12-lead electrocardiography, and Holter electrocardiography are available for functional evaluation in all member institutes. Additionally, blood gas analysis, transthoracic echocardiography, electromyography, muscle magnetic resonance imaging, muscle biopsy, 6-min-walk testing, 10-m-timed walk testing, and timed up-and-go testing are available in more than 90 % of member institutes. Institutional review boards have been established in all member institutes.

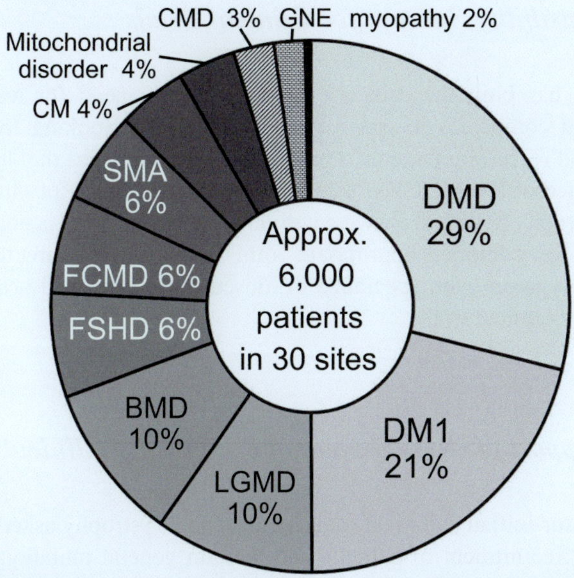

Fig. 12.3 Composition of overall patient cohort under the auspices of the MDCTN. As of December 2014, approximately 6000 patients with neuromuscular diseases were visiting the 30 MDCTN member hospitals annually. *BMD* Becker muscular dystrophy, *CM* congenital myopathy, *CMD* congenital muscular dystrophy excluding Fukuyama type, *DMD* Duchenne muscular dystrophy, *DM1* Myotonic dystrophy type 1, *FCMD* Fukuyama congenital muscular dystrophy, *FSHD* facioscapulohumeral muscular dystrophy, *LGMD* limb-girdle muscular dystrophy, *SMA* spinal muscular atrophy

12.5 The Activities of MDCTN in Japan

12.5.1 Propagation of Information and Education

The MDCTN holds annual workshops to share opinions and information regarding updates in research and current and promising therapies, these workshops being open to network members, pharmaceutical companies, patient advocacy groups, members of regulatory agencies, and anyone else with an interest in MDCTN activities. The MDCTN also has regular meetings with representatives of member institutes for communication purposes. As a component of its working group activities, the MDCTN also holds seminars about neuromuscular diseases and standardized evaluation for physical therapists and clinical research coordinators. These seminars and workshops are generally well received because they provide a great opportunity for communication between physical therapists and clinical research coordinators from different institutes.

12.5.2 Feasibility Surveys for Clinical Trials

The MDCTN has built the capacity to eliminate the need for researchers and pharmaceutical companies to spend their valuable time looking for cooperative researchers and recruiting patients. Pharmaceutical companies that have asked the secretariat office of the MDCTN to investigate the feasibility of clinical trials on muscular dystrophy have had answers within a few weeks. This is possible because the MDCTN has compiled appropriate forms that are sent directly to possible principal investigators who specialize in muscular diseases and are interested in participating in clinical trials.

12.5.3 Support for Recruitment of Patients for Clinical Trials

Two investigator-initiated clinical trials on muscular dystrophy asked the MDCTN for support in recruitment of patients with certain genetic mutations through the patient registry, Remudy [13]. Patient recruitment for one of these studies was completed within only 2 months. However, at the time of writing, the MDCTN was still working on recruitment for the other study because some possible participants were excluded by more detailed exclusion criteria or because they lived too far from the participating site. Otherwise, participants are assigned quickly from the start.

These experiences have demonstrated that tight coordination between the patient registry and clinical trial network greatly facilitates recruitment of patients. The patient registry can be used to rapidly identify and hence recruit participants with specific genotypes and physical conditions who are eligible for the proposed clinical trials.

12.5.4 Collaborative Research

The infrastructures for clinical trials on muscular dystrophy are still inadequate. Nationwide epidemiological information about some ultra-rare diseases is not yet available. It is very hard to establish adequate end points for some gradually progressive diseases, including muscular dystrophy, that lack reliable biomarkers that would enable accurate assessment of disease status. Thus, epidemiological surveys and development of outcome measures are important for improving clinical research into many rare diseases.

The MDCTN's collaborative research program currently includes some ongoing epidemiological studies and a study aimed at developing good outcome measures for muscular dystrophy.

12.6 The Goal of MDCTN, as a Clinical Research Network for Rare Diseases in Japan

The MDCTN was organized for the purpose of serving as "a model of development of pharmaceuticals and medical devices for rare diseases in Japan" and providing infrastructure to support multi-institutional clinical research into promising avenues for improving health care of persons with rare diseases such as muscular dystrophy. This network helps industry–academia collaboration and coordinates connections between muscular disease research specialists. The MDCTN is also working on communication between the patient registry and cooperating sites to enable smooth execution of clinical trials, standardized means of evaluation, and clinical research education. Sharing updates in health-care information and standardization of evaluation among the cooperating sites make it possible to activate quality clinical research even though muscular dystrophy is a rare disease.

Effective use of the clinical research infrastructure provided by the patient registry is a powerful means of recruiting patients with rare diseases and supporting the education of such patients about ongoing clinical research, thus making it easier to gain their consent to participate in clinical trials. This activity will facilitate clinical research with high-quality outcomes and thus contribute to improvements in patient care and treatment options. Moreover, the MDCTN is a useful model for clinical research on rare diseases.

Conflict of Interest The author has no potential conflict of interest concerning this article.

Acknowledgments The author is deeply grateful to the member institutes of the MDCTN, namely, the National Hospital Organization (NHO) Asahikawa Medical Center, NHO Yakumo Hospital, NHO Aomori Hospital, NHO Sendai-Nishitaga National Hospital, NHO Akita National Hospital, NHO Higashisaitama Hospital, NHO Shimoshizu National Hospital, Tokyo Women's Medical University (Department of Pediatrics, Department of Neurology, and Institute of Medical Genetics), National Center of Neurology and Psychiatry, Kitasato University (Department of Orthopedic Surgery), NHO Hakone Hospital, NHO Niigata National Hospital, NHO Iou Hospital, Muscular Dystrophy Network in Nagano Prefecture (representative: Shinshu University), Shinano Iryofukushi Center, Gifu University (Department of Pediatrics), NHO Nagara Medical Center, Nagoya City University (Department of Neonatology and Pediatrics), NHO Suzuka National Hospital, Shiga Medical Center for Children, NHO Utano Hospital, Kyoto City Hospital, NHO Toneyama National Hospital, Osaka University (Department of Neurology), Kobe University (Department of Pediatrics), Hyogo College of Medicine (Department of Pediatrics), Tottori University (Division of Child Neurology), NHO Tokushima National Hospital, Bunyuukai Hara Hospital, NHO Omuta Hospital, Kumamoto University (Department of Pediatrics), and NHO Kumamoto Saishunso National Hospital, as of April 2015. The author is also sincerely grateful to the members of the MDCTN steering committee and secretariat office, especially Dr. Hirofumi Komaki, Dr. En Kimura, Dr. Reiko Shimizu, Dr. Eri Takeshita, Ms. Akemi Tamaura, Ms. Maki Ohata, Ms. Mikiko Shigemori, and Dr. Shin'ichi Takeda (NCNP, Japan). The MDCTN has been supported by Intramural Research Grants (23–6, 26–6) for Neurological and Psychiatric Disorders of NCNP.

References

1. Bushby K, Finkel R, Birnkrant DJ, Case LE, Clemens PR, Cripe L et al (2010) Diagnosis and management of Duchenne muscular dystrophy, part 1: diagnosis, and pharmacological and psychosocial management. Lancet Neurol 9:77–93
2. Leung DG, Wagner KR (2013) Therapeutic advances in muscular dystrophy. Ann Neurol 74:404–411
3. Mendell JR, Rodino-Klapac LR, Sahenk Z, Roush K, Bird L, Lowes LP et al (2013) Eteplirsen for the treatment of Duchenne muscular dystrophy. Ann Neurol 74:637–647
4. Voit T, Topaloglu H, Straub V, Muntoni F, Deconinck N, Campion G et al (2014) Safety and efficacy of drisapersen for the treatment of Duchenne muscular dystrophy (DEMAND II): an exploratory, randomised, placebo-controlled phase 2 study. Lancet Neurol 13:987–996
5. Bushby K, Finkel R, Wong B, Barohn R, Campbell C, Comi GP et al (2014) Ataluren treatment of patients with nonsense mutation dystrophinopathy. Muscle Nerve 50:477–487
6. Rodger S, Lochmüller H, Tassoni A, Gramsch K, König K, Bushby K et al (2013) The TREAT-NMD care and trial site registry: an online registry to facilitate clinical research for neuromuscular diseases. Orphanet J Rare Dis 8:171
7. Sejersen T (2012) Standards of care in neuromuscular disorders. Neuromuscul Disord 22:872
8. TREAT-NMD Neuromuscular Network website. http://www.treat-nmd.eu/. Accessed 1 May 2015
9. The Cooperative International Neuromuscular Research Group website. http://www.cinrgresearch.org/. Accessed 1 May 2015
10. Australasian Neuromuscular Network website. http://www.ann.org.au/. Accessed 1 May 2015
11. Saito T, Tatara K (2012) Database of wards for patients with muscular dystrophy in Japan. In: Hedge M, Ankala A (eds) Muscular dystrophy. Intech, Rijeka, pp 247–260
12. Muscular Dystrophy Clinical Trial Network website. http://www.mdctn.jp/. Accessed 1 May 2015
13. Nakamura H, Kimura E, Mori-Yoshimura M, Komaki H, Matsuda Y, Goto K et al (2013) Characteristics of Japanese Duchenne and Becker muscular dystrophy patients in a novel Japanese national registry of muscular dystrophy (Remudy). Orphanet J Rare Dis 8:60

Chapter 13
Translational Research on DMD in Japan

From Mice to Exploratory Investigator-Initiated Clinical Trial in Human

Shin'ichi Takeda and Tetsuya Nagata

Abstract Currently, antisense oligonucleotides (AONs)-mediated exon skipping therapy is the most promising therapy for Duchenne muscular dystrophy. We performed preclinical studies using dystrophic *mdx52* mice and $CXMD_J$ dystrophic dogs to obtain proof of concept of AONs-mediated exon skipping therapy. Then, Japan participated in the worldwide clinical trials of drisapersen (Phase III). Finally, we developed a new AON targeting exon 53 in collaboration with Nippon Shinyaku Co., Ltd. in Japan and started an investigator-initiated clinical study at the National Center Hospital of NCNP (Phase I). This early phase exploratory study is the first clinical trial of an AON developed in Japan and a good example of translational research for treatment of DMD in Japan. In this chapter, we summarize the long development of the drug and discuss the future direction of splicing therapy for DMD.

Keywords Duchenne muscular dystrophy • Exon 53 • Exon skipping • Morpholino • Reading frame • Dystrophin • Splicing • Investigator-initiated clinical trial

13.1 Mechanisms of Exon Skipping Therapy

Duchenne muscular dystrophy (DMD) is the most common X-linked genetic disease, affecting one in 3500 newborn boys. DMD is caused by mutations in the gene that encodes the 427-kDa cytoskeletal protein dystrophin. Dystrophin protects the muscle cell membrane from damage during muscle contraction. DMD muscle fibers deficient in dystrophin gradually degenerate due to repeated mechanical stress and are lost, resulting in progressive muscle weakness [1]. Cardiomyopathy and respiratory dysfunction are two major causes of premature death of DMD

S. Takeda (✉) • T. Nagata
Department of Molecular Therapy, National Institute of Neuroscience (NIN), National Center of Neurology and Psychiatry (NCNP), 4-1-1 Ogawa-Higashi, 187-8502 Kodaira, Tokyo, Japan
e-mail: takeda@ncnp.go.jp

S. Takeda et al. (eds.), *Translational Research in Muscular Dystrophy*,
DOI 10.1007/978-4-431-55678-7_13

patients. Although prednisolone is proven to slow the deterioration of muscle function in DMD patients to some extent [2], there is no satisfactory therapy for this devastating disease.

Exon skipping by antisense oligonucleotides (AONs) is a strategy to restore the reading frame of the mutated DMD gene by artificial elimination of one or two (or more) exons from pre-mRNAs during the splicing process (not at the genome level) and rescue dystrophin expression. Correctly exon-skipped mRNAs are translated into truncated but still functional dystrophin. The idea of exon skipping by interference with normal splicing of DMD transcripts using AONs was first proposed by Dr. Matsuo at Kobe University [3–5]. Later, Dunckley et al. demonstrated the exon skipping approach in myotube culture of cells derived from *mdx* mice using 2′OMeRNA [6]. In 2001, van Deutekom reported that AONs-induced exon skipping restores dystrophin expression in muscle cells derived from DMD patients [7]. Exon skipping in vivo using AONs has been accomplished in *mdx* mice by local injection [8] and systemic delivery [9, 10].

13.2 AON Chemistry

In current clinical studies, two types of AONs, 2′-*O*-methyl phosphorothioate oligonucleotides (2′OMePSs) and phosphorodiamidate morpholino oligos (PMOs), are being used. The effectiveness of exon skipping by AONs largely depends on chemical modifications of the backbone of the AON. Therefore, new AONs with new chemical modifications and backbones are still under development (Table 13.1).

1. *2′-O-Methyl-phosphorothioate oligonucleotide (2′OMePS)*
   Drisapersen (GSK2402968/PRO051) is a successful example of a 2′OMePS-based AONs targeting exon 51. Although statistically significant improvement in the 6-min walking distance test (6MWT; [12]) was not evident in the Phase III trial of drisapersen, BioMarin and Prosensa have recently announced completion of the submission of a New Drug Application (NDA) for drisapersen to the US Food and Drug Administration (FDA) (http://investors.bmrn.com/releasedetail.cfm?ReleaseID=908731). BioMarin also expressed its intention to submit a marketing authorization application for drisapersen in the European Union in the summer of 2015.
2. *Phosphorodiamidate morpholino oligos (PMOs)*
   Eteplirsen (AVI-4658) (Sarepta Therapeutics, formerly AVI BioPharma, http://www.sarepta.com) is a morpholino-based AONs targeting exon 51 of the DMD gene. Among a variety of AONs tested for exon skipping in animal models, the PMOs is reported to be the safest. For example, *mdx* mice reportedly tolerate a 3-g/kg dose [13]. In human, Sarepta employed a high dose (30 or 50 mg/kg) of eteplirsen for a long period (48 weeks) to cause exon skipping in clinical trials (Phase IIb) on DMD patients without severe side effects [14].

Table 13.1 Comparison of antisense oligonucleotides for clinical and preclinical use

Chemical	Chemical characteristics	Advantages	Disadvantages
2'-O-methylphosphorothioate (2'O-MePS) 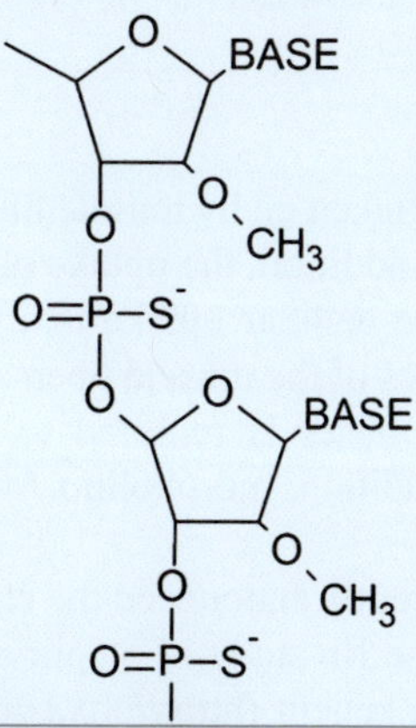	Negatively charged	Good solubility – long half-life Nuclease and RNase H resistant	Do not enter the heart Toxicity
Morpholino (PMO) 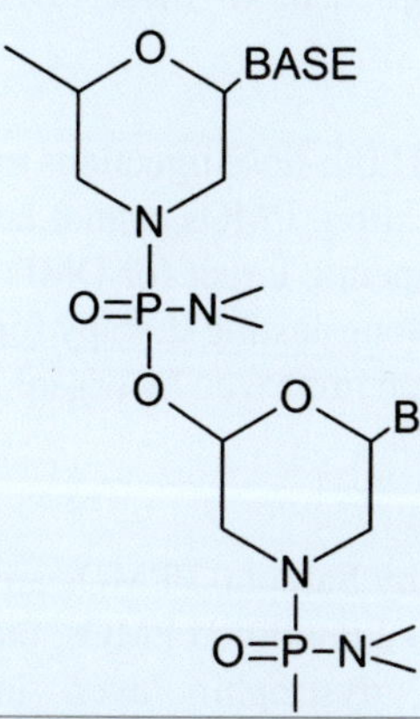	Uncharged	Relatively safe Nuclease and RNase H resistant Stable No interaction with cellular proteins No activation of innate immune responses	Does not enter the heart Rapid renal clearance, Poor cellular uptake
Cell-penetrating peptide-conjugated PMOs (PPMOs)	Conjugation of cell-penetrating peptides to PMOs	Enhanced cellular delivery Effective in vivo delivery Enter cardiac cells	Toxicity
Vivo-morpholinos (vPMOs)	Conjugation of dendrimeric octa-guanidine to PMOs	Enter cardiac muscle Effective at lower dose	Toxicity
Tricycle-DNA (tcDNA)	tc-DNA deviates from natural DNA by	Increased RNA affinity and hydrophobicity Nuclease resistant Do	Toxicity

(continued)

Table 13.1 (continued)

Chemical	Chemical characteristics	Advantages	Disadvantages
	three additional C-atoms between C(5′) and C(3′)	not activate RNase H Enter the heart and cross blood–brain barrier [11]	

Weaknesses of PMOs are that PMOs are poorly taken up by muscle fibers and are excreted in urine soon after administration. In addition, the uptake of PMOs by muscle is not uniform. It is suggested that the cellular uptake is a passive process, probably through leaky plasma membranes of the muscle fibers. Therefore, repeated administration of PMOs in high doses is required to sustain therapeutic levels of dystrophin expression. In addition, morpholino AONs do not enter cardiac cells.

Sarepta has completed Phase IIb studies and recently announced the results of long-term outcomes through 168 weeks of a Phase IIb study of eteplirsen. The results showed a statistically significant treatment benefit (http://phx.corporate-ir.net/mobile.view?c=64231&v=200&d=1&id=2006709). Sarepta now plans to submit an NDA by mid-2015 after collecting more data to meet FDA requirements.

3. *Modified PMOs*

   Unmodified PMOs require frequent (weekly or biweekly) high-dose injections to maintain therapeutic levels of dystrophin protein. In addition, PMOs cannot be delivered to cardiac muscle, which is an important therapeutic target for DMD. To avoid frequent administration and lower the dose for long-lasting therapy for DMD boys and hopefully target the heart, PMOs have been improved by organic chemists.

   - *Cell-penetrating peptide-conjugated PMOs (PPMOs)*

     AVI-5038, targeting exon 50, is a PPMO developed by Sarepta. PPMOs are actively taken up by the cells. Therefore, compared to unmodified PMOs, far lower doses of PPMOs can restore sufficient dystrophin even in cardiomyocytes. A disadvantage of PPMOs is that they have dose-dependent toxicity. High doses of PPMO caused adverse effects, such as lethargy, weight loss, and tubular degeneration in kidneys of rats [15, 16].
   - *Vivo-morpholinos (vPMOs)*

     vPMOs contain a cell-penetrating moiety, an octa-guanidine dendrimer. Due to this modification, vPMOs are actively taken up by cells. As expected, vPMOs are reported to lead to extensive and prolonged dystrophin expression in the dystrophic *mdx* mouse, an animal model of DMD, at a relatively low dose ([17–19]; Echigoya et al., [20]). vPMOs also effectively induced exon skipping in dystrophic dogs in vivo [21].

4. *Tricycle-DNA (tcDNA) oligomers*
   Goyenvalle et al. reported the development of tricycle-DNA (tcDNA) oligomers, as a promising tool for exon skipping therapy of DMD. *Mdx* mice treated with high doses of tcDNA AONs (200 mg/kg/week for 12 weeks) showed improved cardiac function and reduced freezing response [11], which characterizes the neurological defects of *mdx* mice [22]. The authors also reported that tcDNA has a higher propensity to spontaneously self-assemble into nanoparticles. The authors speculate that this property explains efficient uptake of tcDNA by the cells and therefore efficient exon skipping in vivo.

   To achieve high concentrations of AONs in the muscle, further development of new types of AONs is in progress. Tissue-specific delivery systems for AONs are also important to achieve efficient and safe exon skipping with low doses of AONs.

13.3 Preclinical Studies Using Dystrophic Animal Models

13.3.1 Mdx52 *Mice*

Although many exon skipping studies have been performed on *mdx* mice, which have a nonsense mutation in exon 23, a type of mutation that is rare in human, therefore, we used *mdx52* mice, in which exon 52 has been deleted by a gene targeting technique [23] for preclinical study. We designed more than 10 AONs covering exon 51 of the mouse DMD gene and injected them intramuscularly into *mdx52* mice. The highest splicing efficiency was generated by a two-oligonucleotide cocktail targeting both the 5′ and 3′ splice sites of exon 51. We systemically injected the cocktail into *mdx*52 mice seven times at weekly intervals. This protocol induced 20–30 % of wild-type dystrophin expression in all muscles and was accompanied by amelioration of the dystrophic pathology and improvement of skeletal muscle function [24]. This study provided proof of concept for exon 51 skipping in the DMD animal model. Then, we participated in one of the global trials of exon 51 skipping using drisapersen (Phase III). Exon 51 skipping is estimated to be applicable for up to 13 % of all DMD patients, representing the largest patient population treatable by a single-exon skipping strategy.

13.3.2 CXMD$_J$ Dogs

We established a colony of dystrophic dogs (CXMD$_J$) in Japan [25]. The beagle is smaller and more widely used in pharmaceutical research than the golden retriever. Therefore, the original golden retriever muscular dystrophy dogs (GRMD) were crossed with beagles seven times. Using beagle-CXMD$_J$ dystrophic dogs, which harbor a splice site mutation at the boundary of intron 6 and exon 7, we performed systemic administration of a mixture of AONs simultaneously targeting both exons 6 and 8 of the canine DMD gene. In treated $CXMD_J$ dogs, truncated dystrophin proteins were expressed at the sarcolemma, and the performance of affected dogs was significantly improved without serious side effects [26]. The results convinced us that systemic delivery of PMOs for exon skipping is safe and effective, except to cardiac muscle. We also confirmed that the AONs that were effective in the dystrophic dogs also worked in cells from an exon 7-deleted DMD patient [27].

13.4 Phase I Investigator-Initiated Exploratory Study in NCNP Hospital

In 2009, we started development of AONs, which allow exon 53 skipping of the DMD gene together with Nippon Shinyaku Co., Ltd. (http://www.nippon-shinyaku.co.jp/english/). Targeting exon 53 is applicable to DMD patients with deletions of dystrophin exons 42–52, 45–52, 47–52, 48–52, 49–52, 50–52, and 52. In Japan, 300–400 patients are estimated to be treatable by exon 53 skipping. NS-065/NCNP-01 is a newly developed PMO-based AON that skips exon 53 of the dystrophin gene. After the efficacy and safety were confirmed in preclinical studies, a dose escalation study was designed to evaluate the systemic delivery of NS-065/NCNP-01 by intravenous infusion once per week for 12 weeks to three cohorts. The primary endpoint of the trial was safety, and the secondary endpoints were pharmacokinetics and dystrophin expression. Ten subjects, aged 6–14 years responsive to exon 53 skipping, were recruited through REMUDY (Chap. 11) and randomly allocated to one of the three cohorts. In vitro confirmation of exon 53 skipping and dystrophin recovery in subject-derived cells [27] was one of the inclusion criteria. At the end of 2014, administration to all subjects had been completed. The initial analysis detected dystrophin mRNA with the amino acid reading frame restored by exon 53 skipping in every dose group. Furthermore, the expression of dystrophin protein that appeared to have been translated from such an mRNA was detected in the high-dose group. In addition, no serious adverse event was observed throughout the study, and no subject discontinued administration. Anemia and increases in some renal parameters were observed as general adverse events. The analysis of data from the study is still ongoing and will be published elsewhere. As the next step, ambulatory patients should be treated with dose escalation. Using the results of the investigator-initiated clinical trial, Nippon Shinyaku is preparing for the next stage of clinical development with a view to launching this product in Japan in 2018.

13.4.1 Evaluation of the Efficacy of Exon Skipping

In our Phase I study, we assessed the safety of the drug as the primary endpoint. For approval of the drug, how to evaluate the clinical outcomes remains controversial. Although 6MWT, which measures the distance an individual is able to walk in 6 min on a hard, flat surface, is a well-accepted, widely used measurement of cardiac, respiratory, circulatory, and muscular function in DMD (https://www.thoracic.org/statements/resources/pfet/sixminute.pdf), whether 6MWT is suitable for primary endpoint to meet for future clinical trials for DMD is under discussion.

13.5 Next Strategy for Exon Skipping Therapy

13.5.1 Delivery to Cardiac Muscle

Many DMD patients die due to cardiac dysfunction. Since unmodified PMOs or 2′OMePSs do not enter cardiomyocytes, the development of new AONs that can reach cardiac muscle has been awaited. vPMOs or PPMOs are PMOs modified to be efficiently taken up by cardiac cells. In fact, these modified PMOs show higher efficiency in exon skipping in the heart than unmodified PMOs and 2′OMePSs. Importantly, however, modified PMOs have been reported to be cytotoxic at higher doses [16]. The mechanisms of the side effects of modified PMOs remain to be determined. In addition to AON chemistry, the development of a muscle-specific delivery system is important.

13.5.2 Targeting Minor Exons

Exon skipping is a personalized medicine in that the exon to be skipped is different for each patient. At present, the development of AONs by pharmaceutical companies is focusing on exons that will benefit large numbers of patients, e.g., exon 51 (13 %), 45 (8.1 %), or 53 (7.7 %). For other exons, development is delayed. To accelerate drug development for rare mutations, we should appeal to the regulatory agency to change the rules. In fact, the FDA released "Guidance for Industry Duchenne Muscular Dystrophy Developing Drugs for Treatment over the Spectrum of Disease" on September 4, 2014. It seems that input from the DMD disease community is lowering the hurdles for regulatory approval of candidate drugs to treat DMD.

13.5.3 Targeting Multiple Exons

Multiple exon skipping targeting exons 45–55 (11 exons), the mutation hotspot of the DMD gene, is estimated to be capable of ameliorating the dystrophic symptoms of as many as 63 % of all DMD patients. Several experimental studies reported successful multiple exon skipping by using a cocktail of AONs in murine [17, 20] and canine [21, 28] models. In the near future, multiple exon skipping by a combination of AONs may be tested in DMD patients.

13.6 Perspective on Future Reading Frame-Restoring Therapy for DMD

1. *Genome editing in stem cells*
   Out-of-frame mutations can be transformed into in-frame mutations by using genome editing techniques. Hotta's group at the Center for iPS Cell Research and Application, Kyoto University, showed that TALEN and CRISPR/Cas9 systems can restore the reading frame of the mutated DMD gene (from severe DMD-type to benign Becker-type mutations) by generating small deletions or insertions at the targeted site [29]. The gene-edited patient-derived iPS cells are expected to be useful for stem cell transplantation therapy using autologous cells. It was also possible to completely correct gene mutations by homologous recombination in iPS cells [29]. Recently, to increase the number of DMD patients who benefit from genome editing, Ousterout et al. tested multiplex genome editing by simultaneous targeting exons 45–55. Gene-edited DMD patient myoblasts transplanted into immune-deficient mice expressed human spectrin at the sarcolemma of the host muscle [30].
2. *Genome editing in vivo*
   In vivo restoration of the reading frame of the DMD gene on the level of the genome might be an alternative to AONs-mediated exon skipping during the splicing process. Recently, plasmid vectors [31], adeno-associated virus (AAV) vectors [32], and lentiviral vectors [33] have been used to express Cas9 protein and guide RNA in the target organs of adult mice. A concern of direct gene editing in vivo is off-target mutations and unwanted chromosomal translocations associated with off-target DNA cleavages [34]. Therefore, the safety issues should be examined carefully for each single guide RNA. In addition to the accuracy of gene editing, at present, the efficiency of in-frame correction in vivo was low, and gene correction by a knock-in strategy in vivo using homologous recombination is rather challenging.

13.7 Translational Medicine of Muscular Dystrophies in JAPAN

In the past, there was no functional network to promote translational medicine for muscular dystrophies. In 2008, NCNP established a translational research center and then started a nation-wide registry system named "REMUDY" (Registry of Muscular Dystrophy) (http://www.remudy.jp/). In November 2014, REMUDY installed a web-based registry system (Chap. 11), and as of April 2015, 1385 BMD/DMD patients have been registered. The success of REMUDY for BMD/DMD stimulated registries for other neuromuscular diseases (GNE myopathy, myotonic dystrophy type 1, Fukuyama-type congenital dystrophy, etc.) in Japan. We also established a muscular dystrophy clinical trial network (MDTCN) (Chap. 12) (http://www.mdctn.jp/). The two systems provide a good model for translational research for other rare diseases, linking each other and cooperating with international societies for neuromuscular disorders such as TREAT-NMD (http://www.treat-nmd.eu/) or CINRG (http://www.cinrgresearch.org/).

In February 2015, we started an interdisciplinary scientific society, "Japan Muscle Society" (http://www.asas.or.jp/jms/). This academic society, composed of clinicians, scientists and researchers working in the drug industry, who have different backgrounds, will further facilitate translation of basic research to the bedside for muscular dystrophies/myopathies.

Acknowledgments Grants

ST is supported by the following grants:

1. Health and Labor Sciences Research Grants

– 2012–2014 Grant for Clinical Trial on Development of New Drugs and Medical Devices (Clinical Research and Clinical Trial Coordination/Management)

– 2011–2014 Grant for Comprehensive Research and Development on Disability Health and Welfare (Nervous and Muscular Diseases)

2. Intramural Research Grant for Neurological and Psychiatric Disorders of NCNP

References

1. Ozawa E (2010) Our trails and trials in the subsarcolemmal cytoskeleton network and muscular dystrophy researches in the dystrophin era. Proc Jpn Acad Ser B Phys Biol Sci 86:798–821
2. Takeuchi F, Yonemoto N, Nakamura H, Shimizu R, Komaki H, Mori-Yoshimura M, Hayashi YK, Nishino I, Kawai M, Kimura E, Takeda S (2013) Prednisolone improves walking in Japanese Duchenne muscular dystrophy patients. J Neurol 260:3023–3029
3. Pramono ZA, Takeshima Y, Alimsardjono H, Ishii A, Takeda S, Matsuo M (1996) Induction of exon skipping of the dystrophin transcript in lymphoblastoid cells by transfecting an antisense oligodeoxynucleotide complementary to an exon recognition sequence. Biochem Biophys Res Commun 226:445–449
4. Shiga N, Takeshima Y, Sakamoto H, Inoue K, Yokota Y, Yokoyama M, Matsuo M (1997) Disruption of the splicing enhancer sequence within exon 27 of the dystrophin gene by a

nonsense mutation induces partial skipping of the exon and is responsible for Becker muscular dystrophy. J Clin Invest 100:2204–2210
5. Takeshima Y, Nishio H, Sakamoto H, Nakamura H, Matsuo M (1995) Modulation of in vitro splicing of the upstream intron by modifying an intra-exon sequence which is deleted from the dystrophin gene in dystrophin Kobe. J Clin Invest 95:515–520
6. Dunckley MG, Manoharan M, Villiet P, Eperon IC, Dickson G (1998) Modification of splicing in the dystrophin gene in cultured Mdx muscle cells by antisense oligoribonucleotides. Hum Mol Genet 7:1083–1090
7. van Deutekom JC, Bremmer-Bout M, Janson AA, Ginjaar IB, Baas F, den Dunnen JT, van Ommen GJ (2001) Antisense-induced exon skipping restores dystrophin expression in DMD patient derived muscle cells. Hum Mol Genet 10:1547–1554
8. Lu QL, Mann CJ, Lou F, Bou-Gharios G, Morris GE, Xue SA, Fletcher S, Partridge TA, Wilton SD (2003) Functional amounts of dystrophin produced by skipping the mutated exon in the mdx dystrophic mouse. Nat Med 9:1009–1014
9. Alter J, Lou F, Rabinowitz A, Yin H, Rosenfeld J, Wilton SD, Partridge TA, Lu QL (2006) Systemic delivery of morpholino oligonucleotide restores dystrophin expression bodywide and improves dystrophic pathology. Nat Med 12:175–177
10. Lu QL, Rabinowitz A, Chen YC, Yokota T, Yin H, Alter J, Jadoon A, Bou-Gharios G, Partridge T (2005) Systemic delivery of antisense oligoribonucleotide restores dystrophin expression in body-wide skeletal muscles. Proc Natl Acad Sci U S A 102:198–203
11. Goyenvalle A, Griffith G, Babbs A et al (2015) Functional correction in mouse models of muscular dystrophy using exon-skipping tricyclo-DNA oligomers. Nat Med 21:270–275
12. ATS Committee on Proficiency Standards for Clinical Pulmonary Function Laboratories (2002) ATS statement: guidelines for the six-minute walk test. Am J Respir Crit Care Med 166:111–117
13. Wu B, Lu P, Benrashid E, Malik S, Ashar J, Doran TJ, Lu QL (2010) Dose-dependent restoration of dystrophin expression in cardiac muscle of dystrophic mice by systemically delivered morpholino. Gene Ther 17:132–140
14. Mendell JR, Rodino-Klapac LR, Sahenk Z, Roush K, Bird L, Lowes LP, Alfano L, Gomez AM, Lewis S, Kota J, Malik V, Shontz K, Walker CM, Flanigan KM, Corridore M, Kean JR, Allen HD, Shilling C, Melia KR, Sazani P, Saoud JB, Kaye EM, Eteplirsen Study Group (2013) Eteplirsen for the treatment of Duchenne muscular dystrophy. Ann Neurol 74:637–647
15. Amantana A, Moulton HM, Cate ML, Reddy MT, Whitehead T, Hassinger JN, Youngblood DS, Iversen PL (2007) Pharmacokinetics, biodistribution, stability and toxicity of a cell-penetrating peptide-morpholino oligomer conjugate. Bioconjug Chem 18:1325–1331
16. Moulton HM, Moulton JD (2010) Morpholinos and their peptide conjugates: therapeutic promise and challenge for Duchenne muscular dystrophy. Biochim Biophys Acta 1798:2296–2303
17. Aoki Y, Yokota T, Nagata T, Nakamura A, Tanihata J, Saito T, Duguez SM, Nagaraju K, Hoffman EP, Partridge T, Takeda S (2012) Bodywide skipping of exons 45–55 in dystrophic mdx52 mice by systemic antisense delivery. Proc Natl Acad Sci U S A 109:13763–13768
18. Widrick JJ, Jiang S, Choi SJ, Knuth ST, Morcos PA (2011) An octaguanidine-morpholino oligo conjugate improves muscle function of mdx mice. Muscle Nerve 44:563–570
19. Wu B, Li Y, Morcos PA, Doran TJ, Lu P, Lu QL (2009) Octa-guanidine morpholino restores dystrophin expression in cardiac and skeletal muscles and ameliorates pathology in dystrophic mdx mice. Mol Ther 17:864–871
20. Echigoya Y, Yokota T (2014) Skipping multiple exons of dystrophin transcripts using cocktail antisense oligonucleotides. Nucleic Acid Ther 24:57–68
21. Yokota T, Nakamura A, Nagata T, Saito T, Kobayashi M, Aoki Y, Echigoya Y, Partridge T, Hoffman EP, Takeda S (2012) Extensive and prolonged restoration of dystrophin expression with vivo-morpholino- mediated multiple exon skipping in dystrophic dogs. Nucleic Acid Ther 22:306–315

22. Sekiguchi M, Zushida K, Yoshida M, Maekawa M, Kamichi S, Yoshida M, Sahara Y, Yuasa S, Takeda S, Wada K (2009) A deficit of brain dystrophin impairs specific amygdala GABAergic transmission and enhances defensive behaviour in mice. Brain 132:124–135
23. Araki E, Nakamura K, Nakao K, Kameya S, Kobayashi O, Nonaka I, Kobayashi T, Katsuki M (1997) Targeted disruption of exon 52 in the mouse dystrophin gene induced muscle degeneration similar to that observed in Duchenne muscular dystrophy. Biochem Biophys Res Commun 238:492–497
24. Aoki Y, Nakamura A, Yokota T, Saito T, Okazawa H, Nagata T, Takeda S (2010) In-frame dystrophin following exon 51- skipping improves muscle pathology and function in the exon 52-deficient mdx mouse. Mol Ther 18:1995–2005
25. Shimatsu Y, Katagiri K, Furuta T, Nakura M, Tanioka Y, Yuasa K, Tomohiro M, Kornegay JN, Nonaka I, Takeda S (2003) Canine X-linked muscular dystrophy in Japan ($CXMD_J$). Exp Anim 52:93–97
26. Yokota T, Lu QL, Partridge T, Kobayashi M, Nakamura A, Takeda S, Hoffman E (2009) Efficacy of systemic morpholino exon-skipping in Duchenne dystrophy dogs. Ann Neurol 65:667–676
27. Saito T, Nakamura A, Aoki Y, Yokota T, Okada T, Osawa M, Takeda S (2010) Antisense PMO found in dystrophic dog model was effective in cells from exon 7-deleted DMD patient. PLoS One 5(8), e12239
28. Yokota T, Hoffman E, Takeda S (2011) Antisense oligo-mediated multiple exon skipping in a dog model of Duchenne muscular dystrophy. Methods Mol Biol 709:299–312
29. Li HL, Fujimoto N, Sasakawa N, Shirai S, Ohkame T, Sakuma T, Tanaka M, Amano N, Watanabe A, Sakurai H, Yamamoto T, Yamanaka S, Hotta A (2015) Precise correction of the dystrophin gene in Duchenne muscular dystrophy patient induced pluripotent stem cells by TALEN and CRISPR-Cas9. Stem Cell Rep 4:143–154
30. Ousterout DG, Kabadi AM, Thakore PI, Majoros WH, Reddy TE, Gersbach CA (2015) Multiplex CRISPR/Cas9-based genome editing for correction of dystrophin mutations that cause Duchenne muscular dystrophy. Nat Commun 6:6244
31. Yin H, Xue W, Chen S, Bogorad RL, Benedetti E, Grompe M, Koteliansky V, Sharp PA, Jacks T, Anderson DG (2014) Genome editing with Cas9 in adult mice corrects a disease mutation and phenotype. Nat Biotechnol 32:551–553
32. Swiech L, Heidenreich M, Banerjee A, Habib N, Li Y, Trombetta J, Sur M, Zhang F (2015) In vivo interrogation of gene function in the mammalian brain using CRISPR-Cas9. Nat Biotechnol 33:102–106
33. Blasco RB, Karaca E, Ambrogio C, Cheong TC, Karayol E, Minero VG, Voena C, Chiarle R (2014) Simple and rapid in vivo generation of chromosomal rearrangements using CRISPR/Cas9 technology. Cell Rep 9:1219–1227
34. Cho SW, Kim S, Kim Y, Kweon J, Kim HS, Bae S, Kim JS (2014) Analysis of off-target effects of CRISPR/Cas-derived RNA-guided endonucleases and nickases. Genome Res 24:132–141

MIX
Papier aus verantwortungsvollen Quellen
Paper from responsible sources
FSC® C105338

If you have any concerns about our products,
you can contact us on
ProductSafety@springernature.com

In case Publisher is established outside the EU,
the EU authorized representative is:
Springer Nature Customer Service Center GmbH
Europaplatz 3, 69115 Heidelberg, Germany

Printed by Libri Plureos GmbH
in Hamburg, Germany